TAKING SIDES

Clashing Views on Controversial

Bioethical Issues

NINTH EDITION

Selected, Edited, and with Introductions by

Carol Levine
United Hospital Fund

McGraw-Hill/Dushkin
A Division of The McGraw-Hill Companies

For Hannah, Amy, Asher, and Madeleine

Photo Acknowledgment
Cover image: © 2001 by PhotoDisc, Inc.

Cover Art Acknowledgment
Charles Vitelli

Copyright © 2001 by McGraw-Hill/Dushkin,
A Division of The McGraw-Hill Companies, Inc., Guilford, Connecticut 06437

Copyright law prohibits the reproduction, storage, or transmission in any form by any means of any portion of this publication without the express written permission of McGraw-Hill/Dushkin and of the copyright holder (if different) of the part of the publication to be reproduced. The Guidelines for Classroom Copying endorsed by Congress explicitly state that unauthorized copying may not be used to create, to replace, or to substitute for anthologies, compilations, or collective works.

Taking Sides ® is a registered trademark of McGraw-Hill/Dushkin

Manufactured in the United States of America

Ninth Edition

123456789BAHBAH4321

Library of Congress Cataloging-in-Publication Data
Main entry under title:
Taking sides: clashing views on controversial bioethical issues/selected, edited, and with introductions by Carol Levine.—9th ed.
Includes bibliographical references and index.
1. Bioethics. I. Levine, Carol, *comp.*
174.957′4
0-07-243082-6
1091-8809

Printed on Recycled Paper

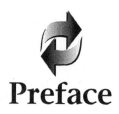

Preface

This is a book about choices—hard and tragic choices. The choices are hard not only because they often involve life and death but also because there are convincing arguments on both sides of the issues. An ethical dilemma, by definition, is one that poses a conflict not between good and evil but between one good principle and another that is equally good. The choices are hard because the decisions that are made—by individuals, groups, and public policymakers—will influence the kind of society we have today and the one we will have in the future.

Although the views expressed in the selections in this volume are strong —even passionate—they are also subtle, concerned with the nuances of the particular debate. *How* one argues matters in bioethics; you will see and have to weigh the significance of varying rhetorical styles and appeals throughout this volume.

Although there are no easy answers to any of the issues in the book, the questions will be answered in some fashion—partly by individual choices and partly by decisions that are made by professionals and government. We must make them the best answers possible, and that can only be done by informed and thoughtful consideration. This book, then, can serve as a beginning for what ideally will become an ongoing process of examination and reflection.

Changes to this edition Many popular issues and the basic structure of the book remain from the previous edition. There are seven parts: Medical Decision Making; Death and Dying; Choices in Reproduction; Children and Bioethics; Genetics; Human and Animal Experimentation; and Bioethics and Public Policy. There are four completely new issues: *Should Genes for Human Diseases Be Patented?* (Issue 11); *Is Sham Surgery Ethically Acceptable in Clinical Research?* (Issue 16); *Should Health Insurance Be Based on Employment?* (Issue 17); and *Should Doctors-in-Training Be Unionized?* (Issue 21). In addition, the YES selection in Issue 13 (*Should Information From Genetic Testing Be Available to Employers and Insurers?*); the NO selection in Issue 19 (*Should Patient-Centered Medical Ethics Govern Managed Care?*); and both selections in Issue 4 (*Should Physicians Be Allowed to Assist in Patient Suicide?*) have been replaced to bring debates up-to-date. In all, there are 12 new selections. Part introductions, issue introductions, and postscripts have been revised as necessary. Also, the *On the Internet* page that begins each part offers relevant Internet site addresses (URLs) that should prove useful as starting points for further research.

A word to the instructor An *Instructor's Manual With Test Questions* (multiple-choice and essay) is available through the publisher, and a general guidebook, *Using Taking Sides in the Classroom*, which discusses methods and techniques for using the pro-con approach in any classroom setting, is also available. An online version of *Using Taking Sides in the Classroom* and a correspondence service for *Taking Sides* adopters can be found at http://www.dushkin.com/usingts/.

Taking Sides: Clashing Views on Controversial Bioethical Issues is only one title in the Taking Sides series. If you are interested in seeing the table of contents for any of the other titles, please visit the Taking Sides Web site at http://www.dushkin.com/takingsides/.

Acknowledgments I received helpful comments and suggestions from the many users of *Taking Sides* across the United States and Canada. Their suggestions have enhanced the quality of this edition of the book and are reflected in the new selections and issues.

Special thanks go to those who responded with specific suggestions for the ninth edition:

James G. Anderson
Purdue University–Lafayette

Linda Benson
Clarion University

Barry Brock
Barry University

Thomas E. Brown
Atlantic Community College

Joan M. Chapdelaine
Salve Regina College

Margaret Curran
Northern Illinois University

Sarah Dean
Eckerd College

Cheryl Slaughter Ellis
Middle Tennessee State University

Robert Farmer
Barry University

Samuel D. Fohr
University of Pittsburgh

Michelle J. Grooter
Northwestern Michigan College

Beverly Hawkins
Widener University

Lawrence Krupka
Michigan State University

Chris Lewis
University of Colorado

James V. Makowski
Messiah College

James C. Marker
University of Wisconsin–Green Bay

Steven McCullagh
Kennesaw State College

James McGregor
Salem State College

J. Mosca
Monmouth University

David Mowry
Ohio University

Paul Muscari
Adirondack Community College

Betty Odello
Los Angeles Pierce College

Michael Rackover
Philadelphia College of Textiles

Mark Sheldon
Indiana University–Northwest

Natalie C. Shiras
Fairfield University

Edward Stevens
Regis College

Ruth Stuckel
Avila College

Milburn Thompson
St. Joseph College

Julio Turrens
University of South Alabama

Claire Tynan
Holy Name Hospital School of Nursing

Duane Westfield
Endicott College

Erleen Whitney
Clark College

Nancy Williams
University of Connecticut

For this edition, Alexis Kuerbis prepared the *Instructor's Manual*. Both of us have benefited immeasurably from Dillan Siegler's, Ben Munisteri's, and Lauri Posner's careful work on previous editions. For their assistance in previous editions, which gave me a solid base from which to proceed, I want to thank Paul Homer, Eric Feldman, and Arthur Caplan. I would particularly like to thank Daniel Callahan, director of the Hastings Center, and Willard Gaylin, both now retired, for their early encouragement in this project.

Carol Levine
United Hospital Fund

Contents In Brief

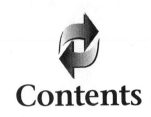

Contents

Physician Robert M. Arnold and professor of psychiatry and sociology Charles W. Lidz assert that informed consent in clinical care is an essential process that promotes good communication and patient autonomy despite the obstacles of implementation. Professor of medical ethics Robert M. Veatch argues that informed consent is a transitional concept that is useful only for moving toward a more radical framework in which physicians and patients are paired on the basis of shared deep social, moral, and institutional values.

John Hardwig, an associate professor of medical ethics, argues that the prevalent ethic of patient autonomy ignores family interests in medical treatment decisions. He maintains that physicians should recognize these interests as legitimate. Bioethicist Jeffrey Blustein contends that although families can be an important resource in helping patients make better decisions about their care, the ultimate decision-making authority should remain with the patient.

Physician Steven H. Miles maintains that physicians' duty to follow patients' wishes ends when the requests are inconsistent with what medical care can reasonably be expected to achieve. Philosopher Felicia Ackerman contends that decisions involving personal values, such as those regarding quality of life, should be made by the patient or family, not by the physician.

Physician M. LeRoy Sprang and osteopathic physician Mark G. Neerhof assert that late-term abortion is needlessly risky, inhumane, and ethically unacceptable. They state that all abortions of 23 weeks or later should be considered unethical unless the fetus has a lethal condition or the mother's life is endangered. While acknowledging that early abortion is safer, simpler, and less controversial, physician David A. Grimes contends that late-term abortion is fundamentally important to women's health because some medical conditions of both women and fetuses cannot be diagnosed early in pregnancy and because of the prevalence of incest and rape.

In a case involving a pregnant woman's use of crack cocaine, a majority of the Supreme Court of South Carolina ruled that a state legislature may impose additional criminal penalties on pregnant drug-using women without violating their constitutional right of privacy. Law professor Alexander Morgan Capron argues that the Supreme Court of South Carolina's decision may lead society to punish pregnant women who expose fetuses to many different types of risk, including women who have multiple births due to fertility drugs.

Ethicist Robert F. Weir and pediatrician Charles Peters assert that adolescents with normal cognitive and developmental skills have the capacity to make decisions about their own health care. Advance directives, if used appropriately, can give older pediatric patients a voice in their care. Pediatrician Lainie Friedman Ross counters that parents should be responsible for making their child's health care decisions. Children need to develop virtues, such as self-control, that will enhance their long-term, not just immediate, autonomy.

Issue 10.   Do Parents Harm Their Children When They Refuse Medical Treatment on Religious Grounds?   166

The Committee on Bioethics of the American Academy of Pediatrics states that all children deserve medical treatment that is likely to prevent substantial harm, suffering, or death, regardless of the parents' religious objections to treatment. Professor of philosophy Mark Sheldon assesses the case of Jehovah's Witness parents who refuse to allow their children to undergo blood transfusions and concludes that they cannot be said to be truly harming or neglecting their children. Rather, they are placing their children's spiritual interests above worldly ones.

PART 5   GENETICS   183

Issue 11.   Should Genes for Human Diseases Be Patented?   184

Bioethicist Glenn McGee argues that disease gene patents are not patents on products of nature but on scientific innovations. He asserts that correctly framed and issued disease-related gene patents will not preclude access to genetic material for educational and scientific uses. Bioethicists Jon F. Merz and Mildred K. Cho counter that disease genes are not patentable because they are indeed products of nature that exist independent of the ingenuity, innovation, and manufacture of humans.

Issue 12.   Should Human Cloning Be Banned?   198

Law professor George J. Annas contends that human cloning devalues people by depriving them of their uniqueness and would radically alter what it means to be human. Law professor John A. Robertson asserts that regulatory policy should avoid a ban on cloning, but should ensure that it is performed in a responsible manner.

Columnist Andrew Sullivan sees no ethical difference between using genetic information to predict future workplace performance and using other means to do so. Sullivan argues that genetic information is more reliable and less discriminatory than other types of information. Thomas H. Murray, a professor of biomedical ethics, contends that actuarial fairness— the insurance industry's standard—fails to accomplish the social goals of health insurance and that genetic tests should not be used to deny people access to health insurance.

Mary Z. Pelias, attorney and professor of genetics, argues that parental autonomy and family privacy should govern decisions about whether or not to test children for genetic predispositions to disease and that physicians and genetic counselors have an obligation to disclose full information. Law professor Diane E. Hoffmann and pediatrician Eric A. Wulfsberg assert that caution and restraint should govern decisions on testing for genetic predispositions in children and that safeguards should be adopted to diminish the potentially negative effects of testing and to protect children's best interests.

Jerod M. Loeb and his colleagues, representing the American Medical Society's Group on Science and Technology, assert that concern for animals cannot impede the development of methods to improve the welfare of humans. Philosopher Tom Regan argues that those who support animal research fail to show proper respect for animals' inherent value.

Physician Thomas B. Freeman and his colleagues contend that their study of fetal-tissue transplantation, which used imitation, or sham, surgery in one group of patients, will establish whether this treatment is beneficial or not. Furthermore, this treatment will benefit thousands of patients with Parkinson's disease if proven effective. Philosopher Ruth Macklin concludes that sham surgery is ethically unacceptable, particularly in the case of fetal-tissue transplantation, because it does not minimize harm to subjects, a fundamental principle underlying research ethics.

PART 7   BIOETHICS AND PUBLIC POLICY   289

Insurance and policy analysts William S. Custer, Charles N. Kahn III, and Thomas F. Wildsmith IV assert that the employment-based health care system in the United States offers a solid, proven foundation on which to base any reform, and that attempts to break the link between employment and health insurance coverage may greatly increase the number of uninsured Americans. Economist Uwe E. Reinhardt argues that, on balance, the debits of the employer-based health insurance system outweigh the credits, and that a parallel system detached from the workplace could eventually absorb the current system.

Physician Andrew C. Yacht argues that doctors-in-training, like other workers, should have the right to organize and to bargain collectively for better working conditions in hospitals so that they can provide enhanced care for their patients. Physician and medical educator Jordan J. Cohen asserts that doctors-in-training are primarily students, not employees, and that union activities would negatively affect the educational experience.

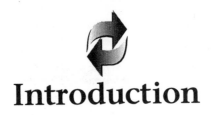

Introduction

Medicine and Moral Arguments

Carol Levine

In the fall of 1975 a 21-year-old woman lay in a New Jersey hospital—as she had for months—in a coma, the victim of a toxic combination of barbiturates and alcohol. Doctors agreed that her brain was irreversibly damaged and that she would never recover. Her parents, after anguished consultation with their priest, asked the doctors and hospital to disconnect the respirator that was artificially maintaining their daughter's life. When the doctors and hospital refused, the parents petitioned the court to be made her legal guardian so that they could authorize the withdrawal of treatment. After hearing all the arguments, the court sided with the parents, and the respirator was removed. Contrary to everyone's expectations, however, the young woman did not die but began to breathe on her own (perhaps because, in anticipation of the court order, the nursing staff had gradually weaned her from total dependence on the respirator). She lived for 10 years until her death in June 1985—comatose, lying in a fetal position, and fed with tubes—in a New Jersey nursing home.

The young woman's name was Karen Ann Quinlan, and her case brought national attention to the thorny ethical questions raised by modern medical technology: When, if ever, should life-sustaining technology be withdrawn? Is the sanctity of life an absolute value? What kinds of treatment are really beneficial to a patient in a "chronic vegetative state" like Karen's? And, perhaps the most troubling question, who shall decide? These and similar questions are at the heart of the growing field of biomedical ethics, or (as it is usually called) *bioethics.*

Ethical dilemmas in medicine are, of course, nothing new. They have been recognized and discussed in Western medicine since a small group of physicians —led by Hippocrates—on the Isle of Cos in Greece, around the fourth century B.C., subscribed to a code of practice that newly graduated physicians still swear to uphold today. But unlike earlier times, when physicians and scientists had only limited abilities to change the course of disease, today they can intervene in profound ways in the most fundamental processes of life and death. Moreover, ethical dilemmas in medicine are no longer considered the sole province of professionals. Professional codes of ethics, to be sure, offer some guidance, but they are usually unclear and ambiguous about what to do in specific situations. More important, these codes assume that whatever decision is to be made is up to the professional, not the patient. Today, to an ever-greater degree, laypeople—patients, families, lawyers, clergy, and others—want to and have become involved in ethical decision making not only in individual cases, such as the Quinlan case, but also in large societal decisions, such as how to allocate scarce medical resources, including high-technology machinery, newborn intensive care units, and the expertise of physicians. While questions about the physician-patient relationship and individual cases are still prominent in bioethics (see, for example, the issues on truth telling and assisting dying patients in suicide), today the field covers a broad range of other decisions as well, such as the use of reproductive technology, the harvesting and transplantation of organs, equity in access to health care, and the future of animal experimentation.

This involvement is part of broader social trends: a general disenchantment with the authority of all professionals and, hence, a greater readiness to challenge the traditional belief that "doctor knows best"; the growth of various civil rights movements among women, the aged, and minorities—of which the patients' rights movement is a spin-off; the enormous size and complexity of the health care delivery system, in which patients and families often feel alienated from the professional; the increasing cost of medical care, much of it at public expense; and the growth of the "medical model," in which conditions that used to be considered outside the scope of physicians' control, such as alcoholism and behavioral problems, have come to be considered diseases.

Bioethics began in the 1950s as an intellectual movement among a small group of physicians and theologians who started to examine the questions raised by the new medical technologies that were starting to emerge as the result of the heavy expenditure of public funds in medical research after World War II. They were soon joined by a number of philosophers who had become disillusioned with what they saw as the arid abstractions of much analytic philosophy at the time and by lawyers who sought to find principles in the law that would guide ethical decision making or, if such principles were not there, to develop them by case law and legislation or regulation. Although these four disciplines—medicine, theology, philosophy, and law—still dominate the field, today bioethics is an interdisciplinary effort, with political scientists, economists, sociologists, anthropologists, nurses, allied health professionals, policymakers, psychologists, and others contributing their special perspectives to the ongoing debates.

The issues discussed in this volume attest to the wide range of bioethical dilemmas, their complexity, and the passion they arouse. But if bioethics today is at the frontiers of scientific knowledge, it is also a field with ancient roots. It goes back to the most basic questions of human life: What is right? What is wrong? How should people act toward others? And why?

While the *bio* part of *bioethics* gives the field its urgency and immediacy, we should not forget that the root word is *ethics*.

Applying Ethics to Medical Dilemmas

To see where bioethics fits into the larger framework of academic inquiry, some definitions are in order. First, *morality* is the general term for an individual's or a society's standards of conduct, both actual and ideal, and of the character traits that determine whether people are considered "good" or "bad." The scientific study of morality is called *descriptive ethics*; a scientist—generally an anthropologist, sociologist, or historian—can describe in empirical terms what the moral beliefs, judgments, or actions of individuals or societies are and what reasons are given for the way they act or what they believe. The philosophical study of morality, on the other hand, approaches the subject of morality in one of two different ways: either as an analysis of the concepts, terms, and methods of reasoning (*metaethics*) or as an analysis of what those standards or moral judgments ought to be (*normative ethics*). Metaethics deals with meanings of moral terms and logic; normative ethics, with which the issues in this volume are concerned, reflects on the kinds of actions and principles that will promote moral behavior.

Because normative ethics accepts the idea that some acts and character traits are more moral than others (and that some are immoral), it rejects the rather popular idea that ethics is relative. Because different societies have different moral codes and values, ethical relativists have argued that there can be no universal moral judgments: What is right or wrong depends on who does it and where, and whether or not society approves. Although it is certainly true that moral values are embedded in a social, cultural, and political context, it is also true that certain moral judgments are universal. We think it is wrong, for example, to sell people into slavery—whether or not a certain society approved or even whether or not a person wanted to be a slave. People may not agree about what these universal moral values are or ought to be, but it is hard to deny that some such values exist.

The other relativistic view rejected by normative ethics is the notion that whatever feels good *is* good. In this view, ethics is a matter of personal preference, weightier than one's choice of which automobile to buy, but not much different in kind. Different people, having different feelings, can arrive at equally valid moral judgments, according to the relativistic view. Just as we should not disregard cultural factors, we should not overlook the role of emotion and personal experience in arriving at moral judgments. But to give emotion ultimate authority would be to consign reason and rationality—the bases of moral argument—to the ethical trash heap. At the very least, it would be impossible to develop a just policy concerning the care of vulnerable persons, like the mentally retarded or newborns, who depend solely on the vagaries of individual caretakers.

Thus, if normative ethics is one branch of philosophy, bioethics is one branch of normative ethics; it is normative ethics applied to the practice of medicine and science. There are other branches—business ethics, legal ethics, journalism ethics, and military ethics, for example. One common term for the entire grouping is *applied and professional ethics*, because these ethics deal with the ethical standards of the members of a particular profession and how they are applied in the professionals' dealings with each other and the rest of society. Bioethics is based on the belief that some solutions to the dilemmas that arise in medicine and science are more moral than others and that these solutions can be determined by moral reasoning and reflection.

Ethical Theories

If the practitioners of bioethics do not rely solely on cultural norms and emotions, what are their sources of determining what is right or wrong? The most comprehensive source is a theory of ethics—a broad set of moral principles (or perhaps just one overriding principle) that is used in measuring human conduct. Divine law is one such source, of course, but even in the Western religious traditions of bioethics (both the Jewish and Catholic religions have rich and comprehensive commentaries on ethical issues, and the Protestant religion has a less cohesive but still important tradition) the law of God is interpreted in terms of human moral principles. A theory of ethics must be acceptable to many groups, not just the followers of one religious tradition. Most writers outside the religious traditions (and some within them) have looked to one of three major traditions in ethics: teleological theories, deontological theories, and natural law theories.

Teleological Theories

Teleological theories are based on the idea that the end or purpose (from the Greek *telos,* or end) of the action determines its rightness or wrongness. The most prominent teleological theory is *utilitarianism.* In its simplest formulation, an act is moral if it brings more good consequences than bad ones. Utilitarian theories are derived from the works of two English philosophers: Jeremy Bentham (1748–1832) and John Stuart Mill (1806–1873). Rejecting the absolutist religious morality of his time, Bentham proposed that "utility"—the greatest good for the greatest number—should guide the actions of human beings. Invoking the hedonistic philosophy of Epicurean Greeks, Bentham said that pleasure (*hedon* in Greek) is good and pain is bad. Therefore, actions are right if they promote more pleasure than pain and wrong if they promote more pain than pleasure. Mill found the highest utility in "happiness," rather than pleasure. (Mill's philosophy is echoed in the Declaration of Independence's espousal of "life, liberty, and the pursuit of happiness.") Other utilitarians have looked to a range of utilities, or goods (including friendship, love, devotion, and the like) that they believe ought to be weighed in the balance—the utilitarian calculus.

Utilitarianism has a pragmatic appeal. It is flexible, and it seems impartial. However, its critics point out that utilitarianism can be used to justify suppression of individual rights for the good of society ("the ends justify the means") and that it is difficult to quantify and compare "utilities," however they are defined.

Utilitarianism, in its many forms, has had a powerful influence on bioethical discussion, partly because it is the closest to the case-by-case risk/benefit ratio that physicians use in clinical decision making. Joseph Fletcher, a Protestant theologian who was one of the pioneers in bioethics in the 1950s, developed utilitarian theories that he called *situation ethics.* He argued that a true Christian morality does not blindly follow moral rules but acts from love and sensitivity to the particular situation and the needs of those involved. He has enthusiastically supported most modern technologies on the grounds that they lead to good ends.

Writers in this volume who use utilitarian theories to arrive at their moral judgments are Thomas B. Freeman and colleagues, who support the use of placebos in surgery trials; Bernard C. Meyer, who defends withholding the truth from dying patients on the grounds that it leads to better consequences than truth telling; and Jerod M. Loeb and his colleagues, who defend animal experimentation.

Deontological Theories

The second major type of ethical theory is *deontological* (from the Greek *deon*, or duty). The rightness or wrongness of an act, these theories hold, should be judged on whether or not it conforms to a moral principle or rule, not on whether it leads to good or bad consequences. The primary exponent of a deontological theory was Immanuel Kant (1724–1804), a German philosopher. Kant declared that there is an ultimate norm, or supreme duty, which he called the "Moral Law." He held that an act is moral only if it springs from a "good will," the only thing that is good without qualification.

We must do good things, said Kant, because we have a duty to do them, not because they result in good consequences or because they give us pleasure (although that can happen as well). Kant constructed a formal "Categorical Imperative," the ultimate test of morality: "I ought never to act except in such a way that I can also will that my maxim should become universal law." Recognizing that this formulation was far from clear, Kant said the same thing in three other ways. He explained that a moral rule must be one that can serve as a guide for everyone's conduct; it must be one that permits people to treat each other as ends in themselves, not solely as means to another's ends; and it must be one that each person can impose on himself by his own will, not one that is solely imposed by the state, one's parents, or God. Kant's Categorical Imperative, in the simplest terms, says that all persons have equal moral worth and that no rule can be moral unless all people can apply it autonomously to all other human beings. Although on its own Kant's Categorical Imperative is merely a formal statement with no moral content at all, he gave some examples of what he meant: "Do not commit suicide," and "Help others in distress."

Kantian ethics is criticized by many who note that Kant gives little guidance on what to do when ethical principles conflict, as they often do. Moreover, they say, his emphasis on autonomous decision making and individual will neglects the social and communal context in which people live and make decisions. It leads to isolation and unreality. These criticisms notwithstanding, Kantian ethics has stimulated much current thinking in bioethics. In this volume, the idea that certain actions are in and of themselves right or wrong underlies, for example, George J. Annas's opposition to human cloning, Sissela Bok's appeal to truth telling, and Mary Z. Pelias's support of physicians' always disclosing the availability of genetic testing to parents.

Two modern deontological theorists are philosophers John Rawls and Robert M. Veatch. In *A Theory of Justice* (1971), Rawls places the highest value on equitable distribution of society's resources. He believes that society has a fundamental obligation to correct the inequalities of historical circumstance and natural endowment of its least well off members. According to this theory, some action is good only if it benefits the least well off. (It can also benefit others, but that is secondary.) His social justice theory has influenced bioethical writings concerning the allocation of scarce resources.

Veatch has applied Rawlsian principles to medical ethics. In his book *A Theory of Medical Ethics* (1981), he offers a model of social contract among professionals, patients, and society that emphasizes mutual respect and responsibilities. This contract model will, he hopes, avoid the narrowness of professional codes of ethics and the generalities and ambiguities of more broadly based ethical theories. In Issue 1 of this volume, Veatch challenges current concepts of informed consent as outmoded.

Natural Law Theory

The third strain of ethical theory that is prominent in bioethics is *natural law theory*, first developed by St. Thomas Aquinas (1223–1274). According to this theory, actions are morally right if they accord with our nature as human beings. The attribute that is distinctively human is the ability to reason and to exercise intelligence. Thus, argues this theory, we can know the good, which is objective and can be learned through reason. References to natural law theory are prominent in the works of Catholic theologians and writers; they see natural law as ultimately derived from God but knowable through the efforts of human beings. The influence of natural law theory can be seen in the issue on human cloning.

Theory of Virtue

The *theory of virtue*, another ethical theory with deep roots in the Aristotelian tradition, has recently been revived in bioethics. This theory stresses not the morality of any particular actions or rules but the disposition of individuals to act morally, to be virtuous. In its modern version, its primary exponent is Alasdair MacIntyre, whose book *After Virtue* (1980) urges a return to the Aristotelian model. Gregory Pence has applied the theory of virtue directly to medicine in *Ethical Options in Medicine* (1980); he lists temperance in personal life, compassion for the suffering patient, professional competence, justice, honesty, courage, and practical judgment as the virtues that are most desirable in physicians. Although this theory has not yet been as fully developed in bioethics as the utilitarian or deontological theories, it is likely to have particular appeal for physicians—many of whom have resisted formal ethics education on the grounds that moral character is the critical factor and that one can best learn to be a moral physician by emulating one's mentors. Although not explicit, assumptions about the qualities of a virtuous physician underlie the discussion in Issue 21 on the unionization of doctors-in-training.

Although various authors, in this volume and elsewhere, appeal in rather direct ways to either utilitarian or deontological theories, often the various types are combined. One may argue both that a particular action is immoral in and of itself and that it will have bad consequences (some commentators say even Kant used this argument). In fact, probably no single ethical theory is adequate to deal with all the ramifications of the issues. In that case we can turn to a middle level of ethical discussion. Between the abstractions of ethical theories (Kant's Categorical Imperative) and the specifics of moral judgments (always obtain informed consent from a patient) is a range of concepts—ethical principles—that can be applied to particular cases.

Ethical Principles

In its four years of deliberation, the National Commission for the Protection of Human Subjects of Biomedical and Behavioral Research grappled with some of the most difficult issues facing researchers and society: When, if ever, is it ethical to do research on fetuses, on children, or on people in mental institutions? This commission—which was composed of people from various religious backgrounds, professions, and social strata—was finally able to agree on specific recommendations on these questions, but only after they had finished their work did the commissioners try to determine what ethical principles they had used in reaching a consensus. In their Belmont Report (1978), named after the conference center where they met to discuss this question, the commissioners outlined what they considered to be the three most important ethical principles (respect for persons, beneficence, and justice) that should govern the conduct of research with human beings. These three principles, they believed, are generally accepted in our cultural tradition and can serve as basic justifications for the many particular ethical prescriptions and evaluations of human action. Because of the principles' general acceptance and widespread applicability, they are at the basis of most bioethical discussion. Although philosophers argue about whether other principles—preventing harm to others or loyalty, for example—ought to be accorded equal weight with these three or should be included under another umbrella, they agree that these principles are fundamental.

Respect for Persons

Respect for persons incorporates at least two basic ethical convictions, according to the Belmont Report. Individuals should be treated as autonomous agents, and persons with diminished autonomy are entitled to protection. The derivation from Kant is clear. Because human beings have the capacity for rational action and moral choice, they have a value independent of anything that they can do or provide to others. Therefore, they should be treated in a way that respects their independent choices and judgments. Respecting autonomy means giving weight to autonomous persons' considered opinions and choices, and refraining from interfering with their choices unless those choices are clearly detrimental to others. However, since the capacity for autonomy varies with age, mental disability, or other circumstances, those people whose autonomy is diminished must be protected—but only in ways that serve their interests and do not interfere with the level of autonomy that they do possess. This subject is discussed in Issue 9 on adolescent life-and-death decision making.

Two important moral rules are derived from the ethical principle of respect for persons: informed consent and truth telling. Persons can exercise autonomy only when they have been fully informed about the range of options open to them, and the process of informed consent is generally considered to include the elements of information, comprehension, and voluntariness. Thus, a person can give informed consent to some medical procedure only if he or she has full information about the risks and benefits, understands them, and agrees voluntarily—that is, without being coerced or pressured into agreement. Although the principle of informed consent has become an accepted moral rule (and a legal one as well), it is difficult—some say impossible—to achieve in a real-world setting. It can easily be turned into a legalistic parody or avoided altogether. But as a moral ideal it serves to balance the unequal power of the physician and patient.

Another important moral ideal derived from the principle of respect for persons is truth telling. It held a high place in Kant's theory. In his essay "The Supposed Right to Tell Lies From Benevolent Motives," he wrote: "If, then, we define a lie merely as an intentionally false declaration towards another man, we need not add that it must injure another . . . ; for it always injures another; if not another individual, yet mankind generally. . . . To be truthful in all declarations is therefore a sacred and conditional command of reasons, and not to be limited by any other expediency."

Other important moral rules that are derived from the principle of respect for persons are confidentiality and privacy.

Beneficence

Most physicians would probably consider beneficence (from the Latin *bene,* or good) the most basic ethical principle. In the Hippocratic Oath it is used this way: "I will apply dietetic measures for the benefit of the sick according to my ability and judgment; I will keep them from harm and injustice." And further on, "Whatever houses I may visit, I will comfort and benefit the sick, remaining free of all intentional injustice." The phrase *Primum non nocere* (First, do no harm) is another well-known version of this idea, but it appears to be a much later, Latinized version—not from the Hippocratic period.

Philosopher William Frankena has outlined four elements included in the principle of beneficence: (1) One ought not to inflict evil or harm; (2) one ought to prevent evil or harm; (3) one ought to remove evil or harm; and (4) one ought to do or promote good. Frankena arranged these elements in hierarchical order, so that the first takes precedence over the second, and so on. In this scheme, it is more important to avoid doing evil or harm than to do good. But in the Belmont Report, beneficence is understood as an obligation—first, to do no harm, and second, to maximize possible benefits and minimize possible harms.

The principle of beneficence is at the basis of Marcia Angell's support of allowing physicians to assist some patients in suicide and of Christopher James Ryan's concerns that some advance directives are too risky for patients.

Justice

The third ethical principle that is generally accepted is justice, which means "what is fair" or "what is deserved." An injustice occurs when some benefit to which a person is entitled is denied without good reason or when some burden is imposed unduly, according to the Belmont Report. Another way of interpreting the principle is to say that equals should be treated equally. However, some distinctions—such as age, experience, competence, physical condition, and the like—can justify unequal treatment. Those who appeal to the principle of justice are most concerned about which distinctions can be made legitimately and which ones cannot (see the issue on insurance and genetic testing).

One important derivative of the principle of justice is the recent emphasis on "rights" in bioethics. Given the successes in the 1960s and 1970s of civil rights movements in the courts and political arena, it is easy to understand the appeal of "rights talk." An emphasis on individual rights is part of the American tradition, in a way that emphasis on the "common good" is not. The language of rights has been prominent in the abortion debate, for instance, where the "right to life" has been pitted against the "right to privacy" or the "right to control one's body." The "right to health care" is a potent rallying cry, though it is one that is difficult to enforce legally. Although claims to rights may be effective in marshaling political support and in emphasizing moral ideals, those rights may not be the most effective way to solve ethical dilemmas. Our society, as philosopher Ruth Macklin has pointed out, has not yet agreed on a theory of justice in health care that will determine who has what kinds of rights and—the other side of the coin—who has the obligation to fulfill them.

When Principles Conflict

These three fundamental ethical principles—respect for persons, beneficence, and justice—all carry weight in ethical decision making. But what happens when they conflict? That is what this book is all about.

On each side of the issues included in this volume are writers who appeal, explicitly or implicitly, to one or more of these principles. For example, in Issue 8, Jean Toal sees beneficence as paramount, and she would criminalize drug-using behavior by pregnant women in order to prevent harm to their fetuses. Alexander Morgan Capron finds such a policy unjust because it singles out certain risks and certain women for state intervention.

Some of the issues are concerned with how to interpret a particular principle: Whether, for example, it is more or less beneficent to allow a physician to assist in suicide, or whether society's interest in healthy babies can be promoted by punishing women who expose fetuses to risk.

Will it ever be possible to resolve such fundamental divisions—those that are not merely matters of procedure or interpretation but of fundamental differences in principle? Lest the situation seem hopeless, consider that some consensus does seem to have been reached on questions that seemed equally tangled a few decades ago. The idea that government should play a role in regulating human subjects research was hotly debated, but it is now generally accepted (at least if the research is medical, not social or behavioral in nature, and is federally funded). And the appropriateness of using the criteria of brain death for determining the death of a person (and the possibility of subsequent removal of their organs for transplantation) has largely been accepted and written into state laws. The idea that a hopelessly ill patient has the legal and moral right to refuse treatment that will only postpone dying is also well established (though it is often hard to exercise because hospitals and physicians continue to resist it). Finally, nearly everyone now agrees that health care is distributed unjustly in the United States—a radical idea only a few years ago. There is, of course, sharp disagreement about whose responsibility it is to rectify the situation—the government's or the private sector's.

In the 16 years since the first edition of this book was published, the dominance of principles as the foundation of bioethics has been challenged. Several philosophers have pointed out, as already noted, that the "mid-level" principles are not grounded in a unified moral theory. Other writers have described the philosophical mode of argument as too arid and abstract, and they have called for the inclusion of other forms of discourse, such as public policy, emotion-based reasoning, and narrative, or "storytelling."

Besides the virtue theory, already described, two other candidates have their defenders. The ethics of caring has been presented as an alternative to traditional bioethics reasoning. Women, it is claimed, embody an ethic of caring, which is itself a prime aim of healing relationships. An ethic of caring would focus on relationships rather than autonomy, on reconciliation rather than winning an argument, and on nurturing rather than imposing dominance. While the absence of caring relationships is clearly a problem in modern health care, this view has been severely criticized by many, including women, as failing to provide a sufficient basis for replacing ethical principles.

Another mode of analysis that is being revived is casuistry. Although associated with the Middle Ages and religious thinking, casuistry is simply a way of reaching consensus on principles by focusing on concrete cases—the clearest ones first, and then the harder ones. The casuist reaches principles from the bottom up, rather than deciding cases from the top (principles first) down.

A final form of analysis is clinical ethics. Its practitioners focus on the clinical realities of moral choices as they emerge in ordinary health care. It is not antithetical to principles but brings abstractions back to reality by measuring proposed solutions against the real world in which doctors and patients live and work. Issue 6 on the refusal of treatment on the grounds of "futility" builds on clinical ethics and real cases.

Edmund Pellegrino, a distinguished physician and ethicist, has seen many changes in the 50 years he has been involved in medicine. Looking toward the future, he does not see the death of principles, but he does foresee some changes. "Physicians and other health workers must become familiar with shifts in contemporary moral philosophy," he says, "if they are to maintain a hand in restructuring the ethics of their profession." But clinicians, too, must change, to "provide a reality check on the nihilism and skepticism of contemporary philosophy. Medical ethics is too ancient and too essential . . . to be left entirely to the fortuitous currents of philosophical fashion or the unsupported assertion of clinicians."

Although there is consensus in some areas, in others there is only controversy. This book will introduce you to some of the ongoing debates. Whether or not we will be able to move beyond opposing views to a realm of moral consensus will depend on society's willingness to struggle with these issues and to make the hard choices that are required.

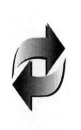

On the Internet . . .

Medical College of Wisconsin: Center for the Study of Bioethics

This site contains a bioethics literature database that is regularly updated. The database contains information on informed consent and other bioethics issues.

http://www.mcw.edu/bioethics/

Agency for Healthcare Research and Quality (AHRQ)

The AHRQ Web site provides research-based information to increase the scientific knowledge needed to enhance consumer and clinical decision making, improve health care quality, and promote efficiency in the organization of public and private systems of health care delivery.

http://www.ahrq.gov

Biomedical Ethics: Readings on the Internet

This site provides an article that outlines the history of patient autonomy and how it has transformed American medicine. Other articles concerning topics in bioethics are also included.

http://www.uwc.edu/fonddulac/faculty/rrigteri/
biomed.htm

PART 1

Medical Decision Making

*I*n *earlier times medical decision making was of concern only to physicians. With their presumed greater knowledge and with patients' best interests at heart, they were entrusted with making life-and-death, as well as critical, decisions. Ironically, although physicians had greater power in those times than they do today, they also had less ability to treat. As medicine has grown more technologically and scientifically sophisticated, the range of people who have an interest in making decisions —and in some cases, a right to do so—among the medical options has grown. Law and ethics have reaffirmed the status of the patient as the primary decision maker. Nevertheless, many ambiguous and troubling situations remain in implementing patients' wishes. It is not even clear that patients have the moral right to make arbitrary decisions about aspects of their care, especially when their preferences impinge on the rights of others, such as family members, physicians, and other patients. This section explores some of the issues that arise when making medical decisions.*

- Is Informed Consent Still Central to Medical Ethics?

- Can Family Interests Ethically Outweigh Patient Autonomy?

ISSUE 1

Is Informed Consent Still Central to Medical Ethics?

YES: Robert M. Arnold and Charles W. Lidz, from "Informed Consent: Clinical Aspects of Consent in Health Care," in Warren T. Reich, ed., *Encyclopedia of Bioethics, vol. 3*, rev. ed. (Simon & Schuster, 1995)

NO: Robert M. Veatch, from "Abandoning Informed Consent," *Hastings Center Report* (March–April 1995)

ISSUE SUMMARY

YES: Physician Robert M. Arnold and professor of psychiatry and sociology Charles W. Lidz assert that informed consent in clinical care is an essential process that promotes good communication and patient autonomy despite the obstacles of implementation.

NO: Professor of medical ethics Robert M. Veatch argues that informed consent is a transitional concept that is useful only for moving toward a more radical framework in which physicians and patients are paired on the basis of shared deep social, moral, and institutional values.

Informed consent is undoubtedly one of the best-known and, arguably, one of the least-implemented concepts in modern medicine. Although much of modern medical ethics has ancient roots, the idea of informed consent is relatively recent. Until the mid-twentieth century most medical ethics were firmly based on the obligations of physicians to act for the benefit of their patients. Information was supposed to be managed carefully in order to protect patients from bad news and to keep them hopeful.

The first "Code of Medical Ethics" of the American Medical Association relied heavily on the work of Thomas Percival, a British physician whose book *Medical Ethics* (1803) played a crucial role in the field for more than a century. Percival believed that the patient's right to the truth was less important than the physician's obligation to benefit the patient. Deception, in the interest of doing good, was thus justified. The patient's consent to treatment, informed or otherwise, is not mentioned in early codes of medical ethics, although on

2

a practical level doctors had to have a patient's permission to perform most procedures.

The modern concept of informed consent came to medical ethics through the courts. The earliest influential decision was *Schloendorff v. New York Hospital* (1914), in which the court ruled that a patient's right to "self-determination" obligated a physician to obtain consent. This case laid the basis for further litigation. The most influential series of decisions occurred in the 1950s and 1960s, when rulings went beyond the obligation to obtain consent to include an explicit duty to disclose information relevant to the patient who is making a decision about consent.

While the earlier cases had been based on the patient's right to be free from unwanted bodily intrusion (legally, "battery"), the court in *Natanson v. Kline* (1960) held that physicians who withheld information while obtaining consent were guilty of negligence. Imposing a legal duty on physicians to inform their patients of the risks, benefits, and alternatives to treatment exposed them to the risk of malpractice suits. Another factor that influenced the ascendance of informed consent in medical treatment were parallel discussions about the ethics of research involving human subjects. Voluntary consent to participate in research was a cornerstone of the Nuremberg Code of 1947, which was issued after the trials of Nazi physicians who had performed lethal experiments on nonconsenting prisoners.

Nevertheless, traditions die hard, and little change was seen in actual practice until the resurgence of interest in medical ethics in the 1970s. In 1972 the case of *Canterbury v. Spence* established a far-reaching patient-centered disclosure standard. The ruling stated, "The patient's right of self-decision can be effectively exercised only if the patient possesses enough information to enable an intelligent choice. . . . Social policy does not accept the paternalistic view that the physician may remain silent because divulgence might prompt the patient to forego needed therapy." In the 1980s and 1990s court cases have focused on individuals who lack the competence to provide informed consent, such as comatose patients, children, and mentally ill persons.

Although the physician's duty to obtain informed consent and the patient's right to information are now firmly established in law and grounded in the ethical principle of respect for persons, medical practice varies considerably. In Warren T. Reich, ed., *Encyclopedia of Bioethics* (1995), Tom L. Beauchamp and Ruth R. Faden, philosophers who have studied informed consent extensively, assert, "The overwhelming impression from the empirical literature and from reported clinical experience is that the actual process of soliciting informed consent often falls short of a serious show of respect for the decisional authority of patients."

The following selections illustrate two views of the future of informed consent. Robert M. Arnold and Charles W. Lidz reassert the importance of informed consent and offer ways in which the process can be improved in the clinical setting, despite the many obstacles. Robert M. Veatch argues that the concept of informed consent is inherently inadequate because clinicians can never assess fully, and thus can never recommend, what might be in the patient's best interests.

Robert M. Arnold and
Charles W. Lidz

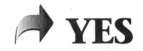

Informed Consent: Clinical Aspects of Consent in Health Care

Health-care decision making is an everyday event, not only for doctors and patients but also for nurses, psychologists, social workers, emergency medical technicians, dentists, and other health professionals. Since the 1960s, however, the cultural ideal of how those decisions should be made has changed considerably. The concept that medical decision making should rely exclusively on the physician's expertise has been replaced by a model in which health-care professionals share information and discuss alternatives with patients who then make the ultimate decisions about treatment. This article reviews the origins in the United States of this ideal in the doctrine of informed consent, discusses various arguments against its use in clinical decision making, and describes a model for effectively incorporating it into clinical practice with competent patients.

The concept of informed consent gained its initial support as part of the general societal trend toward broadening access to decision making during the 1960s. Thus, the initial support for informed consent came from legal and philosophic circles rather than from health-care professionals. In the legal arena, informed consent has been used to develop minimal standards for doctor-patient interactions and clinical decision making (Appelbaum et al., 1987). Although there are some differences by jurisdiction, widely accepted legal standards require that health-care professionals inform patients of the risks, benefits, and alternatives of all proposed treatments and then allow the patient to choose among acceptable therapeutic alternatives. In academia, informed consent has served as a cornerstone for the development of the discipline of bioethics. Based on the importance of autonomy in moral discourse, philosophers have argued that health-care professionals are obligated to engage patients in discussions regarding the goals of therapy and the alternatives for reaching those goals and that patients are the final decision makers regarding all therapeutic decisions.

There also has been some support for informed consent within academic medicine, but there seems to be little enthusiasm for it in routine medical practice (Lidz et al., 1984). Physicians typically think of informed consent as a legal requirement for a signed piece of paper that is at best a waste of time and at worst a bureaucratic, legalistic interference with their care for patients. Rather

From Robert M. Arnold and Charles W. Lidz, "Informed Consent: Clinical Aspects of Consent in Health Care," in Warren T. Reich, ed., *Encyclopedia of Bioethics, vol. 3*, rev. ed. (Simon & Schuster, 1995), pp. 1250–1256. Copyright © 1995 by Warren T. Reich. Reprinted by permission of The Gale Group. References omitted.

than seeing informed consent as a process that promotes good communication and patient autonomy, many health-care professionals view informed consent as a complex, legally prescribed recitation of risks and benefits that only frightens or confuses patients. There are various objections to informed consent that clinicians often make, and it will be useful to review those objections here.

Objections to Informed Consent

Consent cannot be truly "informed."   Many practicing clinicians report that their patients are unable to understand the complex medical information necessary for a fully rational weighing of alternative treatments. There is considerable research support for this view. A variety of studies document that patients recall only a small percentage of the information that professionals present to them (Meisel and Roth, 1981); that they are not as good decision makers when they are sick as at other times (Sherlock, 1986); and that they often make decisions based on medically trivial factors. Informed consent thus appears either to promote uninformed, and thus suboptimal, decisions or to encourage patients to blindly accept health-care professionals' recommendations. In either case informed consent appears to be a charade, and a dangerous one at that.

That patients often do have difficulty understanding important aspects of medical decisions does not mean that health-care professionals are the best decision makers about the patient's treatment. Knowledge about medical facts is not enough. Wise house buyers will have a structural engineer check over an old house, but few would be willing to allow the engineer to choose their house for them. Just as structural engineers cannot decide which house a family should buy because they lack knowledge about the family's pattern of living, personal tastes, and potential family growth, health-care professionals cannot scientifically deduce the best treatment for a specific patient simply from the medical facts. Because what matters to individuals about their health depends on their lifestyles, past experiences, and values, choosing the "optimal therapy" is not a purely "objective" matter. Thus, patients and health-care professionals both contribute essential knowledge to the decision-making process—patients bring their knowledge of their personal situation, goals, and values, and health-care professionals bring their expertise on the nature of the problem and the technology that may be used to meet the patient's goals.

Informed-consent disclosures, even if they are well done, may not lead to what clinicians might consider optimal decisions. Most people make major life decisions, such as whom to marry and which occupation to take up, based on faulty or incomplete information. Patients' lack of understanding of medical information in choosing treatment is probably no worse than their lack of information in choosing a spouse, nor are medical decisions more important than spousal choice. Respecting patient autonomy means allowing individuals to make their own decisions even if the health-care professional disagrees with them. Informed-consent disclosures can improve patient decisions, but they cannot be expected to lead to perfect decisions.

Moreover, although sick persons have some defects in their rational abilities, so do health-care professionals. There are no data that demonstrate that health-care professionals' reasoning abilities are better than patients. In fact, some of the most famous research on the difficulties individuals have with the rational use of probabilistic data involves physicians (Dawson and Ackes, 1987). Health professionals must be careful not to be to pessimistic about patients' ability to become informed decision makers. Patients may not be able to become as technically well-informed as professionals, but they clearly can understand and make decisions based on relevant information. A recent study, for example, showed that patients' decisions regarding life-sustaining treatment changed when they were given accurate information about the therapy's chance of success (Murphy et al., 1994).

Most important, the difficulty of educating sick persons does not justify unilateral decision making. Rather, it places a special obligation on health-care professionals to communicate clearly with patients. Using technical jargon, trying to give all of the available information in one visit, and not asking what the patient wants to know is a recipe for confusing even the most intelligent patient. A growing literature, for example, discusses the problems patients have understanding uncertainty about treatment outcomes and suggests ways to help patients deal with such uncertainty (Katz, 1984). Health-care professionals also need to become more familiar with different cultural patterns of communication in order to talk with patients from different cultural backgrounds. For example, although a simple, factual discussion of depression and its treatment may be acceptable to most middle-class Americans, it would be seen as inappropriate by a first-generation Vietnamese male (Hahn, 1982), whose culture discourages viewing depression as a disease. There is no reason, in principle, why a person who daily makes decisions at home and work cannot, with help, understand the medical data sufficiently to become involved in medical decisions. Health-care professionals must learn how best to present that help.

Patients do not wish to be involved in decision making. Many health-care professionals believe that it is unfair to force patients to make decisions regarding their medical care. After all, they argue, patients pay their health-care professionals to make medical decisions. The empirical literature partially supports the view that patients want professionals to make treatment decisions for them (Steele et al., 1987). For example, in a study of male patients' preferences about medical decision making regarding hypertension, only 53 percent wanted to participate at all in the decision-making process.

There is no reason to force patients to be involved in decisions if they do not want to be. However, unless the health professional asks, he or she cannot know how involved a patient wants to be. Indeed, patients may not always want to be involved in decision making, since many have been socialized into believing that "the doctor knows best." This is particularly true for poorer patients. Studies have shown that physicians wrongly assume that because patients with fewer socioeconomic resources ask fewer questions, they do not want as much information. These patients may in fact want just as much information, but they have been socialized into a different way of interacting with health-care professionals (Waitzkin, 1984).

Patients may choose to allow someone else to make the decision for them. However, when a patient asks, "What would you do if you were me?" the underlying question may be, "As an expert in biomedicine, what alternative do you think will best maximize my values or interest?" If this is the case, the health-care professional should respond by making a recommendation and justifying it in terms of the patient's values or interests. More frequently, the patient is asking, "If you had this disease, what therapy would you choose?" This question presumes that the professional and patient have the same values, needs, and problems, something that is often not true. Health-care professionals should respond by pointing this out and by emphasizing the importance of the patients' values in the decision-making process.

Although many patients do not want to be actively involved in decision making, they almost always want more information concerning their illness than the health-care professional gives them. Health-care professionals should not assume that just because patients do not wish to choose their therapy, they do not want information. Patients may desire information so as to increase compliance or make modifications in other areas of their lives, as well as to make medical decisions.

There are harmful effects of informing patients.   Health-care professionals often justify withholding information from patients because of their belief that informing patients would be psychologically damaging and therefore contrary to the principle of nonmaleficence. Many health-care professionals, however, overestimate potential psychological harm and neglect the positive effects of full disclosure (Faden et al., 1986). Moreover, bad news can often be communicated in a way that ameliorates the psychological effects of the disclosure (Quill and Townsend, 1991). Truth-telling must be distinguished from "truth dumping." Explanation of the care that can be provided, and empathic attention to the patient's fears and uncertainties can often prevent or mitigate otherwise more painful news.

Informed consent takes too much time.   Respecting autonomy and promoting patient well-being, the values served through informed consent, are fundamental to good medicine. However, adhering to the ideals of medical practice takes time, time to help patients understand their illness and work through their emotional reactions to stressful information; to discuss each party's preconceptions and to clarify the therapeutic goals; to decide on a treatment plan; and to elicit questions about diagnosis and treatment.

In U.S. health care, time is money. As many commentators have noted, physicians are less well reimbursed for talking to patients than for performing invasive tests. This may discourage doctors from spending enough time discussing treatment options with patients. Changes in physician reimbursement, such as the Relative-Value Based Scale, which are designed to increase reimbursement for cognitive skills, including the time it takes to discuss diagnosis and treatment with patients, will encourage physicians to discuss patients' preferences with them. The ultimate justification for spending time to facilitate patient decisions, however, is the same as that for spending any time in medical care: that patients will be better cared for.

Clinical Approaches to Informed Consent

Many of the problems in implementing informed consent result at least in part from the way informed consent has been implemented in clinical practice. Informed consent has become synonymous with the "consent form," a legal invention with a legitimate role in documenting that informed consent has taken place, but hardly a substitute for the discussion process leading to informed consent (Andrews, 1984).

A pro forma approach: An event model of informed consent.   In many clinical settings, consent begins when "it is time to get consent," typically just prior to the administration of treatment. The process of getting the patients' consent consists of the recitation by a physician or nurse of the list of material risks and benefits and a request that the patient sign for the proposed treatment. This "conversation" is a very limited one that emphasizes the transfer of information from the physician or nurse to the patient. This procedure does meet the minimal legal requirements for informed consent efficiently. However, it does not meet the higher ethical goal of informed consent, which is to empower patients by educating and involving them in their treatment plans. Instead, it imposes an almost empty ritual on an unchanged relationship between health-care provider and patient (Katz, 1984).

The procedure just described assumes that care involves a series of discrete, circumscribed decisions. In fact, much of clinical medicine consists of a series of frequent, interwoven decisions that must be repeatedly reconsidered as more information becomes available. When "it is time to get consent," there may be nothing left to decide. Consider the operative consent form obtained the evening prior to an operation. After patients have discussed with their families whether to be admitted to the hospital, rearranged their work and child-care schedules for admission, and undergone a long and painful diagnostic workup, the decision to have surgery seems preordained. The evening before the operation, patients do not seriously evaluate the operation's risks and benefits; consent is pro forma. No wonder some health-care professionals feel that "consent" is a waste of time and energy.

The event model for gathering informed consent falls far short of meeting the ethical goal of ensuring patient participation in the decision-making process. Rather than engaging the patient as an active participant in the decision-making process, the patient's role is to agree to or veto the health-care professionals' recommendations. Little attempt is made to elicit patient preferences and to consider how treatment might address them.

A dialogical approach: The process model of informed consent.   Fortunately, it is possible to fulfill legal requirements for informed consent while maximizing active patient participation in the clinical setting. An alternative to the event model described above, which sees informed consent as an aberration from clinical practice, the process model attempts to integrate informed consent into all aspects of clinical care (Appelbaum et al., 1987). The process model of informed consent assumes that each party has something to contribute to the decision-making process. The physician brings technical knowledge and experience in treating patients with similar problems. Patients bring knowledge about their life circumstances and the ability to assess the effect that treatment may have on them. Open discussion makes it possible for the patient and the physician to examine critically their views and to determine what might be optimal treatment.

The process model also recognizes that medical care rarely involves only one decision, made at a single point in time. Decisions about care frequently begin with the suspicion that something is wrong and that treatment may be necessary, and end only when the patient leaves follow-up care. Decisions involve diagnostic as well as therapeutic interventions. Some decisions are made in one visit, while others occur over a prolonged period of time. Although some interactions between health-care professional and patient involve explicit decisions, decisions are made at each interaction, even if the decision is only to continue treatment. The process model also recognizes that various health-care professionals may play a role in making sure that the patients' consent is informed. For example, a woman deciding on various breast cancer treatments may talk with an oncologist and a surgeon about the risks of various treatments, with a nurse about the side effects of medication, with a social worker about financial issues in treatment, and with a patient-support group about her husband's reaction to a possible mastectomy.

Ideally, then, informed consent involves shared decision making over a period of time, that is, a dialogue throughout the course of the patient's relationship with various health-care professionals. Such a dialogue aims to facilitate patient participation and to strengthen the therapeutic alliance.

Tasks Involved in Informed Consent

Consent is a series of interrelated tasks. First, the patient and professional must agree on the problem that will be the focus of their work together (Eisenthal and Lazare, 1976). Most nonemergency consultations involve complex negotiations between health-care professional and patient regarding the definition of the patient's problem. The patient may see the problem as a routine physical examination for a work release, the need for advice, or the investigation of a physical symptom. If professionals are to respond effectively to the patients' goals, they must find out the reason for the visit. Whereas physicians typically focus on biomedical information and its implications, patients typically view the problem in the context of their social situation (Fisher and Todd, 1983). The differences between the patient's perceptions of the problem and the professional's must be explicitly worked through since agreement regarding the focus of the interactions lead to increased patient satisfaction and compliance with further treatment plans (Meichenbaum and Turk, 1987).

Even when the professional and patient have agreed on what the problem is, substantial misunderstanding may arise regarding the treatment goals. The patient may expect the medically impossible, or may expect outcomes based on knowledge of life circumstances about which the physician is unaware. Since assessing the risks and benefits of any treatment option depends on therapeutic goals, the professional and patient must agree on the goals the therapy aims to accomplish.

Finding out what the patient wants is more complicated than merely inquiring, "What do you want?" A patient typically does not come to the professional with well-developed preferences regarding medical therapy except "to get better," with little understanding of what this may involve. As a patient's knowledge and perspective change over the course of an illness, so too may the patient's views regarding the therapeutic goals.

Because clinicians provide much of the medical information needed to ensure that the patient's preferences are grounded in medical possibility, health-care professionals play a significant role in how a patient's preferences evolve. It is important that they understand that patients may reasonably hold different goals from those their practitioners hold. This is particularly true when they come from different economic strata. For example, a physician's emphasis on the most medically sophisticated care may pale in the light of the patient's financial problems. Therapeutic goals, like the definition of the problem, require ongoing clarification and negotiation.

After agreeing upon the problem and the therapeutic goals, the health-care professional and the patient must choose the best way to achieve them. If patients have been involved in the prior two steps, the decision about a treatment plan will more likely reflect their values than if they are merely asked to assent to the clinician's strategy.

Health-care professionals often ask how much information they must supply to ensure that the patient is an informed participant in the decision-making process (Mazur, 1986). There is a more important question: Has the information been provided in a manner that the patient can understand? While the law only requires that health-care professionals inform patients, morally valid consent requires that patients understand the information conveyed. Ensuring patient understanding requires attention to the quality as well as the quantity of information presented (Faden, 1977).

A great deal of empirical data has been collected concerning problems with consent forms. These forms have been criticized, for example, as being unintelligible because of their length and use of technical language (Appelbaum et al., 1987). Health-care professionals thus need to be aware of, and facile in using, a variety of methods to increase patients' comprehension of information; these include verbal techniques, written information, or interactive videodiscs (Stanley et al., 1984).

Still, the question of how much information to present remains. The legal standards regarding information disclosure—what a reasonable patient would find essential to making a decision or what a reasonably prudent physician would disclose—are not particularly helpful. Howard Brody has suggested two important features: (1) The physician must disclose the basis on which the proposed treatment or the alternative possible treatments have been chosen; and (2) the patient must be encouraged to ask questions, suggested by the disclosure about the physician's reasoning, and the questions need to be answered to the patient's satisfaction (Brody, 1989). Health-care professionals must also inform patients when controversy exists about the various therapeutic options. Similarly, patients should also be told the degree to which the recommendation is based on established scientific evidence versus personal experience or educated guesses.

Two other factors will influence the amount of information that should be given: the importance of the decision, given the patient's situation and goals, and the amount of consensus within the health-care professions regarding the agreed-upon therapy. For example, a low-risk intervention, such as giving influenza vaccines to elderly patients, offers a clear-cut benefit with minimal risk. In this case, the professional should describe the intervention and recommend it because of its benefits. A detailed description of the infrequent risks is not needed unless the patient asks or is known to be skeptical of medical interventions. Interventions that present greater risks or a less clear-cut risk-benefit ratio require a longer description—for example, the decision to administer AZT to an HIV (human immunodeficiency virus)-positive, asymptomatic woman with a CD4 count of 400. In neither case is a discussion of pathophysiology or biochemistry necessary. It must be emphasized that there is no formula for deciding how much a patient needs to be told. The amount of information necessary will depend on the patient's individual situation, values, and goals.

Finally, an adequate decision-making process requires continual updating of information, monitoring of expectations, and evaluation of the patient's progress in reaching the chosen or revised goals. Thus the final step in informed consent is follow-up. This step is particularly important for patients with chronic diseases in which modifications of the treatment plan are often necessary.

The process model of informed consent just described has many advantages. Because it assumes many short conversations over time rather than one long interaction, it can be more easily integrated into the professional's ambulatory practice than the event model; it allows patients to be much more involved in decision making and ensures that treatment is more consistent with their values. Furthermore, the continual monitoring of patients' understanding of their disease, the treatment, and its progress is likely to reduce misunderstandings and increase their investment in, and adherence to, the treatment plan. Thus, the process model of informed consent is likely to promote both patient autonomy and well-being.

There are situations in which this approach is not very helpful. Some health-care professionals, anesthesiologists or emergency medical technicians, for example, are not likely to have ongoing relationships with patients. In emergencies, there is not time for a decision to develop through a series of short conversations. In these cases, informed consent may more closely approximate the event model. However, since most medical care is delivered by primary-care practitioners in an ambulatory setting, the process model of informed consent is more helpful.

Robert M. Veatch 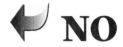 **NO**

Abandoning Informed Consent

Consent has emerged as a concept central to modern medical ethics. Often the term is used with a modifier, such as *informed* or *voluntary* or *full,* as in loosely used phrases like "fully informed and voluntary consent." In some form or another, modern ethics in health care could hardly function without the notion of consent.

While we might occasionally encounter an old-guard retrograde longing for the day when physicians did not have to go through the process of getting consent, by and large consent is now taken as a given, at least at the level of theory. To be sure, we know that actual consent is not obtained in all cases and even when consent is obtained, it may not be adequately informed or autonomous. For purposes of this discussion, we shall not worry about the deviations from the ideal; rather the focus will be on whether consent ought to be the goal.

This consensus in favor of consent may turn out to be all too facile. *Consent* may be what can be called a transition concept, one that appears on the scene as an apparently progressive innovation, but after a period of experience turns out to be only useful as a transition to a more thoroughly revisionary conceptual framework.

This paper will defend the thesis that consent is merely a transitional concept. While it emerged in the field as a liberal, innovative idea, its time may have passed and newer, more enlightened formulations may be needed. Consent means approval or agreement with the actions or opinions of another; terms such as *acquiescence* and *condoning* appear in the dictionary definitions. In medicine, the physician or other health care provider will, after reviewing the facts of the case and attempting to determine what is in the best interest of the patient, propose a course of action for the patient's concurrence. While a few decades ago it might have been considered both radical and innovative to seek the patient's acquiescence in the professional's clinical judgment, by now that may not be nearly enough. It is increasingly clear if one studies the theory of clinical decisionmaking that there is no longer any basis for presuming that the clinician can even guess at what is in the overall best interest of the patient. If that is true, then a model in which the clinician guesses at what he or she believes is best for the patient, pausing only to elicit the patient's concurrence, will no longer be sufficient. Increasingly we will have to go beyond patient

From Robert M. Veatch, "Abandoning Informed Consent," *Hastings Center Report,* vol. 25, no. 2 (March–April 1995). Copyright © 1995 by The Hastings Center. Reprinted by permission.

consent to a model in which plausible options are presented (perhaps with the professional's recommendation regarding a personal preference among them, based on the professional's personally held beliefs and values), but with no rational or "professional" basis for even guessing at which one might truly be in the patient's best interest....

Modern medicine has reluctantly made room for the consent doctrine and has recognized, at least in theory, the right of patients to consent and refuse consent to certain kinds of treatment. Usually explicit consent is reserved for these more complex and exotic decisions. It is still common to hear people distinguish between treatments for which consent is required and those for which it is not. Surely it would be better to speak of those for which consent must be explicit and others that still require consent even though the consent can be implied or presumed. For example, many would probably say that routine blood drawings of modest amounts of blood can be done without consent. This would more appropriately be described as being done without explicit consent and with no specific information needing to be transmitted. The mere extending of the arm should count as an adequate consent.

Likewise, when a physician writes a prescription, he or she is supposed to review the alternatives and choose the best medication, select a brand name or generic equivalent, choose a route of administration, a dosage level, and length of use of the medication. The patient may signal "consent" simply by accepting the prescription and getting it filled at the local pharmacy.

Up until now no one has seriously questioned the adequacy, from the left, of an approach that permits explicit consent for special and complex treatment, including research and surgery, and implicit or presumed consent for more routine procedures. More careful analysis reveals that, in fact, the consent model buys into more of the traditional, authoritarian understanding of clinical decisionmaking than many people realize. As in the days prior to the development of the consent doctrine, the clinician is still supposed to draw on his or her medical knowledge to determine what he or she believes is in the best interest of the patient and propose that course of treatment. Terms such as "doctor's orders" may have been replaced by more appropriate images, but the physician is still expected to determine what is "medically indicated," the "treatment of choice," or what in the "clinical judgment" of the practitioner is best for the patient. The clinician then proposes that course, subject only to the qualification that through either word or action, the patient signals approval of the physician-determined plan.

Consent and the Theory of the Good

Current work on the theory of medical decisionmaking and in axiology [the study of the theory of the good] makes increasingly clear that this pattern no longer makes sense. It still rests on the outdated presumption that the clinician's moral responsibility is to do what is best for the patient, according to his or her ability and judgment, and that there is some reason to hope that the clinician can determine what is in the patient's best interest. The idea in medical ethics of doing what is best for the patient has achieved the status of an unquestioned platitude, but like many platitudes, it may not stand the test of more careful examination. On several levels the problems are beginning to show.

The Best Interest Standard in Surrogate Decisions.   The "best interest standard" has become the standard for surrogate decisionmaking in cases in which the wishes of the patient are not known and substituted judgment based on the patient's beliefs and values is not possible. But the best interest standard, if taken literally, is terribly implausible. In fact, no decisionmaker is held to it in practice.

Two problems arise. First, since such judgments are increasingly recognized to be terribly complex and subjective, it is now widely accepted that the surrogate need not choose literally what is best. It would be extremely difficult to determine whether the absolute best choice has been made. Surely, the opinion of the attending physician cannot serve as a definitive standard. A privately appointed, parochial ethics committee might be better, but still surely is not definitive. If every surrogate decision were taken to court, we still would not have an absolute assurance that the best choice had been made.

Fortunately, we generally do not hold parents and other surrogates to a literal best interest standard when they make decisions for their wards. We expect, tolerate, even encourage a reasonable range of discretion. That is why it makes sense to replace the best interest standard with a "standard of reasonableness" or what could be called a "reasonable interest standard."[1]

There is a second reason why the best interest standard is inappropriate for surrogate decisions. Often surrogates have legitimate moral obligations to people other than the patient. Parents, for example, are pledged to serve the welfare of their other children. When best interests conflict, it is logically impossible to fulfill simultaneously the best interest standard for more than one child at the same time. Surely, all that is expected is that a reasonable balance of the conflicting interests be pursued.

Problems With Best Interest in Clinician Judgments.   Although the problems with the best interest standard in surrogate decisions are more immediately apparent, a more fundamental and important problem with best interest arises when clinicians are held to the best interest standard in an ethic of patient care. For a clinician to guess at what is the best course for the patient, three assumptions must be true regarding a theory of the good. First, the clinician must be expected to determine what will best serve the patient's medical or health interest; second, the clinician must be expected to determine how to trade off health interests with other interests; and third, the clinician must be expected to determine how the patient should relate the pursuit of her best interest to other moral goals and responsibilities, including serving the interests of others and fulfilling any moral duties she may have that happen to conflict with her interest. An examination of the theories of the good and the morally right will reveal that it is terribly implausible to expect a typical clinician to be able to perform any one of these tasks completely correctly, let alone all three of them. If the clinician cannot be expected to guess at what serves the well-being of the patient and determine when patient well-being should be subordinated to other moral requirements, then there is no way that he or she can be expected to propose a course of treatment to which the patient would offer mere consent.

... [W]e can understand what promotes the good for persons better by asking what the elements are that contribute to one's well-being. Another way of putting the question would be to ask in what areas one's limited amount of personal resources—time, money, energy, and material—ought to be invested in order to maximize well-being.

The Main Elements of Well-Being. Several elements can be identified. These would surely include some concern with medicine or what could be called one's organic well-being. Closely related, but distinct, would be psychological well-being. It would be a terrible distortion to assume that well-being involved only the organic and psychological, however. Reasonable persons would devote considerable attention and resources to other elements, including the social, legal, occupational, religious, aesthetic, and other components that together make up one's total well-being. There is no reason to assume that each of these components is the same size. By trading off emphasis on different components one should be able to increase or decrease the size of the whole. Well-being is not a zero-sum game.

The problem is central to the concern about the concept of consent. It is unrealistic to expect experts in any one component to be able to speak knowledgeably about well-being in its other components. If this is true, then it makes no sense to expect them to come up with a proposed intervention that will promote the total well-being of the individual....

Why Experts Should Not Propose a Course for Patient Consent

It should now be clear why it makes no sense to continue to rely on consent as the mode of transaction between professionals and their clients. In order for a physician to make an initial estimate of which treatment best served the patient's interest, he or she would first have to develop a definitive theory of the relationship among various medical goods and pick the course that best served the patient's medical good. Then the clinician would have to estimate correctly the proper relationship between the patient's medical good and all other components of the good so that the patient's overall well-being was served.

Even if this could be done, there is a final problem. In virtually any moral theory the well-being of the individual is only one element. Plausible consequentialist theories (such as utilitarianism) also insist that the good of other parties be taken into account. Plausible nonconsequentialist theories, including Kantian theories, natural law theories, much of biblical ethics, and all other deontological theories, hold that knowing what will be in the best interests of persons does not necessarily settle the question of the right thing to do. Many patients may purposely want to consider options that do not maximize their well-being. A patient may acknowledge, for example, that his well-being would be served if he lived longer, but choose to sacrifice his interests to conserve resources for his offspring. A pregnant woman might conclude, for another example, that her interests would be served if she had an abortion, but that such a course would still be morally wrong. Both of these people would rationally not choose the course of action that admittedly maximized their personal well-being. Even if physicians can figure out what maximizes medical well-being and how medical well-being should be related to other elements of well-being, that still does not necessarily lead to the course that is right, all things considered. To know what is "good medicine" and what should be recommended for the patient's assessment and consent, one needs to know how to answer all three of these questions. There is no basis for assuming that physicians have any special expertise in answering any of them. . . .

Choice: The Liberal Alternative

If consent is no longer adequate as a mechanism for assuring that the patient's beliefs and values will help shape decisions about what a patient ought to do, what are the alternatives? Adherents to medical ethical systems that emphasize autonomy may prefer the concept of choice to that of consent. In this alternative the patient would be presented with a list of plausible treatment options, together with a summary of the potential benefits and risks of each. It is important to emphasize that choice is conceptually different from consent and potentially could replace consent as the basis for patient involvement in health care decisions.

This "liberal" solution, however, faces serious, probably insurmountable problems. First, if the choices that are plausible for the patient are contingent on the beliefs and values of the patient, then the professional cannot be sure that all plausible options are being presented unless he or she has knowledge of the patient's beliefs and values—knowledge that we have argued is normally unavailable. Second, some options (for example, suicide) may be so offensive to some practitioners that they ought not to present them. Third, it is increasingly recognized that even the description of the "facts" necessarily must incorporate certain value judgments, such that even the clinician of good will cannot give a value-free account of the likely outcomes of the alternatives. In short, while the choice alternative may go part of the way toward giving the patient more active control, it is naive to believe it will be able to solve the problems with the consent model.

Pairing Based on "Deep Values"

There is another alternative worth considering. If a clinician is skilled and passionately committed to maximizing the patient's welfare, and knows the belief and value structure and socioeconomic and cultural position of the patient quite well, there would be some more reason to hope for a good guess. Unfortunately, not only is that an ever-vanishing possibility, even knowing the value system of the patient well probably would not be sufficient. The value choices that go into a judgment about what is best for another are so complex and subtle that merely knowing the other's values and trying to empathize will probably not be enough. There is ample evidence that unconscious value distortions will not only influence the clinician's judgment about what is best, but even influence the very interpretation of the scientific data.

There might be more hope if the patient were to choose her cadre of well-being experts (lawyers, accountants, physicians) on the basis of their "deep" value systems. That way when unconscious bias and distortion occur, as inevitably they must, they will tip the decision in the direction of the patient's own system.

I say "deep" value system because I want to make clear that I am not referring to the cursory assessment of the professional's personality, demeanor and short-term tastes. That would hardly suffice. If, however, there were alignments, "value pairings," based on the most fundamental worldviews of the lay person and professional, then there would be some hope. This probably would mean picking providers on the basis of their religious and political affiliations, philosophical and social inclinations, and other deeply penetrating worldviews. To the extent that the provider and patient were of the same mind set, then there is some reason that the technically competent clinician could guess fairly well what would serve the patient's interest.

The difficulty in establishing a convergence of deep values cannot be underestimated. Surely it would not be sufficient, for instance, to pair providers and patients on the basis of their institutional religious affiliations. Not all members of a religious denomination think alike. But there is reason to hope that people can establish an affinity of deep value orientations, at least for certain types of medical services. For example, certain institutionalized health care delivery systems are now organizing around identifiable value frameworks, recruiting professional and administrative staff on the basis of commitment to that value framework, and then announcing that framework to the public so as to attract only those patients who share the basic value commitment of the institution. A hospice is organized around such a constellation of values. It recruits staff committed to those values and attracts patients who share that commitment. When hospice-based health care providers present options to patients they should admit that they do not present all possible options. (They do not propose an aggressive oncology protocol, for instance; most would not present physician-assisted suicide or active mercy killing.) They should also admit that when they explain options and their potential benefits and harms they do so in ways that incorporate a tone of voice or body language that reflects their value judgments. Patients, however, need be less concerned about this value encroachment than if they were discussing options with a provider who was deeply, instinctively committed to maximally aggressive life preservation. There will be biases, but they will be less corrupting of the patient's own perspective.

Other delivery systems are beginning to organize around deep value orientations: feminist health centers, holistic health clinics, and the National Institutes of Health Clinical Center all announce at least their general value orientations to potential patients.

Providing an institutional framework for pairing based on deep value convergence in more routine health care may be more difficult, but not impossible. HMOs could be organized by social and religious groups that could formally articulate certain value commitments. A Catholic HMO, like a Catholic hospital, could articulate to potential members not only a set of values pertaining to obstetrical and gynecological issues, but also a framework for deciding which treatments are morally expendable as disproportionally burdensome. A liberal Protestant health care system would announce a different framework; a libertarian secular system still another. A truly Protestant health care system, for example, would probably reflect the belief that the lay person is capable of having control over the "text." The medical record, accordingly, would plausibly be placed in the patient's hands just as the Bible is.

Such value pairings will obviously not be a total matching, but they should at least place provider and patient in the same general camp. Moreover, organizing health care delivery on the basis of explicit value pairings would put both provider and patient on notice that values are a necessary and essential part of health care decisionmaking, a part that cannot be avoided and cannot be handled adequately by merely obtaining the consent of the patient to a randomly assigned provider's guess about what would be best.

With such an arrangement the problems that arise with use of consent for the normal random pairing of lay people and professionals is mitigated. The clinician has a more plausible basis for guessing what would serve the interests of the patient and, more importantly, will let a system of beliefs and values influence the presentation of medical information in a way that is more defensible. To be sure, such deep value pairing will not eliminate the problem of the necessary influence of beliefs and values on communication of medical facts, but it will structure the communication so that the inevitable influence will resemble the influence that the patient would have brought to the data were he or she to become an authority in medical science.

Barring such radical adjustment in the basis for lay-professional pairings, there is no reason to believe that the process of consent will significantly advance the lay person's role in the medical decisionmaking process. The concept of consent will have to be replaced with a more radical, robust notion of active patient participation in the choice among plausible alternatives—either by getting much greater information to the patient or by actively selecting the professional on the basis of convergence of "deep" value systems.

Reference

1. Robert M. Veatch, "Limits of Guardian Treatment Refusal: A Reasonableness Standard," *American Journal of Law & Medicine* 9, no. 4 (Winter 1984): 427–68; Robert M. Veatch, *Death, Dying, and the Biological Revolution,* rev. ed. (New Haven: Yale University Press, 1989).

POSTSCRIPT

Is Informed Consent Still Central to Medical Ethics?

The Patient Self-Determination Act, a federal law that went into effect in 1991, requires health care institutions to advise patients about their right to accept or refuse medical care and to offer them an opportunity to create an advance directive indicating their medical choices should they become incompetent. Nevertheless, there is considerable evidence that patients and their designated health care proxies are not brought into decision making at the end of life in a timely and effective way. There are also some limits on what kinds of information must be provided to patients. In the 1993 case of *Arato v. Avedon*, the California Supreme Court supported information sharing and patient-centered decision making but ruled that doctors need not supply explicit statistical information about life expectancy to patients. See George J. Annas, "Informed Consent, Cancer, and Truth in Prognosis," *The New England Journal of Medicine* (January 20, 1994).

Nonetheless, the concept of informed consent, from Western political and ethical theories that place a high value on individual self-determination, remains a central principle in the United States. Cultural groups who have different traditions may not share this value. Two articles in the *Journal of the American Medical Association* (September 13, 1995)—"Western Bioethics on the Navajo Reservation," by Joseph A. Carrese and Lorna A. Rhodes, and "Ethnicity and Attitudes Toward Patient Autonomy," by Leslie J. Blackhall—suggest that disclosing negative information and involving patients in decision making may be contrary to the beliefs of certain ethnic populations.

The most comprehensive account of informed consent is *A History and Theory of Informed Consent* by Ruth L. Faden, Tom L. Beauchamp, and Nancy M. P. King (Oxford University Press, 1986). Another useful volume, particularly in terms of psychiatric treatment, is *Informed Consent: Legal Theory and Clinical Practice* by Paul S. Appelbaum, Charles W. Lidz, and Alan Meisel (Oxford University Press, 1987). Jay Katz's *The Silent World of Doctor and Patient* (Free Press, 1984) is an insightful discussion of the reasons physicians may be reluctant to disclose information to their patients. And Christine Laine and Frank Davidoff describe the evolution from physician-based medicine in "Patient-Centered Medicine," *Journal of the American Medical Association* (January 10, 1996).

ISSUE 2

Can Family Interests Ethically Outweigh Patient Autonomy?

YES: John Hardwig, from "What About the Family?" *Hastings Center Report* (March–April 1990)

NO: Jeffrey Blustein, from "The Family in Medical Decisionmaking," *Hastings Center Report* (May–June 1993)

ISSUE SUMMARY

YES: John Hardwig, an associate professor of medical ethics, argues that the prevalent ethic of patient autonomy ignores family interests in medical treatment decisions. He maintains that physicians should recognize these interests as legitimate.

NO: Bioethicist Jeffrey Blustein contends that although families can be an important resource in helping patients make better decisions about their care, the ultimate decision-making authority should remain with the patient.

In law and ethics, parents are considered the rightful decision makers for their minor children. Although controversies still arise, no other institution or individual has been identified as having a more legitimate claim to the right to make decisions regarding a minor's welfare. Similarly, when medical decisions need to be made for an incompetent adult, physicians often consult with family members to determine the course of action that seems most appropriate, given the patient's condition and the family's values and history.

Apart from these significant exceptions (which consume a major portion of the biomedical ethics literature), the family has until very recently been viewed primarily as a source of emotional support for the patient and an endorser of physician recommendations. The competent patient's right to make an autonomous decision remains a central ethical principle. Health care providers seldom involve family members directly in making decisions or in choosing among various treatment alternatives, even though many medical decisions have an enormous impact on the family. For example, the decision to care for a seriously ill person at home, rather than in a nursing home, has a major effect on those who will be expected to participate in the care and to give up their privacy and space. If the treatment decision involves heavy expenses that are not covered by insurance or a government program, the life goals of other family members—such as a college education for children—may be jeopardized. In some cases, the family may lose a home or members may be forced to leave their jobs or to stop participating in important activities in order to provide care.

As cost-containment efforts rapidly continue to push medical care from its institutional base (in hospitals and nursing homes) to outpatient clinics, community-based services, and the home, these issues are likely to arise with greater frequency. Home care now involves high-technology equipment, such as intravenous chemotherapy, total parenteral nutrition (tube feeding through the stomach), and other invasive procedures. More than 22 million Americans (the majority of whom are women) are currently providing home-based care to a relative or friend who is chronically ill, disabled, or elderly. Most family members want to care for their loved ones, but the "informal" care they provide is neither paid for nor reimbursed by insurance.

The dynamic and ever-changing concept of "family" is a further complication. Today, the medical, legal, and social systems in the United States recognize the nuclear family (comprised of a mother, a father, and minor children) as prototypical, but the reality in which many Americans live is quite different. There are divorced and remarried families; extended, intergenerational families; families of affiliation, such as gay and lesbian couples; and families of loosely related kin and friends. While self-defined families include many people outside traditional definitions, the options for participating in medical decision making or representing a particular person's interests remain narrow unless an individual has been legally designated as a health care proxy.

The multiple structures of family also mean that there is no single strategy for resolving conflicts among family members or between family members and health care providers. Differing perspectives may create disagreement even among well-intentioned family members, and, in more extreme circumstances, a family member may advocate a certain path of action for reasons that seem suspect (for instance, a large inheritance may be involved or there may be evidence of abuse or neglect). Sometimes, a representative of the hospital ethics committee is helpful in guiding discussions and resolving conflicts, but in other instances, the courts have to get involved to exclude someone who is unsuitable to participate in making decisions.

The two selections that follow explore the ramifications of including family members as decision makers in the care of a competent patient. John Hardwig asserts that in many cases family members have a greater interest than the patient in which treatment option is chosen and that in those cases the interests of family members should override those of the patient. Jeffrey Blustein declares that the locus of decisional authority should remain with the patient.

John Hardwig

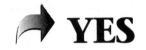 **YES**

What About the Family?

We are beginning to recognize that the prevalent ethic of patient autonomy simply will not do. Since demands for health care are virtually unlimited, giving autonomous patients the care they want will bankrupt our health care system. We can no longer simply buy our way out of difficult questions of justice by expanding the health care pie until there is enough to satisfy the wants and needs of everyone. The requirements of justice and the needs of other patients must temper the claims of autonomous patients.

But if the legitimate claims of other patients and other (non-medical) interests of society are beginning to be recognized, another question is still largely ignored: To what extent can the patient's family legitimately be asked or required to sacrifice their interests so that the patient can have the treatment he or she wants?

This question is not only almost universally ignored, it is generally implicitly dismissed, silenced before it can even be raised. This tacit dismissal results from a fundamental assumption of medical ethics: medical treatment ought always to serve the interests of the patient. This, of course, implies that the interests of family members should be irrelevant to medical treatment decisions or at least ought never to take precedence over the interests of the patient. All questions about fairness to the interests of family members are thus precluded, regardless of the merit or importance of the interests that will have to be sacrificed if the patient is to receive optimal treatment.

Yet there is a whole range of cases in which important interests of family members are dramatically affected by decisions about the patient's treatment; medical decisions often should be made with those interests in mind. Indeed, in many cases family members have a greater interest than the patient in which treatment option is exercised. In such cases, the interests of family members often ought to *override* those of the patient.

The problem of family interests cannot be resolved by considering other members of the family as "patients," thereby redefining the problem as one of conflicting interests among *patients*. Other members of the family are not always ill, and even if ill, they still may not be patients. Nor will it do to define the whole family as one patient. Granted, the slogan "the patient is the family" was coined partly to draw attention to precisely the issues I wish to raise, but

From John Hardwig, "What About the Family?" *Hastings Center Report*, vol. 20 (March–April 1990). Copyright © 1990 by The Hastings Center. Reprinted by permission.

the idea that the whole family is one patient is too monolithic. The conflicts of interests, beliefs, and values among family members are often too real and run too deep to treat all members as "the patient" Thus, if I am correct, it is sometimes the moral thing to do for a physician to sacrifice the interests of her patient to those of nonpatients—specifically, to those of the other members of the patient's family.

But what is the "family"? As I will use it here, it will mean roughly "those who are close to the patient" "Family" so defined will often include close friends and companions. It may also exclude some with blood or marriage ties to the patient. "Closeness" does not, however, always mean care and abiding affection, nor need it be a positive experience—one can hate, resent, fear, or despise a mother or brother with an intensity not often directed toward strangers, acquaintances, or associates. But there are cases where even a hateful or resentful family member's interests ought to be considered.

This use of "family" gives rise to very sensitive ethical—and legal—issues in the case of legal relatives with no emotional ties to the patient that I cannot pursue here. I can only say that I do not mean to suggest that the interests of legal relatives who are not emotionally close to the patient are always to be ignored. They will sometimes have an important financial interest in the treatment even if they are not emotionally close to the patient. But blood and marriage ties can become so thin that they become *merely* legal relationships. (Consider, for example, "couples" who have long since parted but who have never gotten a divorce, or cases in which the next of kin cannot be bothered with making proxy decisions.) Obviously, there are many important questions about just whose interests are to be considered in which treatment decisions and to what extent.

Connected Interests

There is no way to detach the lives of patients from the lives of those who are close to them. Indeed, the intertwining of lives is part of the very meaning of closeness. Consequently, there will be a broad spectrum of cases in which the treatment options will have dramatic and different impacts on the patient's family.

I believe there are many, many such cases. To save the life of a newborn with serious defects is often dramatically to affect the rest of the parents' lives and, if they have other children, may seriously compromise the quality of their lives, as well... The husband of a woman with Alzheimer's disease may well have a life totally dominated for ten years or more by caring for an increasingly foreign and estranged wife... The choice between aggressive and palliative care or, for that matter, the difference between either kind of care and suicide in the case of a father with terminal cancer or AIDS may have a dramatic emotional and financial impact on his wife and children... Less dramatically, the choice between two medications, one of which has the side effect of impotence, may radically alter the life a couple has together... The drug of choice for controlling high blood pressure may be too expensive (that is, requires too many sacrifices) for many families with incomes just above the ceiling for Medicaid...

Because the lives of those who are close are not separable, to be close is to no longer have a life entirely your own to live entirely as you choose. To be part of a family is to be morally required to make decisions on the basis of thinking about what is best for all concerned, not simply what is best for yourself. In healthy families, characterized by genuine care, one wants to make decisions on this basis, and many people do so quite naturally and automatically. My own grandfather committed suicide after his heart attack as a final gift to his wife—he had plenty of life insurance but not nearly enough health insurance, and he feared that she would be left homeless and destitute if he lingered on in an incapacitated state. Even if one is not so inclined, however, it is irresponsible and wrong to exclude or to fail to consider the interests of those who are close. Only when the lives of family members will not be importantly affected can one rightly make exclusively or even predominantly self-regarding decisions.

Although "what is best for all concerned" sounds utilitarian, my position does not imply that the right course of action results simply from a calculation of what is best for all. No, the seriously ill may have a right to special consideration, and the family of an ill person may have a duty to make sacrifices to respond to a member's illness. It is one thing to claim that the ill deserve special consideration; it is quite another to maintain that they deserve exclusive or even overriding consideration. Surely we must admit that there are limits to the right to special treatment by virtue of illness. Otherwise, everyone would be morally required to sacrifice all other goods to better care for the ill. We must also recognize that patients too have moral obligations, obligations to try to protect the lives of their families from destruction resulting from their illnesses.

Thus, unless serious illness excuses one from all moral responsibility—and I don't see how it could—it is an oversimplification to say of a patient who is part of a family that "it's his life" or "after all, it's his medical treatment," as if his life and his treatment could be successfully isolated from the lives of the other members of his family. It is more accurate to say "it's their lives" or "after all, they're all going to have to live with his treatment." Then the really serious moral questions are not *whether* the interests of family members are relevant to decisions about a patient's medical treatment or *whether* their interests should be included in his deliberations or in deliberations about him, but how far family and friends can be asked to support and sustain the patient. What sacrifices can they be morally required to make for his health care? How far can they reasonably be asked to compromise the quality of their lives so that he will receive the care that would improve the quality of his life? To what extent can he reasonably expect them to put their lives "on hold" to preoccupy themselves with his illness to the extent necessary to care for him?

The Anomaly of Medical Decisionmaking

The way we analyze medical treatment decisions by or for patients is plainly anomalous to the way we think about other important decisions family members make. I am a husband, a father, and still a son, and no one would argue that I should or even responsibly could decide to take a sabbatical, another job, or even a weekend trip *solely* on the basis of what I want for myself. Why should decisions about my medical treatment be different? Why should we have even *thought* that medical treatment decisions might be different?

Is it because medical decisions, uniquely, involve life and death matters? Most medical decisions, however, are not matters of life and death, and we as a society risk or shorten the lives of other people—through our toxic waste disposal decisions, for example—quite apart from considerations of whether that is what they want for themselves.

Have we been misled by a preoccupation with the biophysical model of disease? Perhaps it has tempted us to think of illness and hence also of treatment as something that takes place *within* the body of the patient. What happens in my body does not—barring contagion—affect my wife's body, yet it usually does affect her.

Have we tacitly desired to simplify the practice and the ethics of medicine by considering only the *medical* or health-related consequences of treatment decisions? Perhaps, but it is obvious that we need a broader vision of and sensitivity to *all* the consequences of action, at least among those who are not simply technicians following orders from above. Generals need to consider more than military consequences, businessmen more than economic consequences, teachers more than educational consequences, lawyers more than legal consequences.

Does the weakness and vulnerability of serious illness imply that the ill need such protection that we should serve only their interests? Those who are sick may indeed need special protection, but this can only mean that we must take special care to see that the interests of the ill are duly considered. It does not follow that their interests are to be served exclusively or even that their interests must always predominate. Moreover, we must remember that in terms of the dynamics of the family, the patient is not always the weakest member, the member most in need of protection.

Does it make *historical,* if not logical, sense to view the wishes and interests of the patient as always overriding? Historically, illnesses were generally of much shorter duration; patients got better quickly or died quickly. Moreover, the costs of the medical care available were small enough that rarely was one's future mortgaged to the costs of the care of family members. Although this was once truer than it is today, there have always been significant exceptions to these generalizations.

None of these considerations adequately explains why the interests of the patient's family have been thought to be appropriately excluded from consideration. At the very least, those who believe that medical treatment decisions are morally anomalous to other important decisions owe us a better account of how and why this is so.

Limits of Public Policy

It might be thought that the problem of family interests *is* a problem only because our society does not shelter families from the negative effects of medical decisions. If, for example, we adopted a comprehensive system of national health insurance and also a system of public insurance to guarantee the incomes of families, then my sons' chances at a college education and the quality of the rest of their lives might not have to be sacrificed were I to receive optimal medical care.

However, it is worth pointing out that we are still moving primarily in the *opposite* direction. Instead of designing policies that would increasingly shelter family members from the adverse impact of serious and prolonged illnesses, we are still attempting to shift the burden of care to family members in our efforts to contain medical costs. A social system that would safeguard families from the impact of serious illness is nowhere in sight in this country. And we must not do medical ethics as if it were.

It is perhaps even more important to recognize that the lives of family members could not be sheltered from all the important ramifications of medical treatment decisions by *any* set of public policies. In any society in which people get close to each other and care deeply for each other, treatment decisions about one will often and *irremediably* affect more than one. If a newborn has been saved by aggressive treatment but is severely handicapped, the parents may simply not be emotionally capable of abandoning the child to institutional care. A man whose wife is suffering from multiple sclerosis may simply not be willing or able to go on with his own life until he sees her through to the end. A woman whose husband is being maintained in a vegetative state may not feel free to marry or even to see other men again, regardless of what some revised law might say about her marital status.

Nor could we desire a society in which friends and family would quickly lose their concern as soon as continuing to care began to diminish the quality of their own lives. For we would then have alliances for better but not for worse, in health, but not in sickness, until death appears on the horizon. And we would all be poorer for that. A man who can leave his wife the day after she learns she has cancer, on the grounds that he has his own life to live, is to be deplored. The emotional inability or principled refusal to separate ourselves and our lives from the lives of ill or dying members of our families is *not* an unfortunate fact about the structure of our emotions. It is a desirable feature, not to be changed even if it could be; not to be changed even if the resulting intertwining of lives debars us from making exclusively self-regarding treatment decisions when we are ill.

Our present individualistic medical ethics is isolating and destructive. For by implicitly suggesting that patients make "their own" treatment decisions on a self-regarding basis and supporting those who do so, such an ethics encourages each of us to see our lives as simply our own. We may yet turn ourselves into beings who are ultimately alone.

Fidelity or Fairness?

Fidelity to the interests of the patient has been a cornerstone of both traditional codes and contemporary theories of medical ethics. The two competing paradigms of medical ethics—the "benevolence" model and the "patient autonomy" model—are simply different ways of construing such fidelity. Both must be rejected or radically modified. The admission that treatment decisions often affect more than just the patient thus forces major changes on both the theoretical and the practical level. Obviously, I can only begin to explore the needed changes here.

Instead of starting with our usual assumption that physicians are to serve the interests of the patient, we must build our theories on a very different assumption: The medical and nonmedical interests of both the patient and other members of the patient's family are to be considered. It is only in the special case of patients without family that we can simply follow the patient's wishes or pursue the patient's interests. In fact, I would argue that we must build our theory of medical ethics on the presumption of equality: the interests of patients and family members are morally to be weighed equally; medical and nonmedical interests of the same magnitude deserve equal consideration in making treatment decisions. Like any other moral presumption, this one can, perhaps, be defeated in some cases. But the burden of proof will always be on those who would advocate special consideration for any family member's interests, including those of the ill.

Even where the presumption of equality is not defeated, life, health, and freedom from pain and handicapping conditions are extremely important goods for virtually everyone. They are thus very important considerations in all treatment decisions. In the majority of cases, the patient's interest in optimal health and longer life may well be strong enough to outweigh the conflicting interests of other members of the family. But even then, some departure from the treatment plan that would maximize the patient's interests may well be justified to harmonize best the interests of all concerned or to require significantly smaller sacrifices by other family members. That the patient's interests may often outweigh the conflicting interests of others in treatment decisions is no justification for failing to recognize that an attempt to balance or harmonize different, conflicting interests is often morally required. Nor does it justify overlooking the morally crucial cases in which the interests of other members of the family ought to override the interests of the patient. Changing our basic assumption about how treatment decisions are to be made means reconceptualizing the ethical roles of both physician and patient, since our understanding of both has been built on the presumption of patient primacy, rather than fairness to all concerned. Recognizing the moral relevance of the interests of family members thus reveals a dilemma for our understanding of what it is to be a physician: Should we retain a fiduciary ethic in which the physician is to serve the interests of her patient? Or should the physician attempt to weigh and balance all the interests of all concerned? I do not yet know just how to resolve this dilemma. All I can do here is try to envision the options.

If we retain the traditional ethic of fidelity to the interests of the patient, the physician should excuse herself from making treatment decisions that will affect the lives of the family on grounds of a moral conflict of interest, for she is a one-sided advocate. A lawyer for one of the parties cannot also serve as judge in the case. Thus, it would be unfair if a physician conceived as having a fiduciary relationship to her patient were to make treatment decisions that would adversely affect the lives of the patient's family. Indeed, a physician conceived as a patient advocate should not even *advise* patients or family members about which course of treatment should be chosen. As advocate, she can speak only to what course of treatment would be best for the patient, and must remain silent about what's best for the rest of the family or what should be done in light of everyone's interests.

Physicians might instead renounce their fiduciary relationship with their patients. On this view, physicians would no longer be agents of their patients and would not strive to be advocates for their patients' interests. Instead, the physician would aspire to be an impartial advisor who would stand knowledgeably but sympathetically outside all the many conflicting interests of those affected by the treatment options, and who would strive to discern the treatment that would best harmonize or balance the interests of all concerned.

Although this second option contradicts the Hippocratic Oath and most other codes of medical ethics, it is not, perhaps, as foreign as it may at first seem. Traditionally, many family physicians—especially small-town physicians who knew patients and their families well—attempted to attend to both medical and nonmedical interests of all concerned. Many contemporary physicians still make decisions in this way. But we do not yet have an ethical theory that explains and justifies what they are doing.

Nevertheless, we may well question the physician's ability to act as an impartial ethical observer. Increasingly, physicians do not know their patients, much less their patients' families. Moreover, we may doubt physicians' abilities to weigh evenhandedly medical and nonmedical interests. Physicians are trained to be especially responsive to medical interests and we may well want them to remain that way. Physicians also tend to be deeply involved with the interests of their patients, and it may be impossible or undesirable to break this tie to enable physicians to be more impartial advisors. Finally, when someone retains the services of a physician, it seems reasonable that she be able to expect that physician to be *her* agent, pursuing *her* interests, not those of her family.

Autonomy and Advocacy

We must also rethink our conception of the patient. On one hand, if we continue to stress patient autonomy, we must recognize that this implies that patients have moral responsibilities. If, on the other hand, we do not want to burden patients with weighty moral responsibilities, we must abandon the ethic of patient autonomy.

Recognizing that moral responsibilities come with patient autonomy will require basic changes in the accepted meanings of both "autonomy" and "advocacy." Because medical ethics has ignored patient responsibilities, we have come to interpret "autonomy" in a sense very different from [German philosopher Immanuel] Kant's original use of the term. It has come to mean simply the patient's freedom or right to choose the treatment he believes is best for himself. But as Kant knew well, there are many situations in which people can achieve autonomy and moral well-being only by sacrificing other important dimensions of their well-being, including health, happiness, even life itself. For autonomy is the *responsible* use of freedom and is therefore diminished whenever one ignores, evades, or slights one's responsibilities. Human dignity, Kant concluded, consists in our ability to refuse to compromise our autonomy to achieve the kinds of lives (or treatments) we want for ourselves.

If, then, I am morally empowered to make decisions about "my" medical treatment, I am also morally required to shoulder the responsibility of making very difficult moral decisions. The right course of action for me to take will not always be the one that promotes my own interests.

Some patients, motivated by a deep and abiding concern for the well-being of their families, will undoubtedly consider the interests of other family members. For these patients, the interests of their family are *part* of their interests. But not all patients will feel this way. And the interests of family members are not relevant *if* and *because* the patient wants to consider them; they are not relevant because they are *part* of the patient's interests. They are relevant *whether or not* the patient is inclined to consider them. Indeed, the *ethics* of patient decisions is most poignantly highlighted precisely when the patient is inclined to decide without considering the impact of his decision on the lives of the rest of his family.

Confronting patients with tough ethical choices may be part and parcel of treating them with respect as fully competent adults. We don't, after all, think it's right to stand silently by while other (healthy) adults ignore or shirk their moral responsibilities. If, however, we believe that most patients, gripped as they often are by the emotional crisis of serious illness, are not up to shouldering the responsibility of such decisions or should not be burdened with it, then I think we must simply abandon the ethic of patient autonomy. Patient autonomy would then be appropriate only when the various treatment options will affect only the patient's life.

The responsibilities of patients imply that there is often a conflict between patient autonomy and the patient's interests (even as those interests are defined by the patient). And we will have to rethink our understanding of patient advocacy in light of this conflict: Does the patient advocate try to promote the patient's (self-defined) *interests*? Or does she promote the patient's *autonomy* even at the expense of those interests? Responsible patient advocates can hardly encourage patients to shirk their moral responsibilities. But can we really expect health care providers to promote patient autonomy when that means encouraging their patients to sacrifice health, happiness, sometimes even life itself?

If we could give an affirmative answer to this last question, we would obviously thereby create a third option for reinterpreting the role of the physician: The physician could maintain her traditional role as patient advocate without being morally required to refrain from making treatment decisions whenever interests of the patient's family are also at stake *if* patient advocacy were understood as promoting patient autonomy *and* patient autonomy were understood as the responsible use of freedom, not simply the right to choose the treatment one wants.

Much more attention needs to be paid to all of these issues. However, it should be clear that absolutely central features of our theories of medical ethics

—our understanding of physician and patient, and thus of patient advocacy as well as patient dignity, and patient autonomy—have presupposed that the interests of family members should be irrelevant or should always take a back seat to the interests of the patient. Basic conceptual shifts are required once we acknowledge that this assumption is not warranted.

Who Should Decide?

Such basic conceptual shifts will necessarily have ramifications that will be felt throughout the field of medical ethics, for a host of new and very different issues are raised by the inclusion of family interests. Discussions of privacy and confidentiality, of withholding/withdrawing treatment, and of surrogate decisionmaking will all have to be reconsidered in light of the interests of the family. Many individual treatment decisions will also be affected, becoming much more complicated than they already are. Here, I will only offer a few remarks about treatment decisions, organized around the central issue of who should decide.

There are at least five answers to the question of who should make treatment decisions in cases where important interests of other family members are also at stake: the patient, the family, the physician, an ethics committee, or the courts. The physician's role in treatment decisions has already been discussed. Resort to either the courts or to ethics committees for treatment decisions is too cumbersome and time-consuming for any but the most troubling cases. So I will focus here on the contrast between the patient and the family as appropriate decisionmakers. It is worth noting, though, that we need not arrive at one, uniform answer to cover all cases. On the contrary, each of the five options will undoubtedly have its place, depending on the particulars of the case at hand.

Should we still think of a patient as having the right to make decisions about "his" treatment? As we have seen, patient autonomy implies patient responsibilities. What, then, if the patient seems to be ignoring the impact of his treatment on his family? At the very least, responsible physicians must caution such patients against simply opting for treatments because they want them. Instead, physicians must speak of responsibilities and obligations. They must raise considerations of the quality of many lives, not just that of the patient. They must explain the distinction between making a decision and making it in a self-regarding manner. Thus, it will often be appropriate to make plain to patients the consequences of treatment decisions for their families and to urge them to consider these consequences in reaching a decision. And sometimes, no doubt, it will be appropriate for family members to present their cases to the patient in the hope that his decisions would be shaped by their appeals.

Nonetheless, we sometimes permit people to make bad or irresponsible decisions and *excuse* those decisions because of various pressures they were under when they made their choices. Serious illness can undoubtedly be an extenuating circumstance, and perhaps we should allow some patients to make some self-regarding decisions, especially if they insist on doing so and the negative impact of their decisions on others is not too great.

Alternatively, if we doubt that most patients have the ability to make treatment decisions that are really fair to all concerned, or if we are not prepared to accept a policy that would assign patients the responsibility of doing so, we may conclude that they should not be empowered to make treatment decisions in which the lives of their family members will be dramatically affected. Indeed, even if the patient were completely fair in making the decision, the autonomy of other family members would have been systematically undercut by the fact that the patient alone decided.

Thus, we need to consider the autonomy of all members of the family, not just the patient's autonomy. Considerations of fairness and, paradoxically, of autonomy therefore indicate that the *family* should make the treatment decision, with all competent family members whose lives will be affected participating. Many such family conferences undoubtedly already take place. On this view, however, family conferences would often be morally *required.* And these conferences would not be limited to cases involving incompetent patients; cases involving competent patients would also often require family conferences.

Obviously, it would be completely unworkable for a physician to convene a family conference every time a medical decision might have some ramifications on the lives of family members. However, such discussion need not always take place in the presence of the physician; we can recognize that formal family conferences become more important as the impact of treatment decisions on members of the patient's family grows larger. Family conferences may thus be morally *required* only when the lives of family members would be dramatically affected by treatment decisions.

Moreover, family discussion is often morally *desirable* even if not morally required. Desirable, sometimes, even for relatively minor treatment decisions: After the family has moved to a new town, should parents commit themselves to two-hour drives so that their teenage son can continue to be treated for his acne by the dermatologist he knows and whose results he trusts? Or should he seek treatment from a new dermatologist?

Some family conferences about treatment decisions would be characterized throughout by deep affection, mutual understanding, and abiding concern for the interests of others. Other conferences might begin in an atmosphere charged with antagonism, suspicion, and hostility but move toward greater understanding, reconciliation, and harmony within the family. Such conferences would be significant goods in themselves, as well as means to ethically better treatment decisions. They would leave all family members better able to go on with their lives.

Still, family conferences cannot be expected always to begin with or move toward affection, mutual understanding, and a concern for all. If we opt for joint treatment decisions when the lives of several are affected, we need to face the fact that family conferences will sometimes be bitter confrontations in which past hostilities, anger, and resentments will surface. Sometimes, too, the conflicts of interest between patient and family, and between one family member and another will be irresolvable, forcing families to invoke the harsh perspective of justice, divisive and antagonistic though that perspective may be. Those who favor family decisions when the whole family is affected will have to face the question of whether we really want to put the patient, already frightened and weakened by his illness, through the conflict and bitter confrontations that family conferences may sometimes precipitate.

We must also recognize that family members may be unable or unwilling to press or even state their own interests before a family member who is ill. Such refusal may be admirable, even heroic; it is sometimes evidence of willingness to go "above and beyond the call of duty," even at great personal cost. But not always. Refusal to press one's own interests can also be a sign of inappropriate guilt, of a crushing sense of responsibility for the well-being of others, of acceptance of an inferior or dominated role within the family, or of lack of a sense of self-worth. All of these may well be mobilized by an illness in the family. Moreover, we must not minimize the power of the medical setting to subordinate nonmedical to medical interests and to emphasize the well-being of the patient at the expense of the well-being of others. Thus, it will often be not just the patient, but also other family members who will need an advocate if a family conference is to reach the decision that best balances the autonomy and interests of all concerned.

NO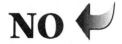

Jeffrey Blustein

The Family in Medical Decisionmaking

Might it be that family members, by virtue of their closeness to the patient, should not only have some special authority to speak on behalf of patients who are incompetent, but should also share decisional authority with patients who are competent?

A recent proposal that speaks to the family's role in medical decision-making has been advanced by John Hardwig. In his provocative essay, "What about the Family?"[1] he contemplates far-reaching changes in medical practice based on a critique of our prevailing patient-centered ethos. My discussion of his proposal is chiefly designed to pave the way for what I call a communitarian account of the role of the family in acute care decisionmaking. This account—which, I hasten to add, I do not endorse—has not to my knowledge been taken seriously as a theoretical possibility in the bioethics literature. Since the label "communitarian" is liable to be misunderstood, I should note at the outset that I am not interested in communitarianism as a political theory. Rather, I want to focus on the family as communitarian political writers sometimes think of it, namely, as a model for their conception of the larger society, and on the basis of this understanding of the family, to mount a challenge to the dominant patient-centered ethos that parallels the communitarian critique of liberal political philosophy. This communitarian position resembles Hardwig's proposal in that it does not regard the competent patient as the ultimate decisionmaker, but takes it as morally significant for the attribution of decisional authority that his or her life is intimately intertwined with the lives of close others. However, as we will see, the communitarian account is philosophically more radical than Hardwig's challenge to the dominant patient-centered medical ethos.

My own position is that the locus of decisional authority should remain the individual patient, but I also argue that family members, by virtue of their closeness to and intimate knowledge of the patient are often uniquely well qualified to shore up the patient's vulnerable autonomy and assist him or her in the exercise of autonomous decisionmaking. Families, in other words, can be an important resource for patients in helping them to make better decisions about their care. Recognition of this fact leads to a broader understanding of the duty to respect patient autonomy than currently prevails in acute care medicine.

From Jeffrey Blustein, "The Family in Medical Decisionmaking," *Hastings Center Report,* vol. 23, no. 3 (May–June 1993). Copyright © 1993 by The Hastings Center. Reprinted by permission. Some references omitted.

Family Decisionmaking and Competent Patients

According to Hardwig, even when the patient is a competent adult, it may be quite appropriate to empower the family, to "make the treatment decision, with all competent family members whose lives will be affected participating." . . .

Particular choices about treatment can seriously affect the lives of family members in many ways, interfering not only with their own personal projects and individual life styles, but with their commitments to other family members as well. In any case, they are "separate" in the sense that they diverge from and possibly conflict with patient interests: they are not to be understood as interests in the interests of patients. Of course, those who love the patient also have a direct interest in the protection and promotion of the patient's interests, assuming that the patient has interests that can be protected and promoted. Indeed, this is part of the very meaning of love. But for Hardwig, there can be closeness without love, and even when there is love, there will usually be other interests of family members as well. When all of these interests are taken into account, it may turn out that what is best for the family as a whole is not what is best for the individual patient.

These other interests may be, and frequently are, quite legitimate, and treatment decisions should not be judged morally better or worse solely from the patient's perspective. Indeed, departures from optimal patient care may be justified "to harmonize best the interests of all concerned or to require significantly smaller sacrifices by other family members." Moreover, and very importantly, Hardwig expresses misgivings about the effectiveness of exhorting the patient to consider the impact of his or her decision on the lives of the rest of the family. Patients who seem to be ignoring their family's stake in the outcome of their decisionmaking process may sometimes respond appropriately to appeals from the physician or other family members, but many patients will be too self-involved to give the interests of others proper consideration or will use their illness as a kind of trump card to dominate the rest of the family. Because of this, Hardwig maintains, we must consider a more radical measure to ensure adequate protection of legitimate family interests, namely, rejection of the prevalent medical ethos according to which the competent patient is always the decisive moral agent. Under this ethos, it is certainly permissible for family members to offer information, counsel, and suasion to patients who must make treatment decisions. But the authority to make the decisions still resides with the competent patient alone, and this Hardwig finds untenable.[2]

The "ethic of patient autonomy" allows the competent patient, and the patient alone, to set the terms and conditions of care. Patients may be frightened and distracted by illness and hence in no position to give careful thought to the interests of others, but if their decisionmaking capacity is judged sufficient for the decision at hand, their wishes prevail. This troubles Hardwig because it amounts to giving patients permission to neglect or slight their moral responsibilities to other family members. Seriously ill patients tend to be self-absorbed and to make exclusively self-regarding choices about care, and in those cases where "the lives of family members would be dramatically affected by treatment decisions." . . .

Hardwig's proposal for greater family involvement in medical decision-making, however, runs up against the problem of patient vulnerability: joint family decisionmaking provides too many opportunities for the exploitation of patient vulnerability: Serious constraints on patient autonomy, such as anxiety depression, fear, and denial, are inherent in the state of being ill.[3] Illness is also frequently disorienting in that patients find themselves thrust into unfamiliar surroundings, unable to pursue customary routines or to enjoy any significant degree of privacy. For these reasons, the ability of patients to assess their medical needs accurately and protect their own interests effectively is limited and precarious. But if those who are ill and those who are healthy already confront each other on an unequal psychological footing, then family conferences, as Hardwig conceives of them, seem especially ill advised. Weakened and confused by their illness, patients are easy prey to manipulation or coercion by other family members and may capitulate to family wishes out of guilt or fear. (Given that Hardwig would allow even hateful or resentful family members to be included in family conferences, this is not an idle worry.) Family members will understandably not want to be seen by the physician as opposing the wishes of the patient and so they might exert pressure on the patient to concur with their opinions about treatment. Of course, even as matters now stand, with decisionmaking not generally thought to belong to the family as a whole, what seems like a patient's autonomous choice often only implements the choice of the others for him or her. But joint family decisionmaking is likely only to exacerbate this problem and to make truly independent choice even more dubious.

Hardwig, it should be noted, does acknowledge that a seriously weakened patient may well need an "advocate," or surrogate participant from outside the family, to take part in the joint family decision. However, this hardly resolves all the difficulties his proposal presents. The presence of an outsider in what is supposed to be a deeply personal and private conference might only create (further) hostility and suspicion among family members. And if consensus in the conference cannot be achieved, the rest of the family could simply overrule the patient's proxy participant, just as it could overrule the patient himself.

From a theoretical point of view, we should, I think, agree with Hardwig about the inadequacy of any view that denies or overlooks the essential interplay between rights and responsibilities. But the practical moral problem as I see it is how to design procedures and structures of decisionmaking that achieve an acceptable balance between rights and responsibilities, between the important values of a patient-centered ethos and the legitimate claims of other family members. If alternative approaches to medical decisionmaking are judged in this light, as Hardwig wants them to be, and not solely in terms of over-all happiness or preference satisfaction or the like, then family decisionmaking for competent patients confronts serious moral objections. For indications are that it will often result not in a mutual accommodation of the autonomy and interests of all affected parties, but rather in a serious erosion of patient autonomy and a subordination of patient interests to the competing interests of other family members.

The Communitarian Defense of Family Decisionmaking

I have focused on the problems that nonideal, less than fully harmonious families pose for Hardwig's proposal. Critics of the patient-as-primary-agent model might instead restrict their attention to those (admittedly infrequent) cases in which patients belong to close-knit and harmonious families, and with this as their conception of the family, offer a defense of family decisionmaking that challenges the patient-centered model in a more radical way than Hardwig does. In ideal families, suspicions, resentments, disagreements, and the like, if they exist, are muted and do not set the tone of family life. But more importantly, it may be claimed, the conception of the person that underlies the theory of patient autonomy is patently inappropriate here. The patient is not, as this theory presupposes, an atomic entity, a free and rational chooser of ends unencumbered by communal and other allegiances. On the contrary, his or her identity is constituted by family relationships, and he or she is united with other family members through common ends and mutual understanding. In these circumstances, the patient is too enmeshed in a network of relations to others to be properly singled out as the one to make treatment decisions.

I call this the communitarian argument for family decisionmaking to distinguish it from the argument from fairness and autonomy discussed in the previous section. When I refer below to what "communitarians" say about medical decisionmaking, I am not thinking of any particular authors who have advanced this position.[4] Rather, I am suggesting that elements of the communitarian view can be taken out of their political context and that a challenge to the prevailing patient-centered ethos can be constructed on the basis of a communitarian conception of the ideal family. Let us look at this challenge more closely.

In acute care settings, the relationship between patients and physicians is, if not exactly adversarial, at least one in which patients should not normally suppose that they and their physicians are participants in a common enterprise with common values and goals. The values involved in medical decisionmaking are by no means exclusively medical values, but also largely normative ones about which patients and physicians frequently disagree. In these circumstances, physicians may attempt to coerce compliance with their wishes, which they are in an advantageous position to do, or to control patient decisions by selective disclosure or nondisclosure of information. In recognition of normative diversity and in the face of various threats to patient autonomy in the caregiving relationship, we invoke the notion of patients' rights. Rights accord patients a protected space in which to make their own choices and pursue their ends free of inappropriate interference from others. Having rights, patients can confront caregivers with the demand that their (possibly conflicting) ends be respected.

Communitarian critics of the traditional ethos of patient autonomy need not deny that patients' rights and patient self-determination play an important role in the caregiving relationship. But, they note, the patient is not always to be thought of simply as the one who is sick or in need of medical attention. If the patient belongs to a close-knit and harmonious family, for example, it is the family as a whole whose values and goals may diverge from those of professional caregivers because such a family is a genuine community, not a mere collection of separate individuals with their own private and possibly conflicting interests. Members of a community have common ends, and these are conceived of and valued as common ends by the members. United by common ends and a common identity, the threats that work against the autonomy of some work against the autonomy of all. Moreover, in these cases the patient would not need to be protected from family pressures for inappropriate treatment. Rather, the family would act as advocate for the patient vis-à-vis the physician, and family decisionmaking would put patients on a much more equal footing with caregivers.

For communitarians the ethics of acute care, focusing as it does on the individual who is the subject of treatment, rests on a conception of the self that is at odds with how persons define and understand themselves in a community. This is a conception for a world of strangers, where the content of each person's good is, to quote Michael Sandel, "largely opaque" to others, where persons have divergent and possibly conflicting plans and interests, and where their capacity for benevolence is extremely limited.[5] But in the community of a close and harmonious family these conditions do not obtain. Rather, the defining features of such a family are mutual sympathy, common ends, a shared identity, love, and spontaneous affection. Of course, it is sheer wishful thinking, and cavalier as well, to assume that all families are like this. Family life may instead be fraught with dissension and interests may diverge and conflict. In these situations questions of justice come to the fore and the importance of individual rights (and individual patient rights) is enhanced. But within the context of a more or less ideal family, the circumstances that make personal autonomy both an appropriate and a pressing concern prevail to a relatively small degree....

The close-knit, harmonious family is a paradigm of community. Here the well-being of one family member does not just have an impact on the well-being of others, for this can happen in families that are no more than associations of individuals (like the ones Hardwig describes). Rather, in families that are genuine communities individuals identify with one another, such that the well-being of one is *part of* the well being of the other. This being so, the communitarian maintains, decisions that importantly affect the well being of one family member are the province of the entire family. To be sure, in the medical cases there is only one family member, the patient, who literally bears the decision in his or her flesh and bones. But this fact alone, it is believed, does not confer upon the patient a unilateral decisionmaking right. The right to make the decision is still a right of the family in ideal circumstance—a group right rather than a right of individuals.

However, since the communitarian argument for family decisionmaking applies only to families that are communities and not to those that are just collections of individuals whose lives affect each other in major ways, its implications for the practice of medicine will not be as significant as those of Hardwig's proposal. Many families, to acknowledge the obvious again, are not ideal. In addition, physicians frequently have only passing acquaintance with the patient's family and no reliable basis for judging the quality of the patient's relationship with other family members. Even if communitarians reveal genuine inadequacies in the prevalent ethos of patient autonomy and patient rights, physicians will often not be in a position to tell whether, in the particular case at hand, the family is harmonious enough to be entrusted with the authority to make decisions for one of its own. On the other hand, physicians will often have enough information to know that the lives of family members will be seriously affected by treatment decisions, and it is on this fact, not on the existence of a harmonious family, that Hardwig premises the case for joint family decisionmaking.

Still, the communitarian critique of the dominant medical ethos of patient autonomy and individual patients' rights raises interesting and important philosophical issues. Practical implications aside, the theoretical challenge it poses deserves a response. In what follows, I will try to indicate why I think this challenge fails.

How the Communitarian Challenge Fails

Even in families that are true communities of love, the harmony that exists among their members may not be so thoroughgoing that invocation of individual decisionmaking rights loses its point. It is not necessary for community that there be complete identity of all ends and unanimity on all matters of value or the good. On the contrary, there is room for significant disagreement about how to rank different components of a common conception of the good, about the proper means and strategies for achieving it, and about whether certain risks are worth taking to achieve common goals. Even if the members of a family are in broad agreement about what is of most importance in life, for example, this does not ensure that they will assess the costs and benefits of particular medical treatments similarly. Indeed, given the diversity of human nature and experience, such disagreements are not just possible but to be expected. Absolute harmony in decisionmaking and thoroughgoing convergence of values are only found in quite extraordinary communities. And this being the case, individual rights can be seen to have an importance the communitarian fails to acknowledge. They are not just claims we fall back on in the unhappy situation where community is lacking or faltering. Additionally, they serve to secure recognition, of the diverse values and ends that persist even in intact and well-functioning communities. This lack of homogeneity is glossed over by talk of family rights.

Individual rights have an important place in community because the existence of community does not eradicate serious disagreement about ends, about the relationship between particular choices and shared ends, and so forth. Individual rights are needed because a significant degree of diversity may exist even in a group united by a common conception of the good. . . .

It may help here to distinguish between having a right and insisting upon or demanding it. The language of demands does seem ill suited to harmonious families. If family members need to insist against one another that they have a right to make their own decisions, then we are probably dealing with a divided and quite antagonistic family. But these observations do not suffice to banish individual rights from harmonious families because the underlying supposition —that rights must always be linked to demands—is false. Rights can be expressed in different ways, and what is divisive and antagonistic to community is not the concept of rights, but only a certain way of expressing them. In harmonious families, rights are typically expressed "as reminders—gentle or forceful, matter-of-fact or emotional—of legitimate expectations and entitlements,"[6] and as such they play a vital role in the moral lives of families.

The implications of these remarks for a communitarian defense of family medical decisionmaking are clear. Even in extremely close families, patients may have different priorities from their loved ones and assess life choices in disparate ways, and these differences may surface in disagreements about how and even whether patients should be treated. Patients need their own rights regarding choice of treatment not just because family members cannot always be trusted to have the patient's best interests at heart, but because, even in families where trust is not an issue and there is a remarkable measure of agreement on ends and deep mutual affection, other family members may not always concur with the wisdom of the patient's choices. Rights protect patient autonomy and patient interests in these circumstances.

Further, rights for patients would be appropriate and useful even in those quite unusual families where the minimal sort of disagreement just mentioned is absent. For decisions about treatment often have dramatic and far-reaching consequences for the shape, quality, and duration of a patient's life, and individuals have an interest in determining for themselves the course their lives take. The interest in directing how one's life will go in accordance with one's values and preferences exists whether these values and preferences are uniquely one's own or shared with other family members, and it calls for recognition even when there is no disagreement between patient and family over the correct treatment decision. This is why patients have rights as individuals even under the unlikely conditions of absolute intrafamilial harmony: they protect the interests that patients have in exercising their agency....

Family Involvement in the Process of Decisionmaking

These responses to the communitarian position do not show that patient choices about treatment always trump the choices of family members, and they do not cut against Hardwig's argument for joint medical decisionmaking by all affected family members. What they show is only that the dominant patient-centered medical ethos cannot be refuted by the sort of all out attack on the notion of individual rights the communitarian launches. To be sure, an adversarial and legalistic conception of individual rights is ill suited to those cases where family relationships are nonadversarial and there are no deep conflicts of interests, preferences, or values among family members. But if this is the basis for the communitarian claim that community renders individual rights (including patient rights) useless or of minor importance, the communitarian betrays a distorted and incomplete understanding of rights.

Should the choices of competent patients trump the choices of family members, except in the rarest of circumstances? "It is an oversimplification to say of a patient who is part of a family," Hardwig notes, that "it's his life" or "after all, it's his medical treatment." Plainly, this by itself hardly shows that patient choices take priority over the choices of others, for when lives are so intertwined that one life cannot be shaped without also shaping the lives of others, it's *their* lives too. Another approach is to argue for a unilateral decisionmaking right for patients on the ground that patients have more to lose than their family members. That is, when we measure the sacrifices that family members must make for a patient's health care and the costs to the patient of not receiving the treatment that, other family members aside, he or she would select, the patient's sacrifices almost always outweigh the family's. Of course, the reverberations of patients' self regarding choices can be so shattering to the lives of other family members that a calculation of relative costs favors the family instead. But familial hardship from this source is usually less of a burden than serious illness, and this difference would be sufficient to establish at least a presumption in favor of patient decisionmaking.

But if the ethos of patient autonomy survives the challenges I have considered in this paper it is nevertheless the case that current medical practice and medical ethics can be faulted for not giving the family a more prominent place in medical decisionmaking for competent patients, and that both family members and patients suffer as a result. For one thing, as we learned from our discussion of Hardwig, because treatment decisions often do have a dramatic impact on family members, procedures need to be devised, short of giving family members a share of decisional authority, that acknowledge the moral weight of their legitimate interests. For another, though patients might well benefit from family involvement in the process of formulating views about medical treatment, under the regime of patient autonomy patients tend to be treated for the most part as if they were solitary decisionmakers, isolated from intimate others.

The ethos of patient autonomy rightly understood takes seriously the impairments of autonomy that affect us when we are ill. Patients are not ideally autonomous agents but anxious, fearful, depressed, often confused, and subject to ill-considered and mistaken ideas. If we are genuinely concerned about ensuring patient self-determination, we will take these factors into account. Here it is necessary to distinguish, as Jay Katz does, between "choices" and "thinking about choices."[7] According to the dominant medical ethos, choices properly belong to the patient alone. At the same time, patients' capacities for reflective thought and effective action are limited and precarious, obliging them to converse and consult with supportive and caring others if they are to make their best choices. Patients' psychological capacities for autonomy can be enhanced by searching conversations with their physicians—the main point of Katz's book —and (I would add) by conversations with other family members.

To explain why this is so, we may turn to a characterization of the family found in Nancy Rhoden's influential law review article, "Litigating Life and

Death."[8] Her argument, which focuses on decisionmaking for incompetent patients, finds within family life features that warrant a legal presumption in favor of family choice. Family members are typically the best decisionmakers partly because of their special epistemic qualifications: they ordinarily have deep and detailed knowledge of one another's lives, characters, values, and desires. This knowledge might be based on specific statements made by one family member to another, for the intimacy of family life encourages and is partly constituted by the unguarded disclosure of one's most private thoughts and deepest feelings. But there may be nothing specific that was said or done to which family members can point as evidence of another member's preferences. Indeed, their knowledge, acquired through long association and the sharing of intense life experiences, is characteristically of the sort that "transcends purely logical evidence." In addition, family members are the best candidates to act as surrogates for an incompetent patient because of their special emotional bonds to the patient. This is important because possessing deep and detailed knowledge of another can put one in an especially good position to frustrate no less than fulfill this person's desires. Family members, however, can be presumed to have a deep emotional commitment to one another, and this makes it likely that they will put their knowledge to the right use—that is, that they will decide as the patient would have wanted.

Those features of families that, in Rhoden's view, justify a legal presumption in favor of family decisionmaking for incompetent patient—intimate knowledge, caring, shared history—also provide good reasons for family involvement in the competent patients' thinking about choices. Family members would have no veto power over a patient's decision and would have to honor the choice ultimately made, no matter how foolish or idiosyncratic. But in family conferences, where the process of making a decision is shared, they could encourage the patient to evaluate different treatment options in terms of their impact on the interests of other family members, and could attempt to persuade the patient that the best choice is one that is fair to all affected parties. In some cases, understanding what a particular treatment decision would cost other family members might give the patient a compelling reason to alter an initial choice.

For the physician, the duty to respect patient autonomy has as its corollary a duty to engage in conversation with patients and to encourage and facilitate conversation between patients and other persons to whom they are close (including family members), unless the physician has reason to think that such conversation will not in fact assist the patient in making autonomous decisions. Current medical practice does not in general reflect a commitment to foster this sort of conversation as an integral part of the physician's professional responsibility. But if, as Katz suggests, genuine respect for patient autonomy is shown not merely in accepting patients' yes or no response to a proposed intervention, but rather in facilitating patients' opportunities for serious reflection on their choices, then promoting discussion and dialogue between patient and family is an important part of the physician's duty to satisfy the patient's right of self-determination.

References

1. John Harding, "What about the Family?" *Hastings Center Report* 10, no. 2 (1996): 5–10.
2. Hardwig's proposal to "reconstruct medical ethics in light of family interests" is novel in that it rejects the model of patient-as-primary-agent for acute care. Others have argued, along lines similar to Hardwig's, that this is not the appropriate model for home care, where family members share heavily in the burdens of care on an ongoing basis. In the view of Bart Collopy, Nancy Dubler, and Connie Zuckerman, for example, "the ethical problem for home care becomes one of gauging the interplay of agents, the relative weight to be granted to the autonomy and interests of the family vis-à-vis those of the elderly recipient of care." While not disputing the value of the patient-centered model in acute care, these writers argue that decisionmaking in home care should be "an interactive process, invoking negotiation, compromise, and the recognition of reciprocal ties." See "The Ethics of Home Care: Autonomy and Accommodation," special supplement, *Hastings Center Report* 20, no. 2 (1990): 1–16, at 9, 10.
3. See Terrence F. Ackerman, "Why Doctors Should Intervene," *Hastings Center Report* 12. no. 4 (1982): 14–17.
4. One author who has advanced something like a communitarian position is James Lindemann Nelson. See his "Taking Families Seriously," *Hastings Center Report* 22, no. 4 (1992): 6–12.
5. Michael Sandel, *Liberalism and the Limits of Justice* (Cambridge: Cambridge University Press, 1982), pp. 170–71.
6. Badhwar, "Circumstances of Justice."
7. Jay Katz, *The Silent World of Doctor and Patient* (New York: Free Press, 1984), p. 111.
8. Nancy Rhoden, "Litigating Life and Death," *Harvard Law Review* 102, no. 2 (1988): 375–446.

POSTSCRIPT

Can Family Interests Ethically Outweigh Patient Autonomy?

Astudy of more than 3,000 seriously ill patients found that those who reported economic hardship as a result of their illnesses were more likely to prefer a goal of maximizing comfort than one of maximizing life expectancy. See Kenneth E. Covinsky et al., "Is Economic Hardship on the Families of the Seriously Ill Associated With Patient and Surrogate Care Preferences?" *Archives of Internal Medicine* (August 12/26, 1996). Of interest is the study's finding that economic hardship on the family does not appear to be a factor in disagreements between patients and surrogates about the goal of care. This study suggests that individual patient autonomy is often influenced by factors other than medical ones and that patients may routinely consider how the risks and benefits of a particular decision would affect others.

Bringing the Hospital Home: Ethical and Social Implications of High-Tech Home Care edited by John D. Arras (Johns Hopkins University Press, 1995) analyzes the impact on family members and patients of introducing high-technology care into a previously private and "homey" setting. The history of long-term care and practice considerations are addressed in *Long-Term Care Decisions: Ethical and Conceptual Dimensions* edited by Laurence B. McCullough and Nancy L. Wilson (Johns Hopkins University Press, 1995). See especially the chapter by Nancy S. Jecker, "What Do Husbands and Wives Owe Each Other in Old Age?"

A Patient in the Family: An Ethics of Medicine and Families by Hilde Lindemann Nelson and James Lindemann Nelson (Routledge, 1995) is one of the first books to deal specifically with the question of families and medical decisions. Mark C. Kuczewski, in "Reconceiving the Family: The Process of Consent in Medical Decisionmaking," *Hastings Center Report* (March–April 1996), argues that bioethicists think about families only in terms of conflicting interests and that this is a mistake resulting from an impoverished notion of informed consent. See also James Lindemann Nelson, "Critical Interests and Sources of Familial Decision-Making Authority for Incapacitated Patients," *Journal of Law, Medicine and Ethics* (vol. 23, no. 2, 1995); Ellen H. Moskowitz, "Moral Consensus in Public Ethics: Patient Autonomy and Family Decisionmaking in the Work of One State Bioethics Commission," *The Journal of Medicine and Philosophy* (vol. 21, no. 2, 1996); and Rosalie A. Kane and Joan D. Penrod, *Family Caregiving in an Aging Society: Policy Perspectives* (Sage Publications, 1995). See also Carol Levine and Connie Zuckerman, "Hands On/Hands Off: Why Health Care Professionals Depend on Families but Keep Them at Arm's Length," *Journal of Law, Medicine & Ethics* (Spring 2000).

On the Internet ...

Choice in Dying

Choice in Dying is a nonprofit organization with a Web site that provides information on advance directives, legal developments, and Internet resources.

http://www.choices.org

Euthanasia and Physician Assisted Suicide: All Sides of the Issues

This site offers a general overview of the controversy concerning physician-assisted suicide as well as statisics and a list of Web sites that represent both sides of the debate.

http://www.religioustolerance.org/euthanas.htm

DeathNET

This site contains many links to biomedical topics, including living wills, "how to" suicide, euthanasia, mercy killing, and legislation regulating the care of the terminally ill.

http://rights.org/deathnet/

PART 2

Death and Dying

*W*hat are the ethical responsibilities associated with death? Doctors are sworn "to do no harm," but this proscription is open to many different interpretations. Death is a natural event that can, in some instances, be hastened to put an end to suffering. Is it ethically necessary to prolong life at all times under all circumstances? Medical personnel as well as families often face these agonizing questions. Even the question of whether or not to tell terminally ill patients the truth about their conditions has great ethical implications. The right of an individual to decide his or her own fate may conflict with society's interest in maintaining the value of human life or in not wasting valuable resources that could be used to save other lives. This conflict is apparent in the matter of physician-assisted suicide and, in a different way, in the question of "futile" treatment. This section examines some of these anguishing questions.

- Are Some Advance Directives Too Risky for Patients?

- Should Physicians Be Allowed to Assist in Patient Suicide?

- Is It Ethical to Withhold the Truth From Dying Patients?

- Should Doctors Be Able to Refuse Demands for "Futile" Treatment?

ISSUE 3

Are Some Advance Directives
Too Risky for Patients?

YES: Christopher James Ryan, from "Betting Your Life: An Argument Against Certain Advance Directives," *Journal of Medical Ethics* (vol. 22, 1996)

NO: Steven Luttrell and Ann Sommerville, from "Limiting Risks by Curtailing Rights: A Response to Dr. Ryan," *Journal of Medical Ethics* (vol. 22, 1996)

ISSUE SUMMARY

YES: Psychiatrist Christopher James Ryan argues that advance directives that refuse active treatment in situations when a patient's incompetence is potentially reversible should be abolished because healthy people are likely to underestimate their desire for treatment should they become ill.

NO: Geriatricians Steven Luttrell and Ann Sommerville assert that respect for the principle of autonomy requires that individuals be permitted to make risky choices about their own lives and that ignoring autonomous choices made by competent adults reinstates the outmoded notion of medical paternalism.

Since ancient times people have drawn up wills to determine what should be done with their property, or who should take custody of their children, after they die. In 1969 Luis Kutner, a law professor, proposed a "living will," a document that would determine the course of medical treatment should the signer become unable to express his or her wishes. A typical living will stated, "If I am permanently unconscious or there is no reasonable expectation for my recovery from a serious incapacitating or lethal illness or condition, I do not wish to be kept alive by artificial means." The proposal came at a time when the public was just beginning to be aware of the use of machines to keep people breathing and their hearts beating even though there was no possibility of regaining consciousness. In 1975 the Karen Ann Quinlan case, involving a young, permanently unconsciousness woman on a ventilator, focused ethical and legal attention on the unwanted use of medical technology.

In 1976, following the Quinlan case, California enacted the nation's first law approving the use of living wills. Nearly every state in the United States followed suit. Sometimes called "natural death acts," these laws and the wills they approved were so vaguely worded and so difficult to interpret that they were hardly ever effective in achieving their goals. It was difficult, for example, to determine what was meant by "reasonable expectation," "artificial means," or even "lethal illness."

In 1983 the President's Commission for the Study of Ethical Problems in Medicine and Biomedical and Behavioral Research recommended an alternative approach. Rather than signing a document that specified certain treatments that should be forgone, patients were encouraged to name a person who would make health care decisions in their place.

There are several types of advance directives. They can be formally written and legally authorized, or they can be informal communications with family members or health care providers. Much of the legal wrangling about withdrawal of life supports has turned on whether or not the patient expressed such desires while competent. The case of Nancy Cruzan, which eventually went to the U.S. Supreme Court, is one example. The parents of this young Missouri woman, who was permanently unconscious after an automobile accident, sued the state to have her life supports removed, claiming that this is what Nancy herself would have wanted. The state argued that there was no clear and convincing evidence that Nancy would have made the same decision. In 1990 the U.S. Supreme Court ruled that states had an interest in preserving life and could require a high standard of evidence of the patient's expressed preference for withdrawing treatment. The case then went back to the Missouri courts, which this time found the evidence convincing and agreed to allow withdrawal of life support.

To add to the weight of the Supreme Court's decision, in 1991 Congress passed the Patient Self-Determination Act (PSDA), which requires all health care providers reimbursed by Medicare to inform patients about their right to sign advance directives. By this measure Congress intended to promote the use of advance directives in hospitals and nursing homes where elderly patients are often treated.

Despite legislative and judicial approval of advance directives and widespread public opinion supporting them, such documents are still rarely signed by competent patients, and even when signed they are still rarely consulted or implemented. Studies have documented barriers such as lack of appropriate communication and physicians' disregard of the wishes expressed in the directives.

The following selections address a more basic issue: the ethical acceptability of a particular kind of advance directive. Christopher James Ryan favors the abolition of advance directives in which a healthy patient chooses withdrawal of active treatment in a future situation in which he or she is incompetent but where the incompetence is potentially reversible. Steven Luttrell and Ann Sommerville assert that advance directives are mostly made by ill patients, who do have a good idea of what they want, and that their autonomous decisions, even when risky, should be respected.

Christopher James Ryan

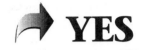 **YES**

Betting Your Life: An Argument Against Certain Advance Directives

Along time ago, in a country far far away, there lived a very wise old king. The king was a very ethical man and his subjects were very happy. Everyone lived together in perfect harmony and times were generally regarded as good.

One day the king introduced a new law. The law allowed his subjects to enter into a mysterious wager. Those who won the wager would receive a rich reward, but those who lost would be put to death. Entry into the wager was entirely voluntary and despite the dire consequences of losing many took up the challenge. To win, a contestant had only correctly to answer an apparently straightforward question. The question was known to all participants before they entered and all who took up the challenge were sure that they knew the answer and could not lose. Strangely, even the king's ethicists had no objection to the introduction of the law and in fact praised the king for his wisdom and progressiveness. The ethicists also believed that the answer to the question was obvious and focused only on the rich reward.

Unfortunately, however, many contestants got the answer wrong. They lost the wager and were put to an early and needless death. The question, that caused so much difficulty, was this: "Even though you are now well and healthy, imagine yourself in a situation where you have a terminal illness and are temporarily confused or unconscious. Imagine that whilst you are in this state your doctors give you a choice; either they will treat you to the best of their ability and you may recover some of your health for some undefined period, or they will treat you conservatively and, though they will ensure that you are in no pain, they will not attempt to save your life. If you were in this situation what would you want the doctors to do?"

Advance directives or living wills frequently require their users to undertake the kind of task set out above; that is, to imagine themselves in a situation where they are required to make a decision about whether or not they should receive active treatment but are incompetent to do so. These have become increasingly popular over the last decade. Legislation giving statutory status to these directives has been enacted in many parts of the Western world and planned in many others. In places where no such legislation exists living wills are thought to have increasing weight in common law.[1-3]

From Christopher James Ryan, "Betting Your Life: An Argument Against Certain Advance Directives," *Journal of Medical Ethics*, vol. 22 (1996), pp. 95–99. Copyright © 1996 by The British Medical Association. Reprinted by permission.

In this paper I oppose a common form of advance directive on ethical grounds. The basis of my argument is my contention that, like the citizens of the country above, many people who take out advance directives do so under the belief that they know the answer to the question above, when in fact they do not. In order [to] support my position I will first provide evidence which supports this contention and then demonstrate the ethical difficulties this creates for advocates of living wills.

I do not intend to provide opposition to all forms of advance directive, but will restrict my discussion to a fairly narrow but not uncommon set of criteria. I will examine only cases where an advance directive demands that the user receive only conservative or palliative care in a situation where he or she is incompetent to consent to such treatment but where that incompetence is potentially reversible.

Getting the Answer Wrong

My argument hinges on the notion that people are likely grossly to underestimate their desire to have medical intervention should they become ill; I will therefore explain why this is likely to be so on theoretical grounds and then provide some empirical evidence that suggests that this actually occurs.

Denial is a strong and largely successful mechanism for dealing with the stressors of everyday life. For the healthy person considering a terminal illness it involves the subconscious decision to reject the possibility that one will suffer in the way one might be expected to if one were to succumb to such an illness. There are two standard ways of going about this. The first is simply to tell yourself that terminal illnesses are things that happen to other people and that they will not happen to you. This method works reasonably well whilst one is still young and all, or most, of the people that get such illnesses are not like you at all. It starts to lose its power, however, as you grow older and terminal illnesses begin to befall your peers. Now the other people begin to look a lot like you and the only-happens-to-others strategy looks increasingly anaemic.

The second option is to use denial in a slightly more complicated manner and when confronted by the suffering of another in the midst of a terminal illness to say that this would not happen to you because, if you were in that situation, you would kill yourself before the suffering became too great. Here you have traded the real and very distressing possibility that you may develop, and suffer at the hands of, a terminal illness for the hypothetical notion of a future early death. As a hypothetical abstract your early death is unpleasant but much more bearable than the realisation that you could become so ill.

Of course once you have developed a terminal illness, this coping strategy will no longer be successful. Now the possibility of your death is no longer hypothetical and you are faced with balancing real dying with the possibility of real suffering. While there is no doubt that some individuals now decide that they would still be better off dead, I believe that the vast majority of people now decide to battle it out. Most people with terminal illnesses do not want to die and are prepared to put up with a certain amount of suffering in order to live a little longer. Now that death is no longer a hypothetical it holds little appeal and frequently denial is used again, this time to maintain hope that a cure will be found.[4]

Human beings are, I suggest, very poor at determining their attitudes to treatment for some hypothetical future terminal illness and very frequently grossly under-estimate their future desire to go on living.

Though based on psychological theorising, there is some evidence to support this contention. The first piece of evidence is admittedly anecdotal but none the less quite powerful. Healthy people frequently believe that if they were suffering a terminal illness and required various forms of medical intervention they would rather be allowed to slip away. This view is so common among healthy people that it can be regarded as perfectly normal. Among terminally ill people, however, the sustained expression of a preference not to receive treatment is very rare. Most palliative care specialists will readily recall one or two patients who persistently requested that they be allowed to die. Some will recall several. However, palliative care physicians do not report that this sustained desire is very common and certainly do not report that it is the norm. This strongly suggests that many people who, when healthy, predict they would refuse treatment in the future, will change their mind when they develop a terminal illness.

This anecdotal evidence is supported by a number of studies in the psychiatric literature. One such study by Owen *et al* found that among patients with cancer the strongest interest in euthanasia was among those patients being offered potentially curative treatment. Patients with poorer prognoses, who were only being offered palliative care, tended to reject the idea of euthanasia as a future option ($p<0.05$).[5] Similarly, a 1994 study by Danis *et al*, which examined the stability of future treatment preferences, found that while preferences for most remained stable over the study's two-year duration, people that had been hospitalised, had an accident or had become immobile were likely to change their health care preferences to opt for more intervention.[6] Both studies suggest that having had an episode of serious illness or a deterioration of an existing illness may make people more likely to want more intervention.

Seale and Addington-Hall asked relatives and friends of people who had died whether the dead person would have benefited from an earlier death. They found that respondents, who were not spouses, were frequently willing to say that an earlier death would have been better for the person even though the person who had died had not expressed a desire to die sooner. That is, the healthy relatives and friends were keener on euthanasia than the terminally ill patient had been. This again suggests that healthy people may view euthanasia differently from terminally ill people or at least that it is hard to empathise with the position of the terminally ill.[7]

Though it is not possible directly to equate suicide with a desire for euthanasia, one might expect that if terminally ill people increasingly wanted to die as they became sicker and sicker then suicide among patients with terminal illness would peak towards the end of their illnesses. This would be the time when pain and suffering was at its worst and when there was little to look forward to. In fact, however, completed suicide is most common in the first year after diagnosis in the terminally ill.[8] It may be that in this situation suicide more often represents an irrational reaction to the crisis of diagnosis than a reasoned decision that life has become intolerable.

Further evidence that a desire for euthanasia is uncommon in the terminally ill comes from a study by Brown and co-workers who found that among forty-four terminally ill patients, the only patients who had experienced a desire for an early death were those who were suffering from a clinical depressive illness.[9]

Arguments in Support of Advance Directives

Advocates of this form of advance directive argue for the documents along two lines. Firstly, they take a deontological position that the directives maximise the affected person's autonomy by allowing her some control over her medical management. They argue that since maximisation of autonomy is a legitimate aim and since living wills seem to facilitate the maximisation of autonomy, then living wills are not only ethically justified but beneficial.[10–12] Second, advocates may take a utilitarian line and argue that the directives help to facilitate the death of people who believe they would be better off dead than alive. By facilitating these deaths the directives not only end people's suffering, but spare them an undignified death. In addition the directive may ease the burden on medical staff and family of the ill individual who may find making these decisions painful. Through all these means, they argue, the directive increases the net utility of the community.[10]

Opponents of this form of advance directive usually base their opposition upon an opposition to euthanasia.[13] However, since most living will legislation throughout the world facilitates only passive euthanasia and since passive euthanasia is rarely objected to, there has been little solid opposition to this form of advance directive legislation.

My objections to these advance directives do not rely on an objection to either active or passive euthanasia. Rather my objections are based on the proposition that these living wills do not necessarily increase the user's autonomy nor society's net utility in the unproblematic way they are imagined to do, because people are much more likely to refuse treatment when faced with a future hypothetical scenario than when faced with a real here and now choice. If this contention is accepted it has a number of consequences for arguments used in support of living wills.

Consequences for the Argument From Autonomy

The principle of a right to autonomy holds that adult human beings have the right to make decisions about their lives and so direct the course of their own fate. The right to autonomy is a powerful maxim. It is the right to autonomy that underlies the notions of consent, the right to freedom and democracy itself. By grounding their support for directives in this principle proponents of living wills set up a strong case.

It is an accepted part of the principle, however, that one cannot properly exercise one's autonomy if one is not in possession of all available information that might influence one's decisions. A patient's consent to a procedure, for example, is only valid if she has been informed of all the risks and consequences. If the psychological reasoning and empirical evidence above is accepted, then a person currently using a living will does not have access to a vital piece of information that may radically alter her decision. Specifically, she does not know that it is highly likely that her decision, made now, that she would rather die if faced with a hypothetical future scenario is not what her decision would have been if she were actually faced with that scenario.

Almost everyone assumes that he knows his own mind and that he would know the choices he would make in the event of a crisis. While there is little doubt that the individual alone is in the best position to know how he would act and it is also true that some people must correctly guess how they would act, nevertheless evidence strongly suggests that many people simply get it wrong. They believe they would not opt for treatment in a hypothetical future circumstance but were they actually to face the circumstance they would opt for treatment. Most people have no experience of their reactions to a life-threatening illness, they can only guess at their reaction and they frequently guess wrong. More importantly for my argument, people do not believe in, or even know of the possibility of, an inaccurate guess. If users of advance directives do not know of the distinct possibility that their choices may be inaccurate, they lack a vital piece of information and that lack prohibits a fully informed and autonomous choice.

Consequences for the Utilitarian Argument

The possibility that a large number of people are dying when they would not have wanted to because of the introduction of advance directives, directly threatens the utilitarian argument offered in support of these directives.

The utilitarian argument draws its strength from the hope that the existence of advance directives will end the suffering of people with terminal illnesses who have decided that they would be better off dead. It is assumed that they have come to this opinion by weighing up the benefits of their continued existence with the pain and suffering of their terminal illness. There is an additional hidden assumption that the affected individuals can accurately estimate this balance from the safety of health and happiness prior to their illness. If this additional assumption is unjustified then the utilitarian argument is undermined.

Conclusions Regarding Living Wills

With the argument from autonomy and the utilitarian argument both undermined, ethical support for living wills of this sort is seriously diminished. The effect this diminution will have upon one's attitudes to living wills will depend on both the seriousness with which one takes the evidence for the inaccuracy of people's choices and one's beliefs about how well this inaccuracy can be addressed through changes to legislation and education.

At a minimum one should require significant changes in legislation to address users' ignorance of their likelihood of wrong decisions. The principle of autonomy demands that the individual making the choice be given all available relevant information, therefore those making living wills must be informed of the apparent likelihood that their decision to refuse treatment now may not accurately reflect the decision they would make in the future, were they competent at the time. To my knowledge, no piece of living will legislation currently refers to this likelihood. Though there are numerous published advance directive forms and more publications to assist in filling them in, none of them inform the potential user of the likely inaccuracy of their current decision.[10,11,14,15]

While such a change may satisfy strong advocates of advance directives that autonomy is now again maximised, I would remain dubious that this were the case. The logistics of giving such warnings to all people filling in living wills will necessarily mean that the warnings will be scant and superficial. The belief that one knows one's own mind now and in the future is understandably held with some vehemence by most of the community. The psychological needs met by the belief that one would rather be dead in a future tragic situation are strong and deeply ingrained. An insignificant warning is unlikely to have any impact upon this belief and many people will continue falsely to believe they definitely know what they would want in the hypothetical scenario.

This kind of reasoning leads me to believe that it will be practically impossible to allow people to make an autonomous choice about this kind of advance directive and therefore on the grounds that such directives will neither increase autonomy nor increase the community's level of utility I believe that this type of living will should be abolished.

It is important to note that this line of argument will not demand the abandonment of all varieties of advance directive. It will not, for example, apply to advance directives where the ability to consent to treatment is irreversibly lost. In this situation there will be no possibility of the person recovering to give carers a more accurate report of her current desire for treatment. Carers would then be justified in taking their best guess as to the affected individual's preferences, no matter how inaccurate it is likely to be. Moreover, this best guess will be substantially improved if the person has taken out a living will. Neither will it affect advance directives made by people who are already critically ill and who are, for example, giving instruction that they should not be resuscitated in the event of cardiac arrest. These people are already critically ill and therefore are able correctly to determine their preferences for what is essentially their current situation.

The argument applies only to advance directives made by essentially healthy individuals who opt for withdrawal of active care in a situation where their inability to consent is potentially reversible. In these situations, patients should be resuscitated and their opinions regarding future treatment sought again now that they are in the scenario that they had previously only imagined. For some no doubt this will lead to considerable hardship, as they must again state their preference that they would rather be allowed to die, but for others, perhaps the majority, it will provide a safety net and a chance to reconsider their decision with all available information.

Those who would have wished to see the King's wager abolished because of the needless deaths it seemed to cause must be similarly troubled by this form of living will.

References

1. Mendelson D. The Medical Treatment (Enduring Power of Attorney) Act and assisted suicide: the legal position in Victoria. *Bioethics News* 1993; **12**: 34–42.
2. Stern K. Living wills in English law. *Palliative Medicine* 1993; **7**: 283–8.
3. Greco PJ, Schulman KA, Lavizzo-Mourey R, Hansen-Flaschen J. The Patient Self-Determination Act and the future of advance directives. *Annals of Internal Medicine* 1991; **115**: 639–43.
4. Kübler-Ross E. *On death and dying.* New York: Macmillan, 1969.
5. Owen C, Tennant C, Levis J, Jones M. Suicide and euthanasia: patient attitudes in the context of cancer. *Psycho-Oncology* 1992; **1**: 79–88.
6. Danis M, Garrett J, Harris R, Patrick DL. Stability of choices about life-sustaining treatments. *Annals of Internal Medicine* 1994; **120**: 567–73.
7. Dillner L. Relatives keener on euthanasia than patients. *British Medical Journal* 1994; *309*: 1107.
8. Allebeck P, Bolund C, Ringback G. Increased suicide rate in cancer patients. *Journal of Clinical Epidemiology* 1989; **42**: 611–6.
9. Brown JH, Henteleff P, Barakat S, Rowe CJ. Is it normal for terminally ill patients to desire death? *American Journal of Psychiatry* 1986; **143**: 208–11.
10. Molloy W, Mepham V, Clarnette R. *Let me decide.* Melbourne: Penguin, 1993.
11. Quill TE. *Death and dignity. Making choices and taking charge.* New York: WW Norton, 1993.
12. Charlesworth M. A good death. In: Kuhse H, ed. *Willing to listen—waiting to die.* Melbourne: Penguin, 1994: 203–16.
13. Marker R. *Deadly compassion. The death of Ann Humphry and the case against euthanisia.* London: Harper Collins, 1994.
14. Humphry D. *Dying with dignity: understanding euthanasia.* New York: Birch Lane Press, 1992.
15. Kennedy L. *Euthanasia.* London: Chatto & Windus, 1990.

NO 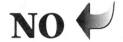 Steven Luttrell and Ann Sommerville

Limiting Risks by Curtailing Rights:
A Response to Dr. Ryan

Decisions about life-sustaining medical treatment should really be left to doctors. That is the core message of "betting your life" by Dr C J Ryan.[1] Although he focuses on only one type of decision—when the patient's mental incompetence is potentially reversible—the implication is that healthy people cannot validly appreciate the dimensions of the risk involved when they seek to limit in advance the scope of their own medical treatment. The danger of such miscalculation is said to be so profound that their right to take the risk must be curtailed for their own good. The general argument is not new. As the House of Lords Select Committee on Medical Ethics noted: "Disabled individuals are commonly more satisfied with their life than able-bodied people expect to be with the disability. The healthy do not choose in the same way as the sick".[2] But does this mean healthy people are to be deprived of the opportunity to make the attempt?

Some of the existing criticism of advance decision-making has been preoccupied with personal identity and the continuity of mind and mental state as the important criteria. According to such arguments, the rupture caused by loss of competence is so great that it makes nonsense of the concept of personal continuity. A competent individual is not making advance decisions for herself but for the future relict of who she once was. Dr Ryan's argument is a variation on this theme and seeks to prove that in advance of disability, people are in such a totally different mind-set that they are "likely to grossly under-estimate their desire for medical intervention should they become ill".[1]

We do not agree with Dr Ryan's view that advance directives dealing with situations where the deterioration in mental capacity is potentially reversible should be abolished and take issue with him on the following points:

(i) His argument hinges on the notion that people are likely to underestimate substantially their desire to have medical intervention should they become ill. The evidence for this is not convincing. Emanuel *et al* following a prospective study of 495 HIV-positive or oncology out-patients and 102 members of the public concluded that most people made moderately stable treatment choices and that recent hospitalisation did not decrease that stability.[3]

From Steven Luttrell and Ann Sommerville, "Limiting Risks by Curtailing Rights: A Response to Dr. Ryan," *Journal of Medical Ethics,* vol. 22 (1996), pp. 100–104. Copyright © 1996 by The British Medical Association. Reprinted by permission.

Even if it is the case that in general the sick do not make the same choices as the healthy, there is evidence that this does not apply to people who have completed an advance directive. Although Danis *et al* found that patients who were hospitalised one or more times between baseline and follow-up interviews were more likely to change their choices and desire more treatment, patients who had a living will were more likely to maintain stable preferences. Indeed, patients who had living wills and chose the least amount of care at their initial interview had extremely stable preferences (96 per cent unchanged).[4]

There appears to be little evidence that healthy people consider making treatment decisions in advance. Even in the United States, where living wills have been in existence much longer than in Britain, there is a wide disparity between the large percentage of people who indicate a desire to die without heroic measures and the small percentage who have made advance directives.[5] The scant UK evidence[6] supports American findings that interest in living wills is primarily shown by people who are educated, articulate and already have a diagnosis. (In the USA, the obligation for hospitals to raise the subject of advance decision-making arose only with patients who were checking in for treatment and therefore, by definition, were not a healthy population.) Part of the increased interest in this mechanism in the UK has been as a result of a small but well-informed population of HIV-positive patients witnessing the terminal treatment of friends and partners. Indeed, one of the limitations of advance statements is their lack of ready accessibility to people with differing levels of education, experience and literacy.

(ii) Dr Ryan states that it is an accepted principle that one cannot properly exercise one's autonomy if one is not in possession of all available information that might influence one's decisions and that a patient's consent to a procedure is only valid if she has been informed of all the risks and consequences. We take issue with this view. It implicitly denies the option of consciously deciding from a knowingly incomplete knowledge base and the option to decide validly to allow another person to decide on one's behalf. It is not necessarily obligatory for an individual to know each and every one of the risks implicit in a course of action. Indeed, if this were the case, no person could ever make a valid decision. As human beings, our motivation is often intuitive or emotional as well as cognitive and we sometimes exercise autonomy by choosing not to know or at least not to recognise the full import of our actions. It is arguably not necessary to examine all the implications in order for a person to be clear that she does not want to go on living indefinitely with a restricted range of competency or mobility, even if some small improvement is possible. If applied to other spheres of medicine, Dr Ryan's principle would mean that people cannot make valid decisions about childbearing without taking account of potentially available genetic information or pre-natal testing.

Arguably, therefore, it cannot be assumed that in real life, people who make advance refusals want to know everything or, if having chosen not to be fully informed of every detail, are incapable of understanding the implications of their decision. Nevertheless, the *Code of Practice on Advance Statements,* published by the British Medical Association, sees health professionals as obliged to make all appropriate efforts to raise patients' awareness at the drafting stage about the risks and disadvantages, as well as the benefits, of advance statements.[7] As a matter of law in the UK, a patient's consent to a procedure is valid if he understands in general terms the nature of the intervention. There is no legal obligation to explain *all* the risks and benefits.[8]

(iii) Even if people do make unwise choices, we believe that this should not be used as a reason to curtail their autonomy. Society generally recognises that individuals sometimes make bad or risky choices in the way they shape their lives. In our society, the libertarian legacy of Mill, however, assumes that individual choices should be permitted, unless they impinge on the rights of others. Mill's famous dictum was that "the sole end for which mankind are warranted, individually or collectively, in interfering with the liberty of action of any of their number is self-protection" and that an individual "cannot rightfully be compelled to do or forbear because it will be better for him to do so, because it will make him happier, because in the opinions of others to do so would be wise or even right".[9] So, does it damage the fabric of society or the rights of other people to allow Jehovah's Witnesses, for example, the right to refuse in advance the administration of blood products in all circumstances, even when their condition is curable? Or should they, as Dr Ryan suggests, be forcibly treated and only then "their opinions regarding future treatment be sought again now that they are in the scenario that they had previously only imagined"?[1]

Common Sense

It is trite to observe that people's views change with their circumstances. The philosopher, Parfit, for example, discussing different stages of individual development, talks about "my most recent self", "one of my earlier selves" and "one of my distant selves"; each of these showing a different degree of psychological connectedness with the present self.[10] From a practical perspective, would this mean that greater weight must automatically be attached to an advance directive made comparatively recently by an individual who is still more or less the same self? Common sense would seem to support such a view even if the individual was completely healthy when making the directive and now is in an altered psychological state. Simply acknowledging varying degrees of psychological continuity or disparity with regard to former and future selves does not answer the question of whether it is morally correct for subsequent selves to be treated in contravention of an advance directive reflecting their former interests.

(iv) We believe that a retreat to medical paternalism is not a practical option in societies increasingly aware of patient charters and consumer rights. Many forms of advance directives offer the drafter a choice of specifying personal instructions and/or nominating a proxy to decide. American surveys show that the option most commonly chosen is for people to select decision-making by a family member or other proxy despite the evidence of a variable correlation between the judgments of nominated proxy decision-makers and the patients' own prior wishes.[11] One study indicated that of 104 patients with life-threatening illness who were offered advance directives, 69 took up the offer and most asked for non-aggressive treatment if "the burdens of treatment outweigh the expected benefits". None, however, gave any other personal instructions,[12] although evidence suggests that proxies are more likely than patients themselves to opt for life-prolonging treatment, ie, to support more conservative choices than the individual would have made if competent and in that situation.[13]

Dr Ryan contests one specific type of advance directive on grounds of utility and autonomy. He argues that it is contrary to utility to permit people to die when their lives could be prolonged and their condition improved. This might be true if utility were a matter of simply prolonging life rather than also a question of maximising happiness and choice and reducing misery, including the misery of families who may see their relative being resuscitated contrary to an informed and competent advance refusal.

Two Autonomies

Nor is autonomy a simple matter. When an individual is conscious but mentally incapacitated, in Dworkin's view, "two autonomies are in play: the autonomy of the demented patient and the autonomy of the person who became demented. These two autonomies can conflict, and the resulting problems are complex and difficult".[14] Of course, some philosophers solve this by attributing no autonomy to the demented person and recognising the "residual interests" of the previously competent individual as paramount. A range of psychological and philosophical questions arise here about our ability to decide now life and death matters for the people we will be in the future when some part of what makes us the individuals we are—our awareness of ourselves, our past and continuity—has been lost. Dworkin seems to support Dr Ryan's approach in seeing the competent person who makes the anticipatory decision as fundamentally different from and other to the incapacitated individual who lives out (or not) the consequences of the decision. It is widely accepted that individuals can only make advance directives for "themselves". A person who becomes severely mentally disordered, however, is in some sense no longer "herself". Nevertheless, despite the lack of continuity, the former, competent "self" should arguably still retain moral rights about how the later, incompetent self is treated.[15] Even if acknowledged as being not quite the same person, the claim of the competent to decide on behalf of the later incompetent self still appears stronger than the claims of other players, especially bearing in mind the above-mentioned tendency for proxy decision-makers to choose options inconsistent with the individual's own values.

There is a danger that health professionals and nominated proxies will not take full account of the complex mixture of reasoning which leads some people to choose to forego treatment even in situations where medicine can offer them an extension of life. Although doctors' decisions about lifesaving treatment correlate with their own estimate of subsequent quality of life, they significantly underestimate their elderly patients' quality of life compared with the views of the patients themselves.[16] For some people, medical views of quality of life or possibility of improvement may not be a central issue. Just as Dr Ryan points out that it is difficult for healthy people convincingly to imagine themselves with disability, so it is often hard for the young or middle-aged to envisage that there may be a stage when we have simply lived long enough and the burdens of further treatment no longer outweigh the benefits. We may then wish to opt out even at the risk of potentially missing out on a slightly prolonged lifespan.

(v) We do not agree that advance directives for conditions of temporary mental incapacity should be less valid than advance directives for conditions of permanent mental incapacity. We question the logic of such a distinction. Dr Ryan concedes that his argument does not apply where loss of mental capacity is permanent. He distinguishes this situation as there "will be no possibility of the person recovering to give carers a more accurate report of her current desire for treatment"[1] and therefore they should be guided by an existing living will. He recognises that an accurate report of individual wishes is of value and therefore should be respected. If, however, a Jehovah's Witness, for example, repeatedly states that under no circumstances does he want a transfusion with blood products, Dr Ryan would urge us to ignore this directive if mental incapacity is temporarily impaired. There is no logical reason why the situation where mental incapacity is temporary should be treated in a different way from the situation where the incapacity is permanent. We feel that in both cases an appropriately worded advance directive should be equally applicable.

Information-Sharing

(vi) Even if Dr Ryan's arguments are accepted, we do not agree that "there is the possibility of large numbers of people dying when they would not have wanted to" although it may be that some will die when doctors would prefer to keep them alive. Doctors hostile to the concept of advance decision-making can limit or otherwise influence patients' choices. The acceptance or refusal of treatment is highly dependent on the amount and manner of information-sharing about the treatment options.[17] Discussion with elderly out-patients about limiting treatment rarely occurs[18] and in Emanuel's survey of patient and public opinion, the lack of physician initiative was the most frequently mentioned perceived barrier to the making of advance directives. In this survey of 405 out-patients and 102 members of the public, 93 per cent of the former and 89 per cent of the latter claimed to desire advance directives but considered their doctors to be reluctant.[19] Yet it is to be strongly advised that advance directives are only made in conjunction with advice and information from health professionals.[20]

Dr Ryan's arguments only apply to advance directives which withhold consent to treatment where there has been a temporary loss of mental capacity. We agree that the greatest value of advance directives is their use in situations where the loss of mental capacity is not reversible, such as in cases of dementia, chronic stroke or chronic brain injury due to trauma.

Nevertheless, we refute his thesis that large numbers of people will die unnecessarily since we believe it unlikely that many people will draft advance directives specifically indicating that they would not want treatment if they were to suffer temporary mental incapacity. Examples of common clinical situations where a reduction in mental capacity is potentially reversible include the acute confusional state in an older person, the early phase of recovery from an acute stroke, and the early stage of recovery from head trauma and psychiatric illness. We agree that the advance directive is of more limited application in these situations as it may be very difficult to envisage what degree of recovery will occur. Certainly, with respect to mental illness, if a patient is detained under a section of the Mental Health Act 1983, treatment under the Act will override any refusal of treatment of mental disorder set out in an advance directive.

If one examines the standard forms for advance directives in the UK, many emphasise that for the decision to be implementable the deterioration in mental capacity must be considered permanent or where life is nearing its end due to a terminal physical illness. People may draft their decisions in any form but many use standard documents which direct attention to irreversible conditions. One of the most common living wills, the Terrence Higgins Trust model, is not unique in allowing drafters the option of choosing to have all available treatment as well as refusing interventions in three situations:

- When there is a life-threatening illness *from which there is no likelihood of recovery* and it is so serious that life is nearing its end;
- When *mental functions become permanently impaired with no likelihood of improvement* and the impairment is so severe that the drafter does not understand what is happening and medical treatment is needed to keep him alive;
- When the drafter is *permanently unconscious* with no likelihood of regaining consciousness.[21]

Dr Ryan's argument is based on the fact that the sick do not make the same choices as the healthy. He does not point out, however, that in many instances advance directives are made by people who are already sick. Indeed, the mechanism is probably most useful for those people who have already been diagnosed as having a chronic illness for which there is no adequate curative treatment and where there is likely to be a predictable pattern of deterioration, for example, patients with AIDS or dementia. Moreover, even if an advance directive is made while the drafter is healthy, he or she will often have the opportunity of revoking or changing it when illness occurs as long as mental capacity is retained.

Conclusion

For the reasons outlined in this paper, we maintain that advance directives refusing treatment during periods of temporary incapacity should be respected. We acknowledge, however, that there are difficulties for healthy people trying to make decisions for future events. It is important that patients are made aware of these difficulties and not discouraged by medical reluctance to discuss the matter so that they draft directives in isolation. Emanuel found that those patients who had discussion with their physicians made the most stable decisions.[3] We would therefore urge any person making an advance directive about medical therapy to discuss the directive with a medical practitioner.

References

1. Ryan J. Betting your life: an argument against certain advance directives. *Journal of Medical Ethics* 1996; **22**: 95-9.
2. House of Lords Select Committee on Medical Ethics. *Report from the Select Committee on Medical Ethics.* London: HMSO, 1994: **1**: 41.
3. Emanuel L, Emanuel E, Stoeckle, *et al.* Advance directives, stability of patient's treatment choices. *Archives of Internal Medicine* 1994; **154**: 209-17.
4. Danis M, Garret J, Harris R, *et al.* Stability of choices about life sustaining treatments. *Annals of Internal Medicine* 1994; **120**: 567-73.
5. Menikoff JA, Sachs GA, Seigler M. Beyond advance directives: health care surrogate laws. *New England Journal of Medicine* 1992; **327**: 1165-9.
6. Meadows P. Use of living wills in HIV infection and AIDS. *Lancet* 1994; **334**: 1509. Calvert GM. The completion of living wills: an examination of the demographics, completion and issues raised by the living will. London: Terrence Higgins Trust, 1994. Schlyter C. *Advance directives and AIDS: an empirical study of the interest in living wills and proxy decision making in the context of HIV/AIDs care.* London: Centre of Medical Law and Ethics, Kings College, 1992.
7. Sommerville A. *Advance statements about medical treatment.* London: BMJ Publishing Group, 1995: 23.
8. Sidaway v Board of Governors of the Bethlem Royal Hospital and the Maudsley Hospital [1985] AC 871.
9. Mill JS. *On liberty.* London: Parker and Son, 1859: 68.
10. Parfit D. Personal identity. In: Honderich T, Burnyeat M, eds. *Philosophy as it is.* Harmondsworth: Pelican, 1979: 186-211.
11. For example see Seckler AB, Meier DE, Mulvihill M, Cammer Paris BE: Substituted judgement: how accurate are proxy predictions? *Annals of Internal Medicine* 1991; **115**: 92-8. Ouslander JG, Tymchuk AJ, Rhabar B. Health care decisions among elderly long care residents and their potential proxies. *Archives of Internal Medicine* 1989; **149**: 1367-72. Emanuel BJ, Emanuel LL. Proxy decision making for incompetent patients: an ethical and empirical analysis. *Journal of the American Medical Association* 1992; **267**: 2067-71.
12. Schneiderman L, *et al.* Effects of offering advance directives on medical treatments and costs. *Annals of Internal Medicine* 1992; **117**: 599-606.
13. See reference 11: Seckler AB, *et al.*
14. Dworkin R. *Life's dominion.* London: Harper Collins, 1993.
15. Sommerville A. Are advance directives the answer? In: Maclean S, ed. *Death, dying and the law.* Aldershot: Dartmouth Press, 1996.
16. Uhlmann RF, Pearlman RA. Perceived quality of life and preferences for life sustaining treatment in older adults. *Archives of Internal Medicine* 1991; **151**: 495-7.
17. Ainslie A, Beisecker A. Changes in treatment decisions by elderly persons based on treatment descriptions. *Archives of Internal Medicine* 1994; **154**: 2225-33. Malloy TR, Wigton RS, Meeske J, Tape TG. The influence of treatment descriptions on advance directive decisions. *Journal of the American Geriatric Society* 1992; **40**: 1255-60.
18. Goold SD, Arnold RM, Siminoff LA. Discussion about limiting treatment in a geriatric clinic. *Journal of the American Geriatric Society* 1993; **41**: 277-81.
19. Emanuel LL, Barry MJ, Stoeckle JD, *et al.* Advance directives for medical care—a case for greater use. *New England Journal of Medicine* 1991; **324**: 889-95.
20. Mower WR, Baraff LJ. Advance directives, effect of type of directive on physicians' therapeutic decisions. *Archives of Internal Medicine* 1993; **153**: 375-81.
21. Living will drawn up by Terrence Higgins Trust and King's College Centre for Medical Ethics and Law.

POSTSCRIPT

Are Some Advance Directives Too Risky for Patients?

In November 1995 a major two-year study indicated that there are substantial shortcomings in the care of seriously ill hospitalized patients, despite an intervention that tried to improve communication between physicians and patients and their families about preferences regarding end-of-life treatment. The Study to Understand Prognoses and Preferences for Outcomes and Risks of Treatment, or SUPPORT study, concluded that the intervention failed to improve care or patient outcomes and that more forceful measures may be needed to change established practices. See "A Controlled Trial to Improve Care for Seriously Ill Hospitalized Patients," *Journal of the American Medical Association* (November 22/29, 1995).

A study of the impact of ethnicity on knowledge about and completion of advance directives found that advance directives seem to fit best with the prevailing beliefs of European Americans. By contrast, African Americans tended to have a positive view of advance directives but less knowledge about them. Mexican Americans tended to have negative attitudes, and Korean Americans were almost completely unaware of advance directives and reported negative reactions to the concept. See Sheila T. Murphy et al., "Ethnicity and Advance Care Directives," *Journal of Law, Medicine and Ethics* (Summer 1996).

Linda Emanuel, in "Structured Advance Planning: Is It Finally Time for Physician Action and Reimbursement?" *Journal of the American Medical Association* (August 9, 1995), suggests that an immediate agenda to bring advance directives into more widespread use would include encouraging physicians to co-sign the documents and reimbursing physicians for time spent discussing advance directives.

Nancy M. P. King argues in favor of advance directives in *Making Sense of Advance Directives,* rev. ed. (Georgetown University Press, 1996). Among her major points are that advance directives are only one procedural mechanism for implementing an individual's constitutional right to make decisions concerning his or her own body. Another book is *Planning for Uncertainty: A Guide to Living Wills and Other Advance Directives for Health Care* by D. J. Doukas and W. Reichel (Johns Hopkins University Press, 1993). In collaboration with the American Medical Association and the American Bar Association, the American Association of Retired Persons has prepared a booklet called *A Matter of Choice: Planning Ahead for Health Care Decisions* (AARP, 1919 K Street, Washington, D.C. 20049). Many hospitals and bioethics groups also have educational materials concerning advance directives that conform to their state laws.

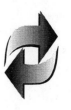

ISSUE 4

Should Physicians Be Allowed to Assist in Patient Suicide?

YES: Marcia Angell, from "The Supreme Court and Physician-Assisted Suicide—The Ultimate Right," *The New England Journal of Medicine* (January 2, 1997)

NO: Kathleen M. Foley, from "Competent Care for the Dying Instead of Physician-Assisted Suicide," *The New England Journal of Medicine* (January 2, 1997)

ISSUE SUMMARY

YES: Physician Marcia Angell asserts that a physician's main duties are to respect patient autonomy and to relieve suffering, even if that sometimes means assisting in a patient's death.

NO: Physician Kathleen M. Foley counters that if physician-assisted suicide becomes legal, it will begin to substitute for interventions that otherwise might enhance the quality of life for dying patients.

Since the early 1980s physicians, lawyers, philosophers, and judges have examined questions about withholding life-sustaining treatment. Their deliberations have resulted in a broad consensus that competent adults have the right to make decisions about their medical care, even if those decisions seem unjustifiable to others and even if they result in death. Furthermore, the right of individuals to name others to carry out their prior wishes or to make decisions if they should become incompetent is now well established. Thirty-eight states now have legislation allowing advance directives (commonly known as "living wills").

The debate in specific cases continues (see, for example, the issue on withholding food and nutrition), but on the whole, patients' rights to self-determination have been bolstered by 80 or more legal cases, dozens of reports, and statements made by medical societies and other organizations.

As often occurs in bioethical debate, the resolution of one issue only highlights the lack of resolution about another. There is clearly no consensus about either euthanasia or physician-assisted suicide.

Like truth telling, euthanasia is an old problem given new dimensions by the ability of modern medical technology to prolong life. The word itself is Greek (literally, *happy death*) and the Greeks wrestled with the question of whether, in some cases, people would be better off dead. But the Hippocratic Oath in this instance was clear: "I will neither give a deadly drug to anybody if asked for it, nor will I make a suggestion to that effect." On the other hand, if the goal of medicine is not simply to prolong life but to reduce suffering, at some point the question of what measures should be taken or withdrawn will inevitably arise. The problem is: When death is inevitable, how far should one go in hastening it?

The majority of cases in which euthanasia is raised as a possibility are among the most difficult ethical issues to resolve, for they involve the conflict between a physician's duty to preserve life and the burden on the patient and the family that is created by fulfilling that duty. One common distinction is between *active* euthanasia (that is, some positive act such as administering a lethal injection) and *passive* euthanasia (that is, an inaction such as deciding not to administer antibiotics when the patient has a severe infection). Another common distinction is between *voluntary* euthanasia (that is, the patient wishes to die and consents to the action that will make it happen) and *involuntary*— or better, *nonvoluntary*—euthanasia (that is, the patient is unable to consent, perhaps because he or she is in a coma).

The two selections that follow address a particularly controversial aspect of this issue. Is it ethical for a physician to assist in a hopelessly ill patient's suicide? Marcia Angell argues that sometimes hastening death should be an option for physicians although "reluctantly as a last resort." Angell states that a physician must consider patient autonomy and suffering when deciding upon care. Kathleen M. Foley contends that the medical profession should take the lead in developing guidelines for the end of life. This means that one must not confuse compassion for a patient's suffering with competence in care.

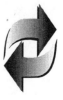

Marcia Angell 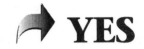 **YES**

The Supreme Court and Physician-Assisted Suicide— The Ultimate Right

The importance and contentious issue of physician-assisted suicide, now being argued before the U.S. Supreme Court, is the subject of the following two editorials. Writing in favor of permitting assisted suicide under certain circumstances is the Journal's executive editor, Dr. Marcia Angell. Arguing against it is Dr. Kathleen Foley, co-chief of the Pain and Palliative Care Service of Memorial Sloan-Kettering Cancer Center in New York. We hope these two editorials, which have in common the authors' view that care of the dying is too often inadequate, will help our readers in making their own judgments.

—Jerome P. Kassirer, M.D.

The U.S. Supreme Court will decide later this year whether to let stand decisions by two appeals courts permitting doctors to help terminally ill patients commit suicide.[1] The Ninth and Second Circuit Courts of Appeals last spring held that state laws in Washington and New York that ban assistance in suicide were unconstitutional as applied to doctors and their dying patients.[2,3] If the Supreme Court lets the decisions stand, physicians in 12 states, which include about half the population of the United States, would be allowed to provide the means for terminally ill patients to take their own lives, and the remaining states would rapidly follow suit. Not since *Roe* v. *Wade* has a Supreme Court decision been so fateful.

The decision will culminate several years of intense national debate, fueled by a number of highly publicized events. Perhaps most important among them is Dr. Jack Kevorkian's defiant assistance in some 44 suicides since 1990, to the dismay of many in the medical and legal establishments, but with substantial public support, as evidenced by the fact that three juries refused to convict him even in the face of a Michigan statute enacted for that purpose. Also since 1990, voters in three states have considered ballot initiatives that would legalize some form of physician-assisted dying, and in 1994 Oregon became the first state to approve such a measure.[4] (The Oregon law was stayed

From Marcia Angell, "The Supreme Court and Physician-Assisted Suicide—The Ultimate Right," *The New England Journal of Medicine*, vol. 336 (January 2, 1997). Copyright © 1997 by The Massachusetts Medical Society. All rights reserved. Reprinted by permission.

pending a court challenge.) Several surveys indicate that roughly two thirds of the American public now support physician-assisted suicide,[5,6] as do more than half the doctors in the United States,[6,7] despite the fact that influential physicians' organizations are opposed. It seems clear that many Americans are now so concerned about the possibility of a lingering, high-technology death that they are receptive to the idea of doctors' being allowed to help them die.

In this editorial I will explain why I believe the appeals courts were right and why I hope the Supreme Court will uphold their decisions. I am aware that this is a highly contentious issue, with good people and strong arguments on both sides. The American Medical Association (AMA) filed an amicus brief opposing the legalization of physician-assisted suicide,[8] and the Massachusetts Medical Society, which owns the *Journal,* was a signatory to it. But here I speak for myself, not the *Journal* or the Massachusetts Medical Society. The legal aspects of the case have been well discussed elsewhere, to me most compellingly in Ronald Dworkin's essay in the *New York Review of Books.*[9] I will focus primarily on the medical and ethical aspects.

I begin with the generally accepted premise that one of the most important ethical principles in medicine is respect for each patient's autonomy, and that when this principle conflicts with others, it should almost always take precedence. This premise is incorporated into our laws governing medical practice and research, including the requirement of informed consent to any treatment. In medicine, patients exercise their self-determination most dramatically when they ask that life-sustaining treatment be withdrawn. Although others may sometimes consider the request ill-founded, we are bound to honor it if the patient is mentally competent—that is, if the patient can understand the nature of the decision and its consequences.

A second starting point is the recognition that death is not fair and is often cruel. Some people die quickly, and others die slowly but peacefully. Some find personal or religious meaning in the process, as well as an opportunity for a final reconciliation with loved ones. But others, especially those with cancer, AIDS, or progressive neurologic disorders, may die by inches and in great anguish, despite every effort of their doctors and nurses. Although nearly all pain can be relieved, some cannot, and other symptoms, such as dyspnea, nausea, and weakness, are even more difficult to control. In addition, dying sometimes holds great indignities and existential suffering. Patients who happen to require some treatment to sustain their lives, such as assisted ventilation or dialysis, can hasten death by having the life-sustaining treatment withdrawn, but those who are not receiving life-sustaining treatment may desperately need help they cannot now get.

If the decisions of the appeals courts are upheld, states will not be able to prohibit doctors from helping such patients to die by prescribing a lethal dose of a drug and advising them on its use for suicide. State laws barring euthanasia (the administration of a lethal drug by a doctor) and assisted suicide for patients who are not terminally ill would not be affected. Furthermore, doctors would not be *required* to assist in suicide; they would simply have that option. Both appeals courts based their decisions on constitutional questions. This is important, because it shifted the focus of the debate from what the majority would approve through the political process, as exemplified by the Oregon initiative, to a matter of fundamental rights, which are largely immune from the political process. Indeed, the Ninth Circuit Court drew an explicit analogy between suicide and abortion, saying that both were personal choices protected by the Constitution and that forbidding doctors to assist would in effect nullify these rights. Although states could regulate assisted suicide, as they do abortion, they would not be permitted to regulate it out of existence.

It is hard to quarrel with the desire of a greatly suffering, dying patient for a quicker, more humane death or to disagree that it may be merciful to help bring that about. In those circumstances, loved ones are often relieved when death finally comes, as are the attending doctors and nurses. As the Second Circuit Court said (in the case of *Quill v. Vacco*), the state has no interest in prolonging such a life. Why, then, do so many people oppose legalizing physician-assisted suicide in these cases? There are a number of arguments against it, some stronger than others, but I believe none of them can offset the overriding duties of doctors to relieve suffering and to respect their patients' autonomy. Below I list several of the more important arguments against physician-assisted suicide and discuss why I believe they are in the last analysis unpersuasive.

Assisted suicide is a form of killing, which is always wrong. In contrast, withdrawing life-sustaining treatment simply allows the disease to take its course. There are three methods of hastening the death of a dying patient: withdrawing life-sustaining treatment, assisting suicide, and euthanasia. The right to stop treatment has been recognized repeatedly since the 1976 case of Karen Ann Quinlan[10] and was affirmed by the U.S. Supreme Court in the 1990 Cruzan decision[11] and the U.S. Congress in its 1990 Patient Self-Determination Act.[12] Although the legal underpinning is the right to be free of unwanted bodily invasion, the purpose of hastening death was explicitly acknowledged. In contrast, assisted suicide and euthanasia have not been accepted; euthanasia is illegal in all states, and assisted suicide is illegal in most of them.

Why the distinctions? Most would say they turn on the doctor's role: whether it is passive or active. When life-sustaining treatment is withdrawn, the doctor's role is considered passive and the cause of death is the underlying disease, despite the fact that switching off the ventilator of a patient dependent on it looks anything but passive and would be considered homicide if done without the consent of the patient or a proxy. In contrast, euthanasia by the injection of a lethal drug is active and directly causes the patient's death. Assisting suicide by supplying the necessary drugs is considered somewhere in between, more active than switching off a ventilator but less active than injecting drugs, hence morally and legally more ambiguous.

I believe, however, that these distinctions are too doctor-centered and not sufficiently patient-centered. We should ask ourselves not so much whether the doctor's role is passive or active but whether the *patient's* role is passive or active. From that perspective, the three methods of hastening death line up quite differently. When life-sustaining treatment is withdrawn from an incompetent patient at the request of a proxy or when euthanasia is performed, the patient may be utterly passive. Indeed, either act can be performed even if the patient is unaware of the decision. In sharp contrast, assisted suicide, by definition, cannot occur without the patient's knowledge and participation. Therefore, it must be active—that is to say, voluntary. That is a crucial distinction, because it provides an inherent safeguard against abuse that is not present with the other two methods of hastening death. If the loaded term "kill" is to be used, it is not the doctor who kills, but the patient. Primarily because euthanasia can be performed without the patient's participation, I oppose its legalization in this country.

Assisted suicide is not necessary. All suffering can be relieved if care givers are sufficiently skillful and compassionate, as illustrated by the hospice movement.   I have no doubt that if expert palliative care were available to everyone who needed it, there would be few requests for assisted suicide. Even under the best of circumstances, however, there will always be a few patients whose suffering simply cannot be adequately alleviated. And there will be some who would prefer suicide to any other measures available, including the withdrawal of life-sustaining treatment or the use of heavy sedation. Surely, every effort should be made to improve palliative care, as I argued 15 years ago,[13] but when those efforts are unavailing and suffering patients desperately long to end their lives, physician-assisted suicide should be allowed. The argument that permitting it would divert us from redoubling our commitment to comfort care asks these patients to pay the penalty for our failings. It is also illogical. Good comfort care and the availability of physician-assisted suicide are no more mutually exclusive than good cardiologic care and the availability of heart transplantation.

Permitting assisted suicide would put us on a moral "slippery slope." Although in itself assisted suicide might be acceptable, it would lead inexorably to involuntary euthanasia.   It is impossible to avoid slippery slopes in medicine (or in any aspect of life). The issue is how and where to find a purchase. For example, we accept the right of proxies to terminate life-sustaining treatment, despite the obvious potential for abuse, because the reasons for doing so outweigh the risks. We hope our procedures will safeguard patients. In the case of assisted suicide, its voluntary nature is the best protection against sliding down a slippery slope, but we also need to ensure that the request is thoughtful and freely made. Although it is possible that we may someday decide to legalize voluntary euthanasia under certain circumstances or assisted suicide for patients who are not terminally ill, legalizing assisted suicide for the dying does not in itself make these other decisions inevitable. Interestingly, recent reports from the Netherlands, where both euthanasia and physician-assisted suicide are permitted, indicate that fears about a slippery slope there have not been borne out.[14,15,16]

Assisted suicide would be a threat to the economically and socially vulnerable. The poor, disabled, and elderly might be coerced to request it.   Admittedly, overburdened families or cost-conscious doctors might pressure vulnerable patients to request suicide, but similar wrongdoing is at least as likely in the case of withdrawing life-sustaining treatment, since that decision can be made by proxy. Yet, there is no evidence of widespread abuse. The Ninth Circuit Court recalled that it was feared *Roe* v. *Wade* would lead to coercion of poor and uneducated women to request abortions, but that did not happen. The concern that coercion is more likely in this era of managed care, although understandable, would hold suffering patients hostage to the deficiencies of our health care system. Unfortunately, no human endeavor is immune to abuses. The question is not whether a perfect system can be devised, but whether abuses are likely to be sufficiently rare to be offset by the benefits to patients who otherwise would be condemned to face the end of their lives in protracted agony.

Depressed patients would seek physician-assisted suicide rather than help for their depression. Even in the terminally ill, a request for assisted suicide might signify treatable depression, not irreversible suffering.   Patients suffering greatly at the end of life may also be depressed, but the depression does not necessarily explain their decision to commit suicide or make it irrational. Nor is it simple to diagnose depression in terminally ill patients. Sadness is to be expected, and some of the vegetative symptoms of depression are similar to the symptoms of terminal illness. The success of antidepressant treatment in these circumstances is also not ensured. Although there are anecdotes about patients who changed their minds about suicide after treatment,[17] we do not have good studies of how often that happens or the relation to antidepressant treatment. Dying patients who request assisted suicide and seem depressed should certainly be strongly encouraged to accept psychiatric treatment, but I do not believe that competent patients should be *required* to accept it as a condition of receiving assistance with suicide. On the other hand, doctors would not be required to comply with all requests; they would be expected to use their judgment, just as they do in so many other types of life-and-death decisions in medical practice.

Doctors should never participate in taking life. If there is to be assisted suicide, doctors must not be involved.   Although most doctors favor permitting assisted suicide under certain circumstances, many who favor it believe that doctors should not provide the assistance.[6,7] To them, doctors should be unambiguously committed to life (although most doctors who hold this view would readily honor a patient's decision to have life-sustaining treatment withdrawn). The AMA, too, seems to object to physician-assisted suicide primarily because it violates the profession's mission. Like others, I find that position too abstract.[18] The highest ethical imperative of doctors should be to provide care in whatever way best serves patients' interests, in accord with each patient's wishes, not with a theoretical commitment to preserve life no matter what the cost in suffering.[19] If a patient requests help with suicide and the doctor believes the request is appropriate, requiring someone else to provide the assistance would be a form of abandonment. Doctors who are opposed in principle need not assist, but they should make their patients aware of their position early in the relationship so that a patient who chooses to select another doctor can do so. The greatest harm we can do is to consign a desperate patient to unbearable suffering—or force the patient to seek out a stranger like Dr. Kevorkian. Contrary to the frequent assertion that permitting physician-assisted suicide would lead patients to distrust their doctors, I believe distrust is more likely to arise from uncertainty about whether a doctor will honor a patient's wishes.

Physician-assisted suicide may occasionally be warranted, but it should remain illegal. If doctors risk prosecution, they will think twice before assisting with suicide. This argument wrongly shifts the focus from the patient to the doctor. Instead of reflecting the condition and wishes of patients, assisted suicide would reflect the courage and compassion of their doctors. Thus, patients with doctors like Timothy Quill, who described in a 1991 *Journal* article how he helped a patient take her life,[20] would get the help they need and want, but similar patients with less steadfast doctors would not. That makes no sense.

People do not need assistance to commit suicide. With enough determination, they can do it themselves. This is perhaps the cruelest of the arguments against physician-assisted suicide. Many patients at the end of life are, in fact, physically unable to commit suicide on their own. Others lack the resources to do so. It has sometimes been suggested that they can simply stop eating and drinking and kill themselves that way. Although this method has been described as peaceful under certain conditions,[21] no one should count on that. The fact is that this argument leaves most patients to their suffering. Some, usually men, manage to commit suicide using violent methods. Percy Bridgman, a Nobel laureate in physics who in 1961 shot himself rather than die of metastatic cancer, said in his suicide note, "It is not decent for Society to make a man do this to himself."[22]

My father, who knew nothing of Percy Bridgman, committed suicide under similar circumstances. He was 81 and had metastatic prostate cancer. The night before he was scheduled to be admitted to the hospital, he shot himself. Like Bridgman, he thought it might be his last chance. At the time, he was not in extreme pain, nor was he close to death (his life expectancy was probably longer than six months). But he was suffering nonetheless—from nausea and the side effects of antiemetic agents, weakness, incontinence, and hopelessness. Was he depressed? He would probably have freely admitted that he was, but he would have thought it beside the point. In any case, he was an intensely private man who would have refused psychiatric care. Was he overly concerned with maintaining control of the circumstances of his life and death? Many people would say so, but that was the way he was. It is the job of medicine to deal with patients as they are, not as we would like them to be.

I tell my father's story here because it makes an abstract issue very concrete. If physician-assisted suicide had been available, I have no doubt my father would have chosen it. He was protective of his family, and if he had felt he had the choice, he would have spared my mother the shock of finding his body. He did not tell her what he planned to do, because he knew she would stop him. I also believe my father would have waited if physician-assisted suicide had been available. If patients have access to drugs they can take when they choose, they will not feel they must commit suicide early, while they are still able to do it on their own. They would probably live longer and certainly more peacefully, and they might not even use the drugs.

Long before my father's death, I believed that physician-assisted suicide ought to be permissible under some circumstances, but his death strengthened my conviction that it is simply a part of good medical care—something to be done reluctantly and sadly, as a last resort, but done nonetheless. There should be safeguards to ensure that the decision is well considered and consistent, but they should not be so daunting or violative of privacy that they become obstacles instead of protections. In particular, they should be directed not toward reviewing the reasons for an autonomous decision, but only toward ensuring that the decision is indeed autonomous. If the Supreme Court upholds the decisions of the appeals courts, assisted suicide will not be forced on either patients or doctors, but it will be a choice for those patients who need it and those doctors willing to help. If, on the other hand, the Supreme Court overturns the lower courts' decisions, the issue will continue to be grappled with state by state, through the political process. But sooner or later, given the need and the widespread public support, physician-assisted suicide will be demanded of a compassionate profession.

References

1. Greenhouse L. High court to say if the dying have a right to suicide help. New York Times. October 2, 1996:A1.
2. Compassion in Dying v. Washington, 79 F.3d 790 (9th Cir. 1996).
3. Quill v. Vacco, 80 F.3d 716 (2d Cir. 1996).
4. Annas GJ. Death by prescription—the Oregon initiative. N Engl J Med 1994;331:1240-3.
5. Blendon RJ, Szalay US, Knox RA. Should physicians aid their patients in dying? The public perspective. JAMA 1992;267:2658-62.
6. Bachman JG, Alcser KH, Doukas DJ, Lichtenstein RL, Corning AD, Brody H. Attitudes of Michigan physicians and the public toward legalizing physician-assisted suicide and voluntary euthanasia. N Engl J Med 1996;334:303-9.
7. Lee MA, Nelson HD, Tilden VP, Ganzini L, Schmidt TA, Tolle SW. Legalizing assisted suicide—views of physicians in Oregon. N Engl J Med 1996;334:310-5.
8. Gianelli DM. AMA to court: no suicide aid. American Medical News. November 25, 1996:1, 27, 28.
9. Dworkin R. Sex, death, and the courts. New York Review of Books. August 8, 1996.
10. In re: Quinlan, 70 N.J. 10, 355 A.2d 647 (1976).
11. Cruzan v. Director, Missouri Department of Health, 497 U.S. 261, 110 S.Ct. 2841 (1990).
12. Omnibus Budget Reconciliation Act of 1990, P.L. 101-508, sec. 4206 and 4751, 104 Stat. 1388, 1388-115, and 1388-204 (classified respectively at 42 U.S.C. 1395cc(f) (Medicare) and 1396a(w) (Medicaid) (1994)).
13. Angell M. The quality of mercy. N Engl J Med 1982;306:98-9.
14. van der Maas PJ, van der Wal G, Haverkate I, et al. Euthanasia, physician-assisted suicide, and other medical practices involving the end of life in the Netherlands, 1990-1995. N Engl J Med 1996;335:1699-705.
15. van der Wal G, van der Maas PJ, Bosma JM, et al. Evaluation of the notification procedure for physician-assisted death in the Netherlands. N Engl J Med 1996;335:1706-11.
16. Angell M. Euthanasia in the Netherlands—good news or bad? N Engl J Med 1996;335:1676-8.

17. Chochinov HM, Wilson KG, Enns M, et al. Desire for death in the terminally ill. Am J Psychiatry 1995;152:1185–91.
18. Cassel CK, Meier DE. Morals and moralism in the debate over euthanasia and assisted suicide. N Engl J Med 1990;323:750–2.
19. Angell M. Doctors and assisted suicide. Ann R Coll Physicians Surg Can 1991;24:493–4.
20. Quill TE. Death and dignity—a case of individualized decision making. N Engl J Med 1991;324:691–4.
21. Lynn J, Childress JF. Must patients always be given food and water? Hastings Cent Rep 1983;13(5):17–21.
22. Nuland SB. How we die. New York: Alfred A. Knopf, 1994:152.

Kathleen M. Foley

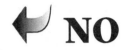 **NO**

Competent Care for the Dying Instead of Physician-Assisted Suicide

While the Supreme Court is reviewing the decisions by the Second and Ninth Circuit Courts of Appeals to reverse state bans on assisted suicide, there is a unique opportunity to engage the public, health care professionals, and the government in a national discussion of how American medicine and society should address the needs of dying patients and their families. Such a discussion is critical if we are to understand the process of dying from the point of view of patients and their families and to identify existing barriers to appropriate, humane, compassionate care at the end of life. Rational discourse must replace the polarized debate over physician-assisted suicide and euthanasia. Facts, not anecdotes, are necessary to establish a common ground and frame a system of health care for the terminally ill that provides the best possible quality of living while dying.

The biased language of the appeals courts evinces little respect for the vulnerability and dependency of the dying. Judge Stephen Reinhardt, writing for the Ninth Circuit Court, applied the liberty-interest clause of the Fourteenth Amendment, advocating a constitutional right to assisted suicide. He stated, "The competent terminally ill adult, having lived nearly the full measure of his life, has a strong interest in choosing a dignified and humane death, rather than being reduced to a state of helplessness, diapered, sedated, incompetent."[1] Judge Roger J. Miner, writing for the Second Circuit Court of Appeals, applied the equal-rights clause of the Fourteenth Amendment and went on to emphasize that the state "has no interest in prolonging a life that is ending."[2] This statement is more than legal jargon. It serves as a chilling reminder of the low priority given to the dying when it comes to state resources and protection.

The appeals courts' assertion of a constitutional right to assisted suicide is narrowly restricted to the terminally ill. The courts have decided that it is the patient's condition that justifies killing and that the terminally ill are special—so special that they deserve assistance in dying. This group alone can receive such assistance. The courts' response to the New York and Washington cases they reviewed is the dangerous form of affirmative action in the name of compassion. It runs the risk of further devaluing the lives of terminally ill patients

From Kathleen M. Foley, "Competent Care for the Dying Instead of Physician-Assisted Suicide," *The New England Journal of Medicine*, vol. 336 (January 2, 1997). Copyright © 1997 by The Massachusetts Medical Society. All rights reserved. Reprinted by permission.

and may provide the excuse for society to abrogate its responsibility for their care.

Both circuit courts went even further in asserting that physicians are already assisting in patients' deaths when they withdraw life-sustaining treatments such as respirators or administer high doses of pain medication that hasten death. The appeals courts argued that providing a lethal prescription to allow a terminally ill patient to commit suicide is essentially the same as withdrawing life-sustaining treatment or aggressively treating pain. Judicial reasoning that eliminates the distinction between letting a person die and killing runs counter to physicians' standards of palliative care.[3] The courts' purported goal in blurring these distinctions was to bring society's legal rules more closely in line with the moral value it places on the relief of suffering.[4]

In the real world in which physicians care for dying patients, withdrawing treatment and aggressively treating pain are acts that respect patients' autonomous decisions not to be battered by medical technology and to be relieved of their suffering. The physician's intent is to provide care, not death. Physicians do struggle with doubts about their own intentions.[5] The courts' arguments fuel their ambivalence about withdrawing life-sustaining treatments or using opioid or sedative infusions to treat intractable symptoms in dying patients. Physicians are trained and socialized to preserve life. Yet saying that physicians struggle with doubts about their intentions in performing these acts is not the same as saying that their intention is to kill. In palliative care, the goal is to relieve suffering, and the quality of life, not the quantity, is of utmost importance.

Whatever the courts say, specialists in palliative care do not think that they practice physician-assisted suicide or euthanasia.[6] Palliative medicine has developed guidelines for aggressive pharmacologic management of intractable symptoms in dying patients, including sedation for those near death.[3,7,8] The World Health Organization has endorsed palliative care as an integral component of a national health care policy and has strongly recommended to its member countries that they not consider legalizing physician-assisted suicide and euthanasia until they have addressed the needs of their citizens for pain relief and palliative care.[9] The courts have disregarded this formidable recommendation and, in fact, are indirectly suggesting that the World Health Organization supports assisted suicide.

Yet the courts' support of assisted suicide reflects the requests of the physicians who initiated the suits and parallels the numerous surveys demonstrating that a large proportion of physicians support the legalization of physician-assisted suicide.[10,11,12,13,14,15] A smaller proportion of physicians are willing to provide such assistance, and an even smaller proportion are willing to inject a lethal dose of medication with the intent of killing a patient (active voluntary euthanasia). These survey data reveal a gap between the attitudes and behavior of physicians; 20 to 70 percent of physicians favor the legalization of physician-assisted suicide, but only 2 to 4 percent favor active voluntary euthanasia, and only approximately 2 to 13 percent have actually aided patients in dying, by either providing a prescription or administering a lethal injection. The limitations of these surveys, which are legion, include inconsistent definitions of physician-assisted suicide and euthanasia, lack of information about nonrespondents, and provisions for maintaining confidentiality that have led to inaccurate reporting.[13,16] Since physicians' attitudes toward alternatives to assisted suicide have not been studied, there is a void in our knowledge about the priority that physicians place on physician-assisted suicide.

The willingness of physicians to assist patients in dying appears to be determined by numerous complex factors, including religious beliefs, personal values, medical specialty, age, practice setting, and perspective on the use of financial resources.[13,16,17,18,19] Studies of patients' preferences for care at the end of life demonstrate that physicians' preferences strongly influence those of their patients.[13] Making physician-assisted suicide a medical treatment when it is so strongly dependent on these physician-related variables would result in a regulatory impossibility.[19] Physicians would have to disclose their values and attitudes to patients to avoid potential conflict.[13] A survey by Ganzini et al. demonstrated that psychiatrists' responses to requests to evaluate patients were highly determined by their attitudes.[13] In a study by Emanuel et al., depressed patients with cancer said they would view positively those physicians who acknowledged their willingness to assist in suicide. In contrast, patients with cancer who were suffering from pain would be suspicious of such physicians.[11]

In this controversy, physicians fall into one of three groups. Those who support physician-assisted suicide see it as a compassionate response to a medical need, a symbol of nonabandonment, and a means to reestablish patients' trust in doctors who have used technology excessively.[20] They argue that regulation of physician-assisted suicide is possible and, in fact, necessary to control the actions of physicians who are currently providing assistance surreptitiously.[21] The two remaining groups of physicians oppose legalization.[19,22,23,24] One group is morally opposed to physician-assisted suicide and emphasizes the need to preserve the professionalism of medicine and the commitment to "do no harm." These physicians view aiding a patient in dying as a form of abandonment, because a physician needs to walk the last mile with the patient, as a witness, not as an executioner. Legalization would endorse justified killing, according to these physicians, and guidelines would not be followed, even if they could be developed. Furthermore, these physicians are concerned that the conflation of assisted suicide with the withdrawal of life support or adequate treatment of pain would make it even harder for dying patients, because there would be a backlash against existing policies. The other group is not ethically opposed to physician-assisted suicide and, in fact, sees it as acceptable in exceptional cases, but these physicians believe that one cannot regulate the unregulatable.[19] On this basis, the New York State Task Force on Life and the Law, a 24-member committee with broad public and professional representation, voted unanimously against the legalization of physician-assisted suicide.[24] All three groups of physicians agree that a national effort is needed to improve the care of the dying. Yet it does seem that those in favor of legalizing physician-assisted suicide are disingenuous in their use of this issue as a wedge. If this form of assistance with dying is legalized, the courts will be forced to broaden the assistance to include active voluntary euthanasia and, eventually, assistance in response to requests from proxies.

One cannot easily categorize the patients who request physician-assisted suicide or euthanasia. Some surveys of physicians have attempted to determine retrospectively the prevalence and nature of these requests.[10] Pain, AIDS, and neurodegenerative disorders are the most common conditions in patients requesting assistance in dying. There is a wide range in the age of such patients, but many are younger persons with AIDS.[10] From the limited data available, the factors most commonly involved in requests for assistance are concern about future loss of control, being or becoming a burden to others, or being unable to care for oneself and fear of severe pain.[10] A small number of recent studies have directly asked terminally ill patients with cancer or AIDS about their desire for death.[25,26,27] All these studies show that the desire for death is closely associated with depression and that pain and lack of social support are contributing factors.

Do we know enough, on the basis of several legal cases, to develop a public policy that will profoundly change medicine's role in society?[1,2] Approximately 2.4 million Americans die each year. We have almost no information on how they die and only general information on where they die. Sixty-one percent die in hospitals, 17 percent in nursing homes, and the remainder at home, with approximately 10 to 14 percent of those at home receiving hospice care.

The available data suggest that physicians are inadequately trained to assess and manage the multifactorial symptoms commonly associated with patients' requests for physician-assisted suicide. According to the American Medical Association's report on medical education, only 5 of 126 medical schools in the United States require a separate course in the care of the dying.[28] Of 7048 residency programs, only 26 percent offer a course on the medical and legal aspects of care at the end of life as a regular part of the curriculum. According to a survey of 1068 accredited residency programs in family medicine, internal medicine, and pediatrics and fellowship programs in geriatrics, each resident or fellow coordinates the care of 10 or fewer dying patients annually.[28] Almost 15 percent of the programs offer no formal training in terminal care. Despite the availability of hospice programs, only 17 percent of the training programs offer a hospice rotation, and the rotation is required in only half of those programs; 9 percent of the programs have residents or fellows serving as members of hospice teams. In a recent survey of 55 residency programs and over 1400 residents, conducted by the American Board of Internal Medicine, the residents were asked to rate their perception of adequate training in care at the end of life. Seventy-two percent reported that they had received adequate training in managing pain and other symptoms; 62 percent, that they had received adequate training in telling patients that they are dying; 38 percent, in describing what the process will be like; and 32 percent, in talking to patients who request assistance in dying or a hastened death (Blank L: personal communication).

The lack of training in the care of the dying is evident in practice. Several studies have concluded that poor communication between physicians and patients, physicians' lack of knowledge about national guidelines for such care, and their lack of knowledge about the control of symptoms are barriers to the provision of good care at the end of life.[23,29,30]

Yet there is now a large body of data on the components of suffering in patients with advanced terminal disease, and these data provide the basis for treatment algorithms.[3] There are three major factors in suffering: pain and other physical symptoms, psychological distress, and existential distress (described as the experience of life without meaning). It is not only the patients who suffer but also their families and the health care professionals attending them. These experiences of suffering are often closely and inextricably related. Perceived distress in any one of the three groups amplifies distress in the others.[31,32]

Pain is the most common symptom in dying patients, and according to recent data from U.S. studies, 56 percent of outpatients with cancer, 82 percent of outpatients with AIDS, 50 percent of hospitalized patients with various diagnoses, and 36 percent of nursing home residents have inadequate management of pain during the course of their terminal illness.[33,34,35,36] Members of minority groups and women, both those with cancer and those with AIDS, as well as the elderly, receive less pain treatment than other groups of patients. In a survey of 1177 physicians who had treated a total of more than 70,000 patients with cancer in the previous six months, 76 percent of the respondents cited lack of knowledge as a barrier to their ability to control pain.[37] Severe pain that is not adequately controlled interferes with the quality of life, including the activities of daily living, sleep, and social interactions.[33,38]

Other physical symptoms are also prevalent among the dying. Studies of patients with advanced cancer and of the elderly in the year before death show that they have numerous symptoms that worsen the quality of life, such as fatigue, dyspnea, delirium, nausea, and vomiting.[36,38]

Along with these physical symptoms, dying patients have a variety of well-described psychological symptoms, with a high prevalence of anxiety and depression in patients with cancer or AIDS and the elderly.[27,39] For example, more than 60 percent of patients with advanced cancer have psychiatric problems, with adjustment disorders, depression, anxiety, and delirium reported most frequently. Various factors that contribute to the prevalence and severity of psychological distress in the terminally ill have been identified.[39] The diagnosis of depression is difficult to make in medically ill patients[3,26,40]; 94 percent of the Oregon psychiatrists surveyed by Ganzini et al. were not confident that they could determine, in a single evaluation, whether a psychiatric disorder was impairing the judgment of a patient who requested assistance with suicide.[13]

Attention has recently been focused on the interaction between uncontrolled symptoms and vulnerability to suicide in patients with cancer or AIDS.[41] Data from studies of both groups of patients suggest that uncontrolled pain contributes to depression and that persistent pain interferes with patients' ability to receive support from their families and others. Patients with AIDS have a high risk of suicide that is independent of physical symptoms. Among New York City residents with AIDS, the relative risk of suicide in men between the ages of 20 and 59 years was 36 times higher than the risk among men without AIDS in the same age group and 66 times higher than the risk in the general population.[41] Patients with AIDS who committed suicide generally did so within nine months after receiving the diagnosis; 25 percent had made a previous suicide attempt,

50 percent had reported severe depression, and 40 percent had seen a psychiatrist within four days before committing suicide. As previously noted, the desire to die is most closely associated with the diagnosis of depression.[26,27] Suicide is the eighth leading cause of death in the United States, and the incidence of suicide is higher in patients with cancer or AIDS and in elderly men than in the general population. Conwell and Caine reported that depression was underdiagnosed by primary care physicians in a cohort of elderly patients who subsequently committed suicide; 75 percent of the patients had seen a primary care physician during the last month of life but had not received a diagnosis of depression.[22]

The relation between depression and the desire to hasten death may vary among subgroups of dying patients. We have no data, except for studies of a small number of patients with cancer or AIDS. The effect of treatment for depression on the desire to hasten death and on requests for assistance in doing so has not been examined in the medically ill population, except for a small study in which four of six patients who initially wished to hasten death changed their minds within two weeks.[26]

There is also the concern that certain patients, particularly members of minority groups that are estranged from the health care system, may be reluctant to receive treatment for their physical or psychological symptoms because of the fear that their physicians will, in fact, hasten death. There is now some evidence that the legalization of assisted suicide in the Northern Territory of Australia has undermined the Aborigines' trust in the medical care system[42]; this experience may serve as an example for the United States, with its multicultural population.

The multiple physical and psychological symptoms in the terminally ill and elderly are compounded by a substantial degree of existential distress. Reporting on their interviews with Washington State physicians whose patients had requested assistance in dying, Back et al. noted the physicians' lack of sophistication in assessing such nonphysical suffering.[10]

In summary, there are fundamental physician-related barriers to appropriate, humane, and compassionate care for the dying. These range from attitudinal and behavioral barriers to educational and economic barriers. Physicians do not know enough about their patients, themselves, or suffering to provide assistance with dying as a medical treatment for the relief of suffering. Physicians need to explore their own perspectives on the meaning of suffering in order to develop their own approaches to the care of the dying. They need insight into how the nature of the doctor-patient relationship influences their own decision making. If legalized, physician-assisted suicide will be a substitute for rational therapeutic, psychological, and social interventions that might otherwise enhance the quality of life for patients who are dying. The medical profession needs to take the lead in developing guidelines for good care of dying patients. Identifying the factors related to physicians, patients, and the health care system that pose barriers to appropriate care at the end of life should be the first step in a national dialogue to educate health care professionals and the public on the topic of death and dying. Death is an issue that society as a whole faces, and it requires a compassionate response. But we should not confuse compassion with competence in the care of terminally ill patients.

References

1. Reinhardt, Compassion in Dying v. State of Washington, 79 F. 3d 790 9th Cir. 1996.
2. Miner, Quill v. Vacco 80 F. 3d 716 2nd Cir. 1996.
3. Doyle D, Hanks GWC, MacDonald N. The Oxford textbook of palliative medicine. New York: Oxford University Press, 1993.
4. Orentlicher D. The legalization of physician-assisted suicide. N Engl J Med 1996;335:663-7.
5. Wilson WC, Smedira NG, Fink C, McDowell JA, Luce JM. Ordering and administration of sedatives and analgesics during the withholding and withdrawal of life support from critically ill patients. JAMA 1992;267:949-53.
6. Foley KM. The relationship of pain and symptom management to patient requests for physician-assisted suicide. J Pain Symptom Manage 1991;6:289-97.
7. Cherny NI, Coyle N, Foley KM. Guidelines in the care of the dying patient. Hematol Oncol Clin North Am 1996;10:261-86.
8. Cherny NI, Portenoy RK. Sedation in the management of refractory symptoms: guidelines for evaluation and treatment. J Palliat Care 1994;10(2):31-8.
9. Cancer pain relief and palliative care. Geneva: World Health Organization, 1989.
10. Back AL, Wallace JI, Starks HE, Pearlman RA. Physician-assisted suicide and euthanasia in Washington State: patient requests and physician responses. JAMA 1996;275:919-25.
11. Emanuel EJ, Fairclough DL, Daniels ER, Clarridge BR. Euthanasia and physician-assisted suicide: attitudes and experiences of oncology patients, oncologists, and the public. Lancet 1996;347:1805-10.
12. Lee MA, Nelson HD, Tilden VP, Ganzini L, Schmidt TA, Tolle SW. Legalizing assisted suicide—views of physicians in Oregon. N Engl J Med 1996;334:310-5.
13. Ganzini L, Fenn DS, Lee MA, Heintz RT, Bloom JD. Attitudes of Oregon psychiatrists toward physician-assisted suicide. Am J Psychiatry 1996;153:1469-75.
14. Cohen JS, Fihn SD, Boyko EJ, Jonsen AR, Wood RW. Attitudes toward assisted suicide and euthanasia among physicians in Washington State. N Engl J Med 1994;331:89-94.
15. Doukas DJ, Waterhouse D, Gorenflo DW, Seid J. Attitudes and behaviors on physician-assisted death: a study of Michigan oncologists. J Clin Oncol 1995;13:1055-61.
16. Morrison S, Meier D. Physician-assisted dying: fashioning public policy with an absence of data. Generations. Winter 1994:48-53.
17. Portenoy RK, Coyle N, Kash K, et al. Determinants of the willingness to endorse assisted suicide: a survey of physicians, nurses, and social workers. Psychosomatics (in press).
18. Fins J. Physician-assisted suicide and the right to care. Cancer Control 1996;3:272-8.
19. Callahan D, White M. The legalization of physician-assisted suicide: creating a regulatory Potemkin Village. U Richmond Law Rev 1996;30:1-83.
20. Quill TE. Death and dignity—a case of individualized decision making. N Engl J Med 1991;324:691-4.
21. Quill TE, Cassel CK, Meier DE. Care of the hopelessly ill—proposed clinical criteria for physician-assisted suicide. N Engl J Med 1992;327:1380-4.
22. Conwell Y, Caine ED. Rational suicide and the right to die—reality and myth. N Engl J Med 1991;325:1100-3.
23. Foley KM. Pain, physician assisted suicide and euthanasia. Pain Forum 1995;4:163-78.

24. When death is sought: assisted suicide and euthanasia in the medical context. New York: New York State Task Force on Life and the Law, May 1994.
25. Brown JH, Henteleff P, Barakat S, Rowe CJ. Is it normal for terminally ill patients to desire death? Am J Psychiatry 1986;143:208–11.
26. Chochinov HM, Wilson KG, Enns M, et al. Desire for death in the terminally ill. Am J Psychiatry 1995;152:1185–91.
27. Breitbart W, Rosenfeld BD, Passik SD. Interest in physician-assisted suicide among ambulatory HIV-infected patients. Am J Psychiatry 1996;153:238–42.
28. Hill TP. Treating the dying patient: the challenge for medical education. Arch Intern Med 1995;155:1265–9.
29. Callahan D. Once again reality: now where do we go. Hastings Cent Rep 1995;25(6):Suppl:S33–S36.
30. Solomon MZ, O'Donnell L, Jennings B, et al. Decisions near the end of life: professional views on life-sustaining treatments. Am J Public Health 1993;83:14–23.
31. Cherny NI, Coyle N, Foley KM. Suffering in the advanced cancer patient: definition and taxonomy. J Palliat Care 1994;10(2):57–70.
32. Cassel EJ. The nature of suffering and the goals of medicine. N Engl J Med 1982;306:639–45.
33. Cleeland CS, Gonin R, Hatfield AK, et al. Pain and its treatment in outpatients with metastatic cancer. N Engl J Med 1994;330:592–6.
34. Breitbart W, Rosenfeld BD, Passik SD, McDonald MV, Thaler H, Portenoy RK. The undertreatment of pain in ambulatory AIDS patients. Pain 1996;65:243–9.
35. The SUPPORT Principal Investigators. A controlled trial to improve care for seriously ill hospitalized patients. JAMA 1995;274:1591–8.
36. Seale C, Cartwright A. The year before death. Hants, England: Avebury, 1994.
37. Von Roenn JH, Cleeland CS, Gonin R, Hatfield AK, Pandya KJ. Physician attitudes and practice in cancer pain management: a survey from the Eastern Cooperative Oncology Group. Ann Intern Med 1993;119:121–6.
38. Portenoy RK. Pain and quality of life: clinical issues and implications for research. Oncology 1990;4:172–8.
39. Breitbart W. Suicide risk and pain in cancer and AIDS patients. In: Chapman CR, Foley KM, eds. Current and emerging issues in cancer pain. New York: Raven Press, 1993.
40. Chochinov H, Wilson KG, Enns M, Lander S. Prevalence of depression in the terminally ill: effects of diagnostic criteria and symptom threshold judgments. Am J Psychiatry 1994;151:537–40.
41. Passik S, McDonald M, Rosenfeld B, Breitbart W. End of life issues in patients with AIDS: clinical and research considerations. J Pharm Care Pain Symptom Control 1995;3:91–111.
42. NT "success" in easing rural fear of euthanasia. The Age. August 31, 1996:A7.

POSTSCRIPT

Should Physicians Be Allowed to Assist in Patient Suicide?

In June 1997 the U.S. Supreme Court overturned lower court decisions and ruled unanimously that there is no constitutional right to physician-assisted suicide. In the states of Washington and New York, as in most others, it is a criminal offense for a physician, or anyone else, to assist another person in committing suicide. Physicians and dying patients have filed lawsuits challenging the bans. Although the Supreme Court decision was unanimous, the Justices seemed to allow for the possibility of future discussions. Their opinions strongly supported access to adequate palliative care (pain relief and symptom control) and did not foreclose state legislative action regulating physician-assisted suicide.

Oregon became the first state to legalize physician-assisted suicide in November 1997 by passing the Death With Dignity Act. Under this law a person who is mentally competent and suffering from a terminal illness (likely to die within six months) may receive lethal drugs froma a physician. The person has to consult two doctors and wait 15 days before obtaining the drugs. In 1999 twenty-seven patients died after taking lethal medications under the law, an increase from sixteen in 1998. See Amy D. Sullivan, Katrina Hedberg, and David Flemming, "Legalized Physician-Assisted Suicide in Oregon—The Second Year," *The New England Journal of Medicine* (February 24, 2000). These authors assert that patients who request assistance with suicide are motivated primarily by their loss of autonomy and a determination to control the way in which they die.

For two analyses of the Supreme Court decision, see David Orentlicher, "The Surpreme Court and Physician-Assisted Suicide: Rejecting Assisted Suicide but Embracing Euthanasia" and Robert A. Burt, "The Supreme Court Speaks: Not Assisted Suicide but a Constitutional Right to Palliative Care," both in the *New England Journal of Medicine* (October 23, 1997). Ezekiel Emanuel and Margaret P. Battin address the economic implications in "What Are the Potential Cost Savings From Legalizing Physician-Assisted Suicide?" *The New England Journal of Medicine* (July 16, 1998). A survey of patients in Washington and Oregon with the neurological disease amyotrophic lateral sclerosis (Lou Gehrig's disease) found that a majority would contemplate physician-assisted suicide. See Linda Ganzini et al., "Attitudes of Patients With ALS and Their Care Givers Toward Assisted Suicide," *The New England Journal of Medicine* (October 1, 1998). See also Arthur L. Caplan, Lois Snyder, and Kathy Feber-Langendoen, "The Role of Guidelines in the Practice of Physician-Assisted Suicide," *Annals of Internal Medicine* (March 21, 2000). The entire issue is devoted to this subject.

ISSUE 5

Is It Ethical to Withhold the Truth From Dying Patients?

YES: Bernard C. Meyer, from "Truth and the Physician," in E. Fuller Torrey, ed., *Ethical Issues in Medicine* (Little, Brown, 1968)

NO: Sissela Bok, from *Lying: Moral Choice in Public and Private Life* (Pantheon Books, 1978)

ISSUE SUMMARY

YES: Physician Bernard C. Meyer argues that physicians must use discretion in communicating bad news to patients. Adherence to a rigid formula of truth telling fails to appreciate the differences in patients' readiness to hear and understand the information.

NO: Philosopher Sissela Bok challenges the traditional physician's view by arguing that the harm resulting from disclosure is less than they think and is outweighed by the benefits, including the important one of giving the patient the right to choose among treatments.

In his powerful short story "The Death of Ivan Ilych," Leo Tolstoy graphically portrays the physical agony and the social isolation of a dying man. However, "What tormented Ivan Ilych most was the deception, the lie, which for some reason they all accepted, that he was not dying but was simply ill, and that he only need keep quiet and undergo a treatment and then something very good would result." Instrumental in setting up the deception is Ivan's doctor, who reassures him to the very end that all will be well. Hearing the banal news from his doctor once again, "Ivan Ilych looks at him as much as to say: 'Are you really never ashamed of lying?' But the doctor does not wish to understand this question."

Unlike many of the ethical issues discussed in this volume, which have arisen as a result of modern scientific knowledge and technology, the question of whether or not to tell dying patients the truth is an old and persistent one. But this debate has been given a new urgency because medical practices today are so complex that it is often difficult to know just what the "truth" really is. A dying patient's life can often be prolonged, although at great financial and personal cost, and many people differ over the definition of a terminal illness.

What must be balanced in this decision are two significant principles of ethical conduct: the obligation to tell the truth and the obligation not to harm others. Moral philosophers, beginning with Aristotle, have regarded truth as either an absolute value or one that, at the very least, is preferable to deception. The great nineteenth-century German philosopher Immanuel Kant argued that there is no justification for lying (although some later commentators feel that his absolutist position has been overstated). Other philosophers have argued that deception is sometimes justified. For example, Henry Sidgwick, an early-twentieth-century British philosopher, believed that it was entirely acceptable to lie to invalids and children to protect them from the shock of the truth. Although the question has been debated for centuries, no clear-cut answer has been reached. In fact, the case of a benevolent lie to a dying patient is often given as the prime example of an excusable deception.

If moral philosophers cannot agree, what guidance is there for the physician torn between the desire for truth and the desire to protect the patient from harm (and the admittedly paternalistic conviction that the doctor knows best what will harm the patient)? None of the early medical codes and oaths offered any advice to physicians on what to tell patients, although they were quite explicit about the physician's obligation to keep confidential whatever a patient revealed. The American Medical Association's (AMA) 1847 "Code of Ethics" did endorse some forms of deception by noting that the physician has a sacred duty "to avoid all things which have a tendency to discourage the patient and to depress his spirits." The most recent (1980) AMA "Principles of Medical Ethics" say only that "a physician shall deal honestly with patients and colleagues." However, the American Hospital Association's "Patient's Bill of Rights," adopted in 1972, is more specific: "The patient has the right to obtain from his physician complete current information concerning his diagnosis, treatment, and prognosis in terms the patient can reasonably be expected to understand. When it is not medically advisable to give such information to the patient, the information should be made available to an appropriate person in his behalf."

In the following selections, Bernard C. Meyer argues for an ethic that transcends the virtue of uttering truth for truth's sake. He asserts that the physician's prime responsibility is contained in the Hippocratic Oath—"So far as possible, do no harm." Sissela Bok counters with evidence that physicians often misread patients' wishes and that withholding the truth can often harm them more than disclosure.

Bernard C. Meyer

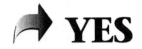 **YES**

Truth and the Physician

Truth does not do so much good in this world as the semblance of it does harm.

— La Rochefoucauld

Among the reminiscences of his Alsatian boyhood, my father related the story of the local functionary who was berated for the crude and blunt manner in which he went from house to house announcing to wives and mothers news of battle casualties befalling men from the village. On the next occasion, mindful of the injunctions to be more tactful and to soften the impact of his doleful message, he rapped gently on the door and, when it opened, inquired, "Is the widow Schmidt at home?"

Insofar as this essay is concerned with the subject of truth it is only proper to add that when I told this story to a colleague, he already knew it and claimed that it concerned a woman named Braun who lived in a small town in Austria. By this time it would not surprise me to learn that the episode is a well-known vignette in the folklore of Tennessee where it is attributed to a woman named Smith or Brown whose husband was killed at the battle of Shiloh. Ultimately, we may find that all three versions are plagiarized accounts of an occurrence during the Trojan War.

Communication Between Physician and Patient

Apocryphal or not, the story illustrates a few of the vexing aspects of the problem of conveying unpalatable news, notably the difficulty of doing so in a manner that causes a minimum amount of pain, and also the realization that not everyone is capable of learning how to do it. Both aspects find their application in the field of medicine where the imparting of the grim facts of diagnosis and prognosis is a constant and recurring issue. Nor does it seem likely that for all our learning we doctors are particularly endowed with superior talents and techniques for coping with these problems. On the contrary, for reasons to be given later, there is cause to believe that in not a few instances, elements

From Bernard C. Meyer, "Truth and the Physician," in E. Fuller Torrey, ed., *Ethical Issues in Medicine* (Little, Brown, 1968). Copyright © 1968 by Little, Brown, and Company, Inc. Reprinted by permission.

in his own psychological makeup may cause the physician to be singularly ill-equipped to be the bearer of bad tidings. It should be observed, moreover, that until comparatively recent times, the subject of communication between physician and patient received little attention in medical curriculum and medical literature.

Within the past decade or so, coincident with an expanded recognition of the significance of emotional factors in all medical practice, an impressive number of books and articles by physicians, paramedical personnel, and others have been published, attesting to both the growing awareness of the importance of the subject and an apparent willingness to face it. An especially noteworthy example of this trend was provided by a three-day meeting in February, 1967, sponsored by the New York Academy of Sciences, on the subject of *The Care of Patients with Fatal Illness.* The problem of communicating with such patients and their families was a recurring theme in most of the papers presented.

Both at this conference and in the literature, particular emphasis has been focused on the patient with cancer, which is hardly surprising in light of its frequency and of the extraordinary emotional reactions that it unleashes not only in the patient and in his kinsmen but in the physician himself. At the same time, it should be noted that the accent on the cancer patient or the dying patient may foster the impression that in less grave conditions this dialogue between patient and physician hardly warrants much concern or discussion. Such a view is unfounded, however, and could only be espoused by someone who has had the good fortune to escape the experience of being ill and hospitalized. Those less fortunate will recall the emotional stresses induced by hospitalization, even when the condition requiring it is relatively banal.

A striking example of such stress may sometimes be seen when the patient who is hospitalized, say, for repair of an inguinal hernia, happens to be a physician. All the usual anxieties confronting a prospective surgical subject tend to become greatly amplified and garnished with a generous sprinkling of hypochondriasis in the physician-turned-patient. Wavering unsteadily between these two roles, he conjures up visions of all the complications of anesthesia, of wound dehiscence or infection, of embolization, cardiac arrest, and whatnot that he has ever heard or read about. To him, lying between hospital sheets, clad in impersonal hospital clothes, divested of his watch and the keys to his car, the hospital suddenly takes on a different appearance from the place he may have known in a professional capacity. Even his colleagues—the anesthetist who will put him to sleep or cause a temporary motor and sensory paralysis of the lower half of his body, and the surgeon who will incise it—appear different. He would like to have a little talk with them, a very professional talk to be sure, although in his heart he may know that the talk will also be different. And if they are in tune with the situation, they too know that it will be different, that beneath the restrained tones of sober and factual conversation is the thumping anxiety of a man who seeks words of reassurance. With some embarrassment he may introduce his anxieties with the phrase, "I suppose this is going to seem a little silly, but..."; and from this point on he may sound like any other individual confronted by the ordeal of surgical experience.[1] Indeed, it would appear that under these circumstances, to say nothing of more ominous ones, most people, regardless of their experience, knowledge, maturity or sophistication, are assailed by more or less similar psychological pressures, from which they seek relief not through pharmacological sedation, but through the more calming influence of the spoken word.

Seen in this light the question of what to tell the patient about his illness is but one facet of the practice of medicine as an art, a particular example of that spoken and mute dialogue between patient and physician which has always been and will always be an indispensable ingredient in the therapeutic process. How to carry on this dialogue, what to say and when to say it, and what not to say, are questions not unlike those posed by an awkward suitor; like him, those not naturally versed in this art may find themselves discomfited and needful of the promptings of some Cyrano who will whisper those words and phrases that ultimately will wing their way to soothe an anguished heart.

Emotional Reactions of Physician

The difficulties besetting the physician under these circumstances, however, cannot be ascribed simply to his mere lack of experience or innate eloquence. For like the stammering suitor, the doctor seeking to communicate with his patient may have an emotional stake in his message. When that message contains an ominous significance, he may find himself too troubled to use words wisely, too ridden with anxiety to be kind, and too depressed to convey hope. An understanding of such reactions touches upon a recognition of some of the several psychological motivations that have led some individuals to choose a medical career. There is evidence that at times that choice has been dictated by what might be viewed as counterphobic forces. Having in childhood experienced recurring brushes with illness and having encountered a deep and abiding fear of death and dying, such persons may embrace a medical career as if it will confer upon them a magical immunity from a repetition of those dreaded eventualities; for them the letters M.D. constitute a talisman bestowing upon the wearer a sense of invulnerability and a pass of safe conduct through the perilous frontiers of life. There are others for whom the choice of a career dedicated to helping and healing appears to have arisen as a reaction formation against earlier impulses to wound and to destroy.[2] For still others among us, the practice of medicine serves as the professional enactment of a long-standing rescue fantasy.

It is readily apparent in these examples (which by no means exhaust the catalogue of motives leading to the choice of a medical career) that confrontation by the failure of one's efforts and by the need to announce it may unloose a variety of inner psychological disturbances: faced by the gravely ill or dying patient the "counterphobic" doctor may feel personally vulnerable again; the "reaction-formation" doctor, evil and guilty; and the "rescuer," worthless and impotent. For such as these, words cannot come readily in their discourse with the seriously or perilously ill. Indeed, they may curtail their communications; and, what is no less meaningful to their patients, withdraw their physical presence. Thus the patient with inoperable cancer and his family may discover that the physician, who at a more hopeful moment in the course of the illness had been both articulate and supportive, has become remote both in his speech and in his behavior. Nor is the patient uncomprehending of the significance of the change in his doctor's attitude. Observers have recorded the verbal expressions of patients who sensed the feelings of futility and depression in their physicians. Seeking to account for their own reluctance to ask questions (a reluctance based partly upon their own disinclination to face a grim reality), one such patient said, "He looked so tired." Another stated, "I don't want to upset him because he has tried so hard to help me"; and another, "I know he feels so badly already and is doing his best" (Abrams, 1966). To paraphrase a celebrated utterance, one might suppose that these remarks were dictated by the maxim: "Ask not what your doctor can do for you; ask what you can do for your doctor."[3]

Adherence to a Formula

In the dilemma created both by a natural disinclination to be a bearer of bad news and by those other considerations already cited, many a physician is tempted to abandon personal judgment and authorship in his discourse with his patients, and to rely instead upon a set formula which he employs with dogged and indiscriminate consistency. Thus, in determining what to say to patients with cancer, there are exponents of standard policies that are applied routinely in seeming disregard of the overall clinical picture and of the personality or psychological makeup of the patient. In general, two such schools of thought prevail; i.e., those that always tell and those that never do. Each of these is amply supplied with statistical anecdotal evidence proving the correctness of the policy. Yet even if the figures were accurate—and not infrequently they are obtained via a questionnaire, itself a rather opaque window to the human mind—all they demonstrate is that more rather than less of a given proportion of the cancer population profited by the policy employed. This would provide small comfort, one might suppose, to the patients and their families that constitute the minority of the sample.

Truth as Abstract Principle

At times adherence to such a rigid formula is dressed up in the vestments of slick and facile morality. Thus a theologian has insisted that the physician has a moral obligation to tell the truth and that his withholding it constitutes a deprivation of the patient's right; therefore it is "theft, therefore unjust, therefore immoral" (Fletcher, 1954). "Can it be," he asks, "that doctors who practice professional deception would, if the roles were reversed, want to be coddled or deceived?" To which, as many physicians can assert, the answer is distinctly *yes*. Indeed so adamant is this writer upon the right of the patient to know the facts of his illness that in the event he refuses to hear what the doctor is trying to say, the latter should "ask leave to withdraw from the case, urging that another physician be called in his place."[4] (Once there were three boy scouts who were sent away from a campfire and told not to return until each had done his good turn for the day. In 20 minutes all three had returned, and curiously each one reported that he had helped a little old lady to cross a street. The scoutmaster's surprise was even greater when he learned that in each case it was the same little old lady, prompting him to inquire why it took the three of them to perform this one simple good deed. "Well, sir," replied one of the boys, "you see she really didn't want to cross the street at all.")

In this casuistry wherein so much attention is focused upon abstract principle and so little upon humanity, one is reminded of the no less specious arguments of those who assert that the thwarting of suicide and the involuntary hospitalization of the mentally deranged constitute violations of personal freedom and human right.[5] It is surely irregular for a fire engine to travel in the wrong direction on a one-way street, but if one is not averse to putting out fires and saving lives, the traffic violation looms as a conspicuous irrelevancy. No less irrelevant is the obsessional concern with meticulous definitions of truth in an enterprise where kindness, charity, and the relief of human suffering are the ethical verities. "The letter killeth," say the Scriptures, "but the spirit giveth life."

Problem of Definition

Nor should it be forgotten that in the healing arts, the matter of truth is not always susceptible to easy definition. Consider for a moment the question of the hopeless diagnosis. It was not so long ago that such a designation was appropriate for subacute bacterial endocarditis, pneumococcal meningitis, pernicious anemia, and a number of other conditions which today are no longer incurable, while those diseases which today are deemed hopeless may cease to be so by tomorrow. Experience has proved, too, the unreliability of obdurate opinions concerning prognosis even in those conditions where all the clinical evidence and the known behavior of a given disease should leave no room for doubt. To paraphrase Clemenceau, to insist that a patient is hopelessly ill may at times be worse than a crime; it may be a mistake.

Problem of Determining Patient's Desires

There are other pitfalls, moreover, that complicate the problem of telling patients the truth about their illness. There is the naive notion, for example, that when the patient asserts that what he is seeking is the plain truth he means just that. But as more than one observer has noted, this is sometimes the last thing the patient really wants. Such assertions may be voiced with particular emphasis by patients who happen to be physicians and who strive to display a professional and scientifically objective attitude toward their own condition. Yet to accept such assertions at their face value may sometimes lead to tragic consequences, as in the following incident.

> A distinguished urological surgeon was hospitalized for a hypernephroma, which diagnosis had been withheld from him. One day he summoned the intern into his room, and after appealing to the latter on the basis of we're-both-doctors-and-grown-up-men, succeeded in getting the unwary younger

man to divulge the facts. Not long afterward, while the nurse was momentarily absent from the room, the patient opened a window and leaped to his death.

Role of Secrecy in Creating Anxiety

Another common error is the assumption that until someone has been formally told the truth he doesn't know it. Such self-deception is often present when parents feel moved to supply their pubertal children with the sexual facts of life. With much embarrassment and a good deal of backing and filling on the subjects of eggs, bees, and babies, sexual information is imparted to a child who often not only already knows it but is uncomfortable in hearing it from that particular source. There is indeed a general tendency to underestimate the perceptiveness of children not only about such matters but where graver issues, notably illness and death, are concerned. As a consequence, attitudes of secrecy and overprotection designed to shield children from painful realities may result paradoxically in creating an atmosphere that is saturated with suspicion, distrust, perplexity, and intolerable anxiety. Caught between trust in their own intuitive perceptions and the deceptions practiced by the adults about them, such children may suffer greatly from a lack of opportunity of coming to terms emotionally with some of the vicissitudes of existence that in the end are inescapable. A refreshing contrast to this approach has been presented in a paper entitled "Who's Afraid of Death on a Leukemia Ward?" (Vernick and Karon, 1965). Recognizing that most of the children afflicted with this disease had some knowledge of its seriousness, and that all were worried about it, the hospital staff abandoned the traditional custom of protection and secrecy, providing instead an atmosphere in which the children could feel free to express their fears and their concerns and could openly acknowledge the fact of death when one of the group passed away. The result of this measure was immensely salutary.

Similar miscalculations of the accuracy of inner perceptions may be noted in dealing with adults. Thus, in a study entitled "Mongolism: When Should Parents Be Told?" (Drillien and Wilkinson, 1964), it was found that in nearly half the cases the mothers declared they had realized before being told that something was seriously wrong with the child's development, a figure which obviously excludes the mothers who refused consciously to acknowledge their suspicions. On the basis of their findings the authors concluded that a full explanation given in the early months, coupled with regular support thereafter, appeared to facilitate the mother's acceptance of and adjustment to her child's handicap.

A pointless and sometimes deleterious withholding of truth is a common practice in dealing with elderly people. "Don't tell Mother" often seems to be an almost reflex maxim among some adults in the face of any misfortune, large or small. Here, too, elaborate efforts at camouflage may backfire, for, sensing that he is being shielded from some ostensibly intolerable secret, not only is the elderly one deprived of the opportunity of reacting appropriately to it, but he is being tacitly encouraged to conjure up something in his imagination that may be infinitely worse.

Discussion of Known Truth

Still another misconception is the belief that if it is certain that the truth is known it is all right to discuss it. How mistaken such an assumption may be was illustrated by the violent rage which a recent widow continued to harbor toward a friend for having alluded to cancer in the presence of her late husband. Hearing her outburst one would have concluded that until the ominous word had been uttered, her husband had been ignorant of the nature of his condition. The facts, however, were different, as the unhappy woman knew, for it had been her husband who originally had told the friend what the diagnosis was.

Denial and Repression

The psychological devices that make such seeming inconsistencies of thought and knowledge possible are the mechanisms of repression and denial. It is indeed the remarkable capacity to bury or conceal more or less transparent truth that makes the problem of telling it so sticky and difficult a matter, and one that is so unsusceptible to simple rule-of-thumb formulas. For while in some instances the maintenance of denial may lead to severe emotional distress, in others it may serve as a merciful shield. For example,

> A physician with a reputation for considerable diagnostic acumen developed a painless jaundice. When, not surprisingly, a laparotomy revealed a carcinoma of the head of the pancreas, the surgeon relocated the biliary outflow so that postoperatively the jaundice subsided. This seeming improvement was consistent with the surgeon's explanation to the patient that the operation had revealed a hepatitis. Immensely relieved, the patient chided himself for not having anticipated the "correct" diagnosis. "What a fool I was!" he declared, obviously alluding to an earlier, albeit unspoken, fear of cancer.

Among less sophisticated persons the play of denial may assume a more primitive expression. Thus a woman who had ignored the growth of a breast cancer to a point where it had produced spinal metastases and paraplegia, attributed the latter to "arthritis" and asked whether the breast would grow back again. The same mental mechanism allowed another woman to ignore dangerous rectal bleeding by ascribing it to menstruation, although she was well beyond the menopause.

In contrast to these examples is a case reported by Winkelstein and Blacher of a man who, awaiting the report of a cervical node biopsy, asserted that if it showed cancer he wouldn't want to live, and that if it didn't he wouldn't believe it (Winkelstein and Blacher, 1967). Yet despite this seemingly unambiguous willingness to deal with raw reality, when the chips were down, as will be described later, this man too was able to protect himself through the use of denial.

From the foregoing it should be self-evident that what is imparted to a patient about his illness should be planned with the same care and executed with the same skill that are demanded by any potentially therapeutic measure. Like the transfusion of blood, the dispensing of certain information must be distinctly indicated, the amount given consonant with the needs of the recipient, and the type chosen with the view of avoiding untoward reactions. This means that only in selected instances is there any justification for telling a patient the precise figures of his blood pressure, and that the question of revealing interesting but asymptomatic congenital anomalies should be considered in light of the possibility of evoking either hypochondriacal ruminations or narcissistic gratification.

Under graver circumstances the choices of confronting the physician rest upon more crucial psychological issues. In principle, we should strive to make the patient sufficiently aware of the facts of his condition to facilitate his participation in the treatment without at the same time giving him cause to believe that such participation is futile. "The indispensable ingredient of this therapeutic approach," write Stehlin and Beach, "is free communication between [physician] and patient, in which the latter is sustained by hope within a framework of reality" (Stehlin and Beach, 1966). What this may mean in many instances is neither outright truth nor outright falsehood but a carefully modulated formulation that neither overtaxes human credulity nor invites despair. Thus a sophisticated woman might be expected to reject with complete disbelief the notion that she has had to undergo mastectomy for a benign cyst, but she may at the same time accept postoperative radiation as a prophylactic measure rather than as evidence of metastasis.

A doctor's wife was found to have ovarian carcinoma with widespread metastases. Although the surgeon was convinced she would not survive for more than three or four months, he wished to try the effects of radiotherapy and chemotherapy. After some discussion of the problem with a psychiatrist, he addressed himself to the patient as follows: to his surprise, when examined under the microscope the tumor in her abdomen proved to be cancerous; he fully believed he had removed it entirely; to feel perfectly safe, however, he intended to give her radiation and chemical therapies over an indeterminate period of time. The patient was highly gratified by his frankness and proceeded to live for nearly three more *years,* during which time she enjoyed an active and a productive life.

A rather similar approach was utilized in the case of Winkelstein and Blacher previously mentioned (Winkelstein and Blacher, 1967). In the presence of his wife the patient was told by the resident surgeon, upon the advice of the psychiatrist, that the biopsy of the cervical node showed cancer; that he had a cancerous growth in the abdomen; that it was the type of cancer that responds well to chemotherapy; that if the latter produced any discomfort he would receive medication for its relief; and finally that the doctors were very hopeful for a successful outcome. The patient, who, it will be recalled, had declared he wouldn't want to live if the doctors found cancer, was obviously gratified. Immediately he telephoned members of his family to tell them the news, gratuitously adding that the tumor was of low-grade malignancy. That night he slept well for the first time since entering the hospital and he continued to do so during the balance of his stay. Just before leaving he confessed that he had known all along about the existence of the abdominal mass but that he had concealed his knowledge to see what the doctors would tell him. Upon arriving home he wrote a warm letter of thanks and admiration to the resident surgeon.

It should be emphasized that although in both of these instances the advice of a psychiatrist was instrumental in formulating the discussion of the facts of the illness, it was the surgeon, not the psychiatrist, who did the talking. The importance of this point cannot be exaggerated, for since it is the surgeon who plays the central and crucial role in such cases, it is to him, and not to some substitute mouthpiece, that the patient looks for enlightenment and for hope. As noted earlier, it is not every surgeon who can bring himself to speak in this fashion to his patient; and for some there may be a strong temptation to take refuge in a sterotyped formula, or to pass the buck altogether. The surgical resident, in the last case cited, for example, was both appalled and distressed when he was advised what to do. Yet he steeled himself, looked the patient straight in the eye and spoke with conviction. When he saw the result, he was both relieved and gratified. Indeed, he emerged from the experience a far wiser man and a better physician.

The Dying Patient

The general point of view expressed in the foregoing pages has been espoused by others in considering the problem of communicating with the dying patient. Aldrich stresses the importance of providing such persons with an appropriately timed opportunity of selecting acceptance or denial of the truth in their efforts to cope with their plight (Aldrich, 1963). Weisman and Hackett believe that for the majority of patients it is likely that there is neither complete acceptance nor total repudiation of the imminence of death (Weismann and Hackett, 1961). "To deny this 'middle knowledge' of approaching death," they assert,

> ... is to deny the responsiveness of the mind to both internal perceptions and external information. There is always a psychological sampling of the physiological stream; fever, weakness, anorexia, weight loss and pain are subjective counterparts of homeostatic alteration.... If to this are added changes in those close to the patient, the knowledge of approaching death is confirmed.

Other observers agree that a patient who is sick enough to die often knows it without being told, and that what he seeks from his physician are no longer statements concerning diagnosis and prognosis, but earnest manifestations of his unwavering concern and devotion. As noted earlier, it is at such times that for reason of their own psychological makeup some physicians become deeply troubled and are most prone to drift away, thereby adding, to the dying patient's physical suffering, the suffering that is caused by a sense of abandonment, isolation, and emotional deprivation.

In contrast, it should be stressed that no less potent than morphine nor less effective than an array of tranquilizers is the steadfast and serious concern of the physician for those often numerous and relatively minor complaints of the dying patient. To this beneficent manifestation of psychological denial, which may at times attain hypochondriacal proportions, the physician ideally should respond in kind, shifting his gaze from the lethal process he is now helpless to arrest to the living being whose discomfort and distress he is still able to assuage. In these, the final measures of the dance of life, it may then appear as if both partners had reached a tacit and a mutual understanding, an unspoken pledge to ignore the dark shadow of impending death and to resume those turns and rhythms that were familiar figures in a more felicitious past. If in this he is possessed of enough grace and elegance to play his part the doctor may well succeed in fulfilling the assertion of Oliver Wendell Holmes that if one of the functions of the physician is to assist at the coming in, another is to assist at the going out.

If what has been set down here should prove uncongenial to some strict moralists, one can only observe that there is a hierarchy of morality, and that ours is a profession which traditionally has been guided by a precept that transends the virtue of uttering truth for truth's sake; that is, "So far as possible, do no harm." Where it concerns the communication between the physician and his patient, the attainment of this goal demands an ear that is sensitive to both what is said and what is not said, a mind that is capable of understanding what has been heard, and a heart that can respond to what has been understood. Here, as in many difficult human enterprises, it may prove easier to learn the words than to sing the tune.

> We did not dare to breathe a prayer
> Or give our anguish scope!
> Something was dead in each of us,
> And what was dead was Hope!

> — Oscar Wilde, *The Ballad of Reading Gaol*

Notes

1. It should be observed, however, that while the emotional conflicts of the sick doctor may contribute to the ambiguity of his position, that ambiguity may be abetted by the treating physician, who in turn may experience difficulty in assigning to his ailing colleague the unequivocal status of patient. Indeed the latter may be more or less tacitly invited to share the responsibility in the diagnosis and care of his own illness to a degree that in some instances he is virtually a consultant on his own case.

   A similar lack of a clear-cut definition of role is not uncommon when members of a doctor's family are ill. Here a further muddying of the waters may be caused by the time-honored practice of extending so-called courtesy—i.e., free care —to physicians and their families, a custom which, however well intentioned, may place its presumed beneficiaries in a moral straitjacket that discourages them from making rather ordinary demands on the treating physician, to say nothing of discharging him. It is not surprising that the care of physicians and their families occasionally evokes an atmosphere of bitterness and rancor.

2. The notion that at heart some doctors are killers is a common theme in literature. It is claimed that when in a fit of despondency Napoleon Bonaparte declared he should have been a physician, Talleyrand commented: *"Toujours assassin."*

3. This aspect of the patient-doctor relationship has not received the attention it deserves. Moreover, aside from being a therapeutic success, there are other ways in which his patients may support the doctor's psychological needs. His self-esteem, no less than his economic well-being, may be nourished by an ever-growing roster of devoted patients, particularly when the latter include celebrities and other persons of prominence. How important this can be may be judged by the not too uncommon indiscretions perpetrated by some physicians (and sometimes by their wives) in leaking confidential matters pertaining to their practice, notably the identity of their patients.

4. The same writer relaxes his position when it concerns psychiatric patients. Here he would sanction the withholding of knowledge "precisely because he may prevent the patient's recovery by revealing it." But in this, too, the writer is in error, in double error, it would seem, for, first, it is artificial and inexact to make a sharp distinction between psychiatric and nonpsychiatric patterns—the seriously sick and the dying are not infrequently conspicuously emotionally disturbed: and second, because it may at times be therapeutically advisable to acquaint the psychiatric patient with the facts of his illness.

5. Proponents of these views have seemingly overlooked the unconscious elements in human behavior and thought. Paradoxical though it may seem, the would-be suicide may wish to live: what he seeks to destroy may be restricted to that part of the self that has become burdensome or hateful. By the same token, despite his manifest combativeness, a psychotic individual is often inwardly grateful for the restraints imposed upon his dangerous aggression. There can be no logical objection to designating such persons as "prisoners," as Szasz would have it, provided we apply the same term to breathless individuals who are "incarcerated" in oxygen tents.

References

Abrams, R.D. The patient with cancer—His changing pattern of communication. *New Eng. J. Med.* 274:317, 1966.

Aldrich, C.K. The dying patient's grief. *J.A.M.A.* 184:329, 1963.

Drillien, C.M., and Wilkinson, E.M. Mongolism: When should parents be told? *Brit. Med. J.* 2:1306, 1964.

Fletcher, J. *Morals and Medicine.* Princeton: Princeton University Press, 1954.

Stehlin, J.S., and Beach, K.A. Psychological aspects of cancer therapy. *J.A.M.A.* 197:100, 1966.

Vernick, J., and Karon, M. Who's afraid of death on a leukemia ward? *Amer. J. Dis. Child,* 109:393, 1965.

Weisman, A.D., and Hackett, T. Predilection to death: Death and dying as a psychiatric problem. *Psychosom. Med.* 23:232, 1961.

Winkelstein, C., and Blacher, R. Personal communication, 1967.

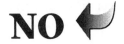
Lies to the Sick and Dying

Deception as Therapy

A forty-six-year-old man, coming to a clinic for a routine physical check-up needed for insurance purposes, is diagnosed as having a form of cancer likely to cause him to die within six months. No known cure exists for it. Chemotherapy may prolong life by a few extra months, but will have side effects the physician does not think warranted in this case. In addition, he believes that such therapy should be reserved for patients with a chance for recovery or remission. The patient has no symptoms giving him any reason to believe that he is not perfectly healthy. He expects to take a short vacation in a week.

For the physician, there are now several choices involving truthfulness. Ought he to tell the patient what he has learned, or conceal it? If asked, should he deny it? If he decides to reveal the diagnosis, should he delay doing so until after the patient returns from his vacation? Finally, even if he does reveal the serious nature of the diagnosis, should he mention the possibility of chemotherapy and his reasons for not recommending it in this case? Or should he encourage every last effort to postpone death?

In this particular case, the physician chose to inform the patient of his diagnosis right away. He did not, however, mention the possibility of chemotherapy. A medical student working under him disagreed; several nurses also thought that the patient should have been informed of this possibility. They tried, unsuccessfully, to persuade the physician that this was the patient's right. When persuasion had failed, the student elected to disobey the doctor by informing the patient of the alternative of chemotherapy. After consultation with family members, the patient chose to ask for the treatment.

Doctors confront such choices often and urgently. What they reveal, hold back, or distort will matter profoundly to their patients. Doctors stress with corresponding vehemence their reasons for the distortion or concealment: not to confuse the sick person needlessly, or cause what may well be unnecessary pain or discomfort, as in the case of the cancer patient; not to leave a patient without hope, as in those many cases where the dying are not told the truth about their condition; or to improve the chances of cure, as where unwarranted optimism is expressed about some form of therapy. Doctors use information

From Sissela Bok, *Lying: Moral Choice in Public and Private Life* (Pantheon Books, 1978). Copyright © 1978 by Sissela Bok. Reprinted by permission of Pantheon Books, a division of Random House, Inc.

as part of the therapeutic regimen; it is given out in amounts, in admixtures, and according to timing believed best for patients. Accuracy, by comparison, matters far less.

Lying to patients has, therefore, seemed an especially excusable act. Some would argue that doctors, and *only* doctors, should be granted the right to ma-nipulate the truth in ways so undesirable for politicians, lawyers, and others. Doctors are trained to help patients; their relationship to patients carries spe-cial obligations, and they know much more than laymen about what helps and hinders recovery and survival.

Even the most conscientious doctors, then, who hold themselves at a dis-tance from the quacks and the purveyors of false remedies, hesitate to forswear all lying. Lying is usually wrong, they argue, but less so than allowing the truth to harm patients. B. C. Meyer echoes this very common view:

> [O]urs is a profession which traditionally has been guided by a precept that transcends the virtue of uttering truth for truth's sake, and that is, "so far as possible, do no harm."

Truth, for Meyer, may be important, but not when it endangers the health and well-being of patients. This has seemed self-evident to many physicians in the past—so much so that we find very few mentions of veracity in the codes and oaths and writings by physicians through the centuries. This absence is all the more striking as other principles of ethics have been consistently and movingly expressed in the same documents....

Given such freedom, a physician can decide to tell as much or as little as he wants the patient to know, so long as he breaks no law. In the case of the man mentioned at the beginning of this chapter, some physicians might feel justified in lying for the good of the patient, others might be truthful. Some may conceal alternatives to the treatment they recommend; others not. In each case, they could appeal to the A.M.A. Principles of Ethics. A great many would choose to be able to lie. They would claim that not only can a lie avoid harm for the patient, but that it is also hard to know whether they have been right in the first place in making their pessimistic diagnosis; a "truthful" statement could therefore turn out to hurt patients unnecessarily. The concern for curing and for supporting those who cannot be cured then runs counter to the desire to be completely open. This concern is especially strong where the prognosis is bleak; even more so when patients are so affected by their illness or their medication that they are more dependent than usual, perhaps more easily depressed or irrational.

Physicians know only too well how uncertain a diagnosis or prognosis can be. They know how hard it is to give meaningful and correct answers regarding health and illness. They also know that disclosing their own uncertainty or fears can reduce those benefits that depend upon faith in recovery. They fear, too, that revealing grave risks, no matter how unlikely it is that these will come about, may exercise the pull of the "self-fulfilling prophecy." They dislike being the bearers of uncertain or bad news as much as anyone else. And last, but not least, sitting down to discuss an illness truthfully and sensitively may take much-needed time away from other patients.

These reasons help explain why nurses and physicians and relatives of the sick and dying prefer not to be bound by rules that might limit their ability to suppress, delay, or distort information. This is not to say that they necessarily plan to lie much of the time. They merely want to have the freedom to do so when they believe it wise. And the reluctance to see lying prohibited explains, in turn, the failure of the codes and oaths to come to grips with the problems of truth-telling and lying.

But sharp conflicts are now arising. Doctors no longer work alone with patients. They have to consult with others much more than before; if they choose to lie, the choice may not be met with approval by all who take part in the care of the patient. A nurse expresses the difficulty which results as follows:

> From personal experience I would say that the patients who aren't told about their terminal illness have so many verbal and mental questions unanswered that many will begin to realize that their illness is more serious than they're being told....

The doctor's choice to lie increasingly involves coworkers in acting a part they find neither humane nor wise. The fact that these problems have not been carefully thought through within the medical profession, nor seriously addressed in medical education, merely serves to intensify the conflicts. Different doctors then respond very differently to patients in exactly similar predicaments. The friction is increased by the fact that relatives often disagree even where those giving medical care to a patient are in accord on how to approach the patient. Here again, because physicians have not worked out to common satisfaction the question of whether relatives have the right to make such requests, the problems are allowed to be haphazardly resolved by each physician as he sees fit.

The Patient's Perspective

The turmoil in the medical profession regarding truth-telling is further augmented by the pressures that patients themselves now bring to bear and by empirical data coming to light. Challenges are growing to the three major arguments for lying to patients: that truthfulness is impossible; that patients do not want bad news; and that truthful information harms them.

The first of these arguments... confuses "truth" and "truthfulness" so as to clear the way for occasional lying on grounds supported by the second and third arguments. At this point, we can see more clearly that it is a strategic move intended to discourage the question of truthfulness from carrying much weight in the first place, and thus to leave the choice of what to say and how to say it up to the physician. To claim that "since telling the truth is impossible, there can be no sharp distinction between what is true and what is false" is to try to defeat objections to lying before even discussing them. One need only imagine how such an argument would be received, were it made by a car salesman or a real estate dealer, to see how fallacious it is.

In medicine, however, the argument is supported by a subsidiary point: even if people might ordinarily understand what is spoken to them, patients are often not in a position to do so. This is where paternalism enters in. When we buy cars or houses, the paternalist will argue, we need to have all our wits about us; but when we are ill, we cannot always do so. We need help in making choices, even if help can be given only by keeping us in the dark. And the physician is trained and willing to provide such help.

It is certainly true that some patients cannot make the best choices for themselves when weakened by illness or drugs. But most still can. And even those who are incompetent have a right to have someone—their guardian or spouse perhaps—receive the correct information.

The paternalistic assumption of superiority to patients also carries great dangers for physicians themselves—it risks turning to contempt. The following view was recently expressed in a letter to a medical journal:

> As a radiologist who has been sued, I have reflected earnestly on advice to obtain Informed Consent but have decided to "take the risks without informing the patient" and trust to "God, judge, and jury" rather than evade responsibility through a legal gimmick. . . .
>
> [I]n a general radiologic practice many of our patients are uninformable and we would never get through the day if we had to obtain their consent to every potentially harmful study. . . .

The argument which rejects informing patients because adequate truthful information is impossible in itself or because patients are lacking in understanding, must itself be rejected when looked at from the point of view of patients. They know that liberties granted to the most conscientious and altruistic doctors will be exercised also in the "Medicaid Mills"; that the choices thus kept from patients will be exercised by not only competent but incompetent physicians; and that even the best doctors can make choices patients would want to make differently for themselves.

The second argument for deceiving patients refers specifically to giving them news of a frightening or depressing kind. It holds that patients do not, in fact, generally want such information, that they prefer not to have to face up to serious illness and death. On the basis of such a belief, most doctors in a number of surveys stated that they do not, as a rule, inform patients that they have an illness such as cancer.

When studies are made of what patients desire to know, on the other hand, a large majority say that they *would* like to be told of such a diagnosis. All these studies need updating and should be done with larger numbers of patients and non-patients. But they do show that there is generally a dramatic divergence between physicians and patients on the factual question of whether patients want to know what ails them in cases of serious illness such as cancer. In most of the studies, over 80 percent of the persons asked indicated that they would want to be told.

Sometimes this discrepancy is set aside by doctors who want to retain the view that patients do not want unhappy news. In reality, they claim, the fact that patients say they want it has to be discounted. The more someone asks to know, the more he suffers from fear which will lead to the denial of the information even if it is given. Informing patients is, therefore, useless; they resist and deny having been told what they cannot assimilate. According to this view, empirical studies of what patients say they want are worthless since they do not probe deeply enough to uncover this universal resistance to the contemplation of one's own death.

This view is only partially correct. For some patients, denial is indeed well established in medical experience. A number of patients (estimated at between 15 percent and 25 percent) will give evidence of denial of having been told about their illness, even when they repeatedly ask and are repeatedly informed. And nearly everyone experiences a period of denial at some point in the course of approaching death. Elisabeth Kübler-Ross sees denial as resulting often from premature and abrupt information by a stranger who goes through the process quickly to "get it over with." She holds that denial functions as a buffer after unexpected shocking news, permitting individuals to collect themselves and to mobilize other defenses. She describes prolonged denial in one patient as follows:

> She was convinced that the X-rays were "mixed up"; she asked for reassurance that her pathology report could not possibly be back so soon and that another patient's report must have been marked with her name. When none of this could be confirmed, she quickly asked to leave the hospital, looking for another physician in the vain hope "to get a better explanation for my troubles." This patient went "shopping around" for many doctors, some of whom gave her reassuring answers, other of whom confirmed the previous suspicion. Whether confirmed or not, she reacted in the same manner; she asked for examination and reexamination....

But to say that denial is universal flies in the face of all evidence. And to take any claim to the contrary as "symptomatic" of deeper denial leaves no room for reasoned discourse. There is no way that such universal denial can be proved true or false. To believe in it is a metaphysical belief about man's condition, not a statement about what patients do and do not want. It is true that we can never completely understand the possibility of our own death, any more than being alive in the first place. But people certainly differ in the degree to which they can approach such knowledge, take it into account in their plans, and make their peace with it.

Montaigne claimed that in order to learn both to live and to die, men have to think about death and be prepared to accept it. To stick one's head in the sand, or to be prevented by lies from trying to discern what is to come, hampers freedom—freedom to consider one's life as a whole, with a beginning, a duration, an end. Some may request to be deceived rather than to see their lives as thus finite; others reject the information which would require them to do so; but most say that they want to know. Their concern for knowing about their condition goes far beyond mere curiosity or the wish to make isolated personal choices in the short time left to them; their stance toward the entire life they have lived, and their ability to give it meaning and completion, are at stake. In lying or withholding the facts which permit such discernment, doctors may reflect their own fears (which, according to one study, are much stronger than those of laymen) of facing questions about the meaning of one's life and the inevitability of death.

Beyond the fundamental deprivation that can result from deception, we are also becoming increasingly aware of all that can befall patients in the course of their illness when information is denied or distorted. Lies place them in a position where they no longer participate in choices concerning their own health, including the choice of whether to be a "patient" in the first place. A terminally ill person who is not informed that his illness is incurable and that he is near death cannot make decisions about the end of his life: about whether or not to enter a hospital, or to have surgery; where and with whom to spend his last days; how to put his affairs in order—these most personal choices cannot be made if he is kept in the dark, or given contradictory hints and clues.

It has always been especially easy to keep knowledge from terminally ill patients. They are most vulnerable, least able to take action to learn what they need to know, or to protect their autonomy. The very fact of being so ill greatly increases the likelihood of control by others. And the fear of being helpless in the face of such control is growing. At the same time, the period of dependency and slow deterioration of health and strength that people undergo has lengthened. There has been a dramatic shift toward institutionalization of the aged and those near death. (Over 80 percent of Americans now die in a hospital or other institution.)

Patients who are severely ill often suffer a further distancing and loss of control over their most basic functions. Electrical wiring, machines, intravenous administration of liquids, all create new dependency and at the same time new distance between the patient and all who come near. Curable patients are often willing to undergo such procedures; but when no cure is possible, these procedures merely intensify the sense of distance and uncertainty and can even become a substitute for comforting human acts. Yet those who suffer in this way often fear to seem troublesome by complaining. Lying to them, perhaps for the most charitable of purposes, can then cause them to slip unwittingly into subjection to new procedures, perhaps new surgery, where death is held at bay through transfusions, respirators, even resuscitation far beyond what most would wish.

Seeing relatives in such predicaments has caused a great upsurge of worrying about death and dying. At the root of this fear is not a growing terror of the *moment* of death, or even the instants before it. Nor is there greater fear of *being* dead. In contrast to the centuries of lives lived in dread of the punishments to be inflicted after death, many would now accept the view expressed by Epicurus, who died in 270 B.C.:

> Death, therefore, the most awful of evils, is nothing to us, seeing that, when
> we are, death is not come, and, when death is come, we are not.

The growing fear, if it is not of the moment of dying nor of being dead, is of all that which now precedes dying for so many: the possibility of prolonged pain, the increasing weakness, the uncertainty, the loss of powers and chance of senility, the sense of being a burden. This fear is further nourished by the loss of trust in health professionals. In part, the loss of trust results from the abuses which have been exposed—the Medicaid scandals, the old-age home profiteering, the commercial exploitation of those who seek remedies for their ailments;

in part also because of the deceptive practices patients suspect, having seen how friends and relatives were kept in the dark; in part, finally, because of the sheer numbers of persons, often strangers, participating in the care of any one patient. Trust which might have gone to a doctor long known to the patient goes less easily to a team of strangers, no matter how expert or well-meaning.

It is with the working out of all that *informed consent*[1] implies and the information it presupposes that truth-telling is coming to be discussed in a serious way for the first time in the health professions. Informed consent is a farce if the information provided is distorted or withheld. And even complete information regarding surgical procedures or medication is obviously useless unless the patient also knows what the condition is that these are supposed to correct.

Bills of rights for patients, similarly stressing the right to be informed, are now gaining acceptance. This right is not new, but the effort to implement it is. Nevertheless, even where patients are handed the most elegantly phrased Bill of Rights, their right to a truthful diagnosis and prognosis is by no means always respected.

The reason why even doctors who recognize a patient's right to have information might still not provide it brings us to the third argument against telling all patients the truth. It holds that the information given might hurt the patient and that the concern for the right to such information is therefore a threat to proper health care. A patient, these doctors argue, may wish to commit suicide after being given discouraging news, or suffer a cardiac arrest, or simply cease to struggle, and thus not grasp the small remaining chance for recovery. And even where the outlook for a patient is very good, the disclosure of a minute risk can shock some patients or cause them to reject needed protection such as a vaccination or antibiotics.

The factual basis for this argument has been challenged from two points of view. The damages associated with the disclosure of sad news or risks are rarer than physicians believe; and the *benefits* which result from being informed are more substantial, even measurably so. Pain is tolerated more easily, recovery from surgery is quicker, and cooperation with therapy is greatly improved. The attitude that "what you don't know won't hurt you" is proving unrealistic; it is what patients do not know but vaguely suspect that causes them corrosive worry.

It is certain that no answers to this question of harm from information are the same for all patients. If we look, first, at the fear expressed by physicians that informing patients of even remote or unlikely risks connected with a drug prescription or operation might shock some and make others refuse the treatment that would have been best for them, it appears to be unfounded for the great majority of patients. Studies show that very few patients respond to being told of such risks by withdrawing their consent to the procedure and that those who do withdraw are the very ones who might well have been upset enough to sue the physician had they not been asked to consent before hand. It is possible that on even rarer occasions especially susceptible persons might manifest physical deterioration from shock; some physicians have even asked whether patients who die after giving informed consent to an operation, but before it actually takes place, somehow expire because of the information given to them. While such questions are unanswerable in any one case, they certainly argue in favor of caution, a real concern for the person to whom one is recounting the risks he or she will face, and sensitivity to all signs of distress.

The situation is quite different when persons who are already ill, perhaps already quite weak and discouraged, are told of a very serious prognosis. Physicians fear that such knowledge may cause the patients to commit suicide, or to be frightened or depressed to the point that their illness takes a downward turn. The fear that great numbers of patients will commit suicide appears to be unfounded. And if some do, is that a response so unreasonable, so much against the patient's best interest that physicians ought to make it a reason for concealment or lies? Many societies have allowed suicide in the past; our own has decriminalized it; and some are coming to make distinctions among the many suicides which ought to be prevented if at all possible, and those which ought to be respected.

Another possible response to very bleak news is the triggering of physiological mechanisms which allow death to come more quickly—a form of giving up or of preparing for the inevitable, depending on one's outlook. Lewis Thomas, studying responses in humans and animals, holds it not unlikely that:

> ... there is a pivotal moment at some stage in the body's reaction to injury or disease, maybe in aging as well, when the organism concedes that it is finished and the time for dying is at hand, and at this moment the events that lead to death are launched, as a coordinated mechanism. Functions are then shut off, in sequence, irreversibly, and, while this is going on, a neural mechanism, held ready for this occasion, is switched on....

Such a response may be appropriate, in which case it makes the moments of dying as peaceful as those who have died and been resuscitated so often testify. But it may also be brought on inappropriately, when the organism could have lived on, perhaps even induced malevolently, by external acts intended to kill. Thomas speculates that some of the deaths resulting from "hexing" are due to such responses. Levi-Strauss describes deaths from exorcism and the casting of spells in ways which suggest that the same process may then be brought on by the community.

It is not inconceivable that unhappy news abruptly conveyed, or a great shock given to someone unable to tolerate it, could also bring on such a "dying response," quite unintended by the speaker. There is every reason to be cautious and to try to know ahead of time how susceptible a patient might be to the accidental triggering—however rare—of such a response. One has to assume, however, that most of those who have survived long enough to be in a situation where their informed consent is asked have a very robust resistance to such accidental triggering of processes leading to death.

When, on the other hand, one considers those who are already near death, the "dying response" may be much less inappropriate, much less accidental, much less unreasonable. In most societies, long before the advent of modern medicine, human beings have made themselves ready for death once they felt its approach. Philippe Aries describes how many in the Middle Ages prepared themselves for death when they "felt the end approach." They awaited death lying down, surrounded by friends and relatives. They recollected all they had lived through and done, pardoning all who stood near their deathbed, calling on God to bless them, and finally praying. "After the final prayer all that remained was to wait for death, and there was no reason for death to tarry."

Modern medicine, in its valiant efforts to defeat disease and to save lives, may be dislocating the conscious as well as the purely organic responses allowing death to come when it is inevitable, thus denying those who are dying the benefits of the traditional approach to death. In lying to them, and in pressing medical efforts to cure them long past the point of possible recovery, physicians may thus rob individuals of an autonomy few would choose to give up.

Sometimes, then, the "dying response" is a natural organic reaction at the time when the body has no further defense. Sometimes it is inappropriately brought on by news too shocking or given in too abrupt a manner. We need to learn a great deal more about this last category, no matter how small. But there is no evidence that patients in general will be debilitated by truthful information about their condition.

Apart from the possible harm from information, we are coming to learn much more about the benefits it can bring patients. People follow instructions more carefully if they know what their disease is and why they are asked to take medication; any benefits from those procedures are therefore much more likely to come about.[2] Similarly, people recover faster from surgery and tolerate pain with less medication if they understand what ails them and what can be done for them.[3]

Respect and Truthfulness

Taken all together, the three arguments defending lies to patients stand on much shakier ground as a counterweight to the right to be informed than is often thought. The common view that many patients cannot understand, do not want, and may be harmed by, knowledge of their condition, and that lying to them is either morally neutral or even to be recommended, must be set aside. Instead, we have to make a more complex comparison. Over against the right of patients to knowledge concerning themselves, the medical and psychological benefits to them from this knowledge, the unnecessary and sometimes harmful treatment to which they can be subjected if ignorant, and the harm to physicians, their profession, and other patients from deceptive practices, we have to set a severely restricted and narrowed paternalistic view—that *some* patients cannot understand, *some* do not want, and *some* may be harmed by, knowledge of their condition, and that they ought not to have to be treated like everyone else if this is not in their best interest.

Such a view is persuasive. A few patients openly request not to be given bad news. Others give clear signals to that effect, or are demonstrably vulnerable to the shock or anguish such news might call forth. Can one not in such cases infer implied consent to being deceived?

Concealment, evasion, withholding of information may at times be necessary. But if someone contemplates lying to a patient or concealing the truth, the burden of proof must shift. It must rest, here, as with all deception, on those who advocate it in any one instance. They must show why they fear a patient may be harmed or how they know that another cannot cope with the truthful knowledge. A decision to deceive must be seen as a very unusual step, to be talked over with colleagues and others who participate in the care of the patient. Reasons must be set forth and debated, alternatives weighed carefully. At all times, the correct information must go to *someone* closely related to the patient.

Notes

1. The law requires that inroads made upon a person's body take place only with the informed voluntary consent of that person. The term "informed consent" came into common use only after 1960, when it was used by the Kansas Supreme Court in Nathanson vs. Kline, 186 Kan. 393, 350, p. 2d, 1093 (1960). The patient is now entitled to full disclosure of risks, benefits, and alternative treatments to any proposed procedure, both in therapy and in medical experimentation, except in emergencies or when the patient is incompetent, in which case proxy consent is required.

2. Barbara S. Hulka, J. C. Cassel, et al. "Communication, Compliance, and Concordance between Physicians and Patients with Prescribed Medications," *American Journal of Public Health*, Sept. 1976, pp. 847–53. The study shows that of the nearly half of all patients who do not follow the prescriptions of the doctors (thus foregoing the intended effect of these prescriptions), many will follow them if adequately informed about the nature of their illness and what the proposed medication will do.

3. See Lawrence D. Egbert, George E. Batitt, et al., "Reduction of Postoperative Pain by Encouragement and Instruction of Patients," *New England Journal of Medicine*, 270, pp. 825–27, 1964.

   See also: Howard Waitzskin and John D. Stoeckle, "The Communication of Information about Illness," *Advances in Psychosomatic Medicine*, Vol. 8, 1972, pp. 185–215.

POSTSCRIPT

Is It Ethical to Withhold the Truth From Dying Patients?

An important, recent legal case concerning truth telling and informed consent is *Arcato v. Avedon.* Mr. Arcato, a California electrical contractor, was operated on in 1980 to remove a kidney that was not functioning. The surgeons also removed a tumor from his pancreas, but neither they nor the oncologist to whom they referred Arcato told him that approximately 95 percent of people with pancreatic cancer die within a year. Arcato died one year after the cancer had been diagnosed. His wife and children sued the doctors, claiming that California's informed-consent doctrine required the disclosure of the withheld information. If he had been told the truth, his family argued, he might not have undergone the difficult and unsuccessful experimental treatment his oncologist offered. The case ultimately went to the California Supreme Court, which in 1993 upheld the trial court's ruling in favor of the physicians. For more on the case, see George Annas, "Informed Consent, Cancer, and Truth in Prognosis," *The New England Journal of Medicine* (January 20, 1994), in which the author argues that the real issue was not the statistics on life expectancy but the impact of the proposed treatment in terms of prospects for long-term survival and quality of life.

Most of the literature on withholding the truth from patients concerns cancer. Drs. Margaret A. Drickamer and Mark S. Lachs address a different disease in their essay "Should Patients With Alzheimer's Disease Be Told Their Diagnosis?" *The New England Journal of Medicine* (April 2, 1992). Although they favor truth telling, they present the case for not telling, including such factors as the difficulty of conclusive diagnosis, the impaired decision-making capacity and competence of patients with Alzheimer's, and the limited therapeutic options. A cultural difference can be seen in Antonella Surbone's "Truth Telling to the Patient," *Journal of the American Medical Association* (October 7, 1992), in which she describes the practice of withholding information from seriously ill patients in Italy. The same issue contains an accompanying editorial by Edmund D. Pellegrino. Benjamin Freedman offers a middle ground argument in "Offering Truth: One Ethical Approach to the Uninformed Cancer Patient," *Annals of Internal Medicine* (March 8, 1993).

Many articles on truth telling are found in the nursing literature. See, for example, Anthony Tuckett, "Nursing Practice: Compassionate Deception and the Good Samaritan," *Nursing Ethics* (September 1999).

ISSUE 6

Should Doctors Be Able to Refuse Demands for "Futile" Treatment?

YES: Steven H. Miles, from "Informed Demand for 'Non-Beneficial' Medical Treatment," *The New England Journal of Medicine* (August 15, 1991)

NO: Felicia Ackerman, from "The Significance of a Wish," *Hastings Center Report* (July–August 1991)

ISSUE SUMMARY

YES: Physician Steven H. Miles maintains that physicians' duty to follow patients' wishes ends when the requests are inconsistent with what medical care can reasonably be expected to achieve, when they violate community standards of care, and when they consume an unfair share of collective resources.

NO: Philosopher Felicia Ackerman contends that it is ethically inappropriate for physicians to decide what kind of life is worth prolonging and that decisions involving personal values should be made by the patient or family.

In the typical controversy involving life-prolonging treatment, it is the patient or patient's family who wants to stop treatment and the doctor or hospital administrator who wants to continue it. That line of cases began, most prominently, with *In re Quinlan* (1976) and was decided again in *Cruzan v. Director of Missouri Department of Health* (1990). Another scenario, however, is emerging. What happens when the patient or family demands that treatment be continued past the point that doctors or hospital administrators feel it is warranted? Families may hope for a miracle and want "everything possible" done to preserve life. In the case of "Baby L," described by John Paris, Robert K. Crone, and Frank Reardon in *The New England Journal of Medicine* (April 5, 1990), pediatricians refused a mother's request to start ventilator treatment for a severely compromised, blind, deaf, and neurologically impaired child who had spent all 28 months of her life in intensive care.

In other cases, patients or families may act out of religious convictions that life is a God-given gift that must be preserved at all costs. In her book *Ethics on Call* (Crown Publishers, 1992), Nancy Dubler describes the case of "Joseph," a devoutly religious man who interpreted Jewish law to mean that life can be taken only by God, and that he must take whatever measures are available to sustain his life, no matter what suffering was entailed. There may even be cases in which a criminal prosecution may hinge on whether a patient dies or not, or there may be financial motivations to preserving life.

These cases stretch the limits of patient autonomy and come to a full stop when they reach the boundaries of professional responsibility. Just as patients are moral agents, so too are physicians. Their professional ethic begins with the Hippocratic injunction "First, do no harm." Beyond avoiding harm, they are guided by the obligation to do good—to provide benefit to patients within the limits of their expertise. Since ancient times physicians have felt it is their prerogative to determine whether or not treatment is justified. The writings of Hippocrates and Plato warn physicians to acknowledge when their art is doomed to fail.

In modern times the Vatican's 1980 *Declaration on Euthanasia* places a strong emphasis on physician judgment, pointing out that "[doctors] may... judge that the investment in instruments and personnel is disproportionate to the results foreseen; they may also judge that the techniques applied impose on the patient strain or suffering out of proportion with the benefits." The U.S. President's Commission for the Study of Bioethical Problems in Medicine concluded in 1983 that "health care professionals or institutions may decline to provide a particular option because that choice may violate their conscience or professional judgement, though, in doing so they may not abandon a patient." Even more recently (December 1990), the Society of Critical Care Medicine declared that "treatments that offer no benefit and serve to prolong the dying process should not be employed."

As frequently happens in bioethics, one case—not necessarily the first to arise—serves to focus the arguments. In the area of demands for "nonbeneficial" treatment, that case involved the treatment of Helga Wanglie, an elderly Minnesota woman who suffered a series of medical problems, culminating in a year and a half spent unconscious on a respirator in a persistent vegetative state. Her physicians asked her husband to consent to withdrawing treatment; his refusal set off a chain of events described in the following selections.

Steven H. Miles, a gerontologist and ethics consultant to Mrs. Wanglie's physicians, argues that Mrs. Wanglie was "overmastered" by her disease and that continued intensive care was inappropriate and inconsistent with reasonable medical expectations of benefit. Felicia Ackerman maintains that decisions about what lives are worth living properly fall to those who share the values of the patient—in this case, the family.

Steven H. Miles

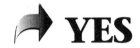 **YES**

Informed Demand for "Non-Beneficial" Medical Treatment

An 85-year-old woman was taken from a nursing home to Hennepin County Medical Center on January 1, 1990, for emergency treatment of dyspnea [shortness of breath] from chronic bronchiectasis [widening of the air passages]. The patient, Mrs. Helga Wanglie, required emergency intubation [insertion of a tube] and was placed on a respirator. She occasionally acknowledged discomfort and recognized her family but could not communicate clearly. In May, after attempts to wean her from the respirator failed, she was discharged to a chronic care hospital. One week later, her heart stopped during a weaning attempt; she was resuscitated and taken to another hospital for intensive care. She remained unconscious, and a physician suggested that it would be appropriate to consider withdrawing life support. In response, the family transferred her back to the medical center on May 31. Two weeks later, physicians concluded that she was in a persistent vegetative state.... She was maintained on a respirator, with repeated courses of antibiotics, frequent airway suctioning, tube feedings, an air flotation bed, and biochemical monitoring.

In June and July of 1990, physicians suggested that life-sustaining treatment be withdrawn since it was not benefiting the patient. Her husband, daughter, and son insisted on continued treatment. They stated their view that physicians should not play God, that the patient would not be better off dead, that removing life support showed moral decay in our civilization, and that a miracle could occur. Her husband told a physician that his wife had never stated her preferences concerning life-sustaining treatment. He believed that the cardiac arrest would not have occurred if she had not been transferred from Hennepin County Medical Center in May. The family reluctantly accepted a do-not-resuscitate order based on the improbability of Mrs. Wanglie's surviving a cardiac arrest. In June, an ethics committee consultant recommended continued counseling for the family. The family declined counseling, including the counsel of their own pastor, and in late July asked that the respirator not be discussed again. In August, nurses expressed their consensus that continued life support did not seem appropriate, and I, as the newly appointed ethics consultant, counseled them.

From Steven H. Miles, "Informed Demand for 'Non-Beneficial' Medical Treatment," *The New England Journal of Medicine*, vol. 325, no. 7 (August 15, 1991), pp. 512–515. Copyright © 1991 by The Massachusetts Medical Society. All rights reserved. Reprinted by permission.

In October 1990, a new attending physician consulted with specialists and confirmed the permanence of the patient's cerebral and pulmonary conditions. He concluded that she was at the end of her life and that the respirator was "non-beneficial," in that it could not heal her lungs, palliate her suffering, or enable this unconscious and permanently respirator-dependent woman to experience the benefit of the life afforded by respirator support. Because the respirator could prolong life, it was not characterized as "futile."[1] In November, the physician, with my concurrence, told the family that he was not willing to continue to prescribe the respirator. The husband, an attorney, rejected proposals to transfer the patient to another facility or to seek a court order mandating this unusual treatment. The hospital told the family that it would ask a court to decide whether members of its staff were obliged to continue treatment. A second conference two weeks later, after the family had hired an attorney, confirmed these positions, and the husband asserted that the patient had consistently said she wanted respirator support for such a condition.

In December, the medical director and hospital administrator asked the Hennepin County Board of Commissioners (the medical center's board of directors) to allow the hospital to go to court to resolve the dispute. In January, the county board gave permission by a 4-to-3 vote. Neither the hospital nor the county had a financial interest in terminating treatment. Medicare largely financed the $200,000 for the first hospitalization at Hennepin County; a private insurer would pay the $500,000 bill for the second. From February through May of 1991, the family and its attorney unsuccessfully searched for another health care facility that would admit Mrs. Wanglie. Facilities with empty beds cited her poor potential for rehabilitation.

The hospital chose a two-step legal procedure, first asking for the appointment of an independent conservator to decide whether the respirator was beneficial to the patient and second, if the conservator found it was not, for a second hearing on whether it was obliged to provide the respirator. The husband cross-filed, requesting to be appointed conservator. After a hearing in late May, the trial court on July 1, 1991, appointed the husband, as best able to represent the patient's interests. It noted that no request to stop treatment had been made and declined to speculate on the legality of such an order.[2] The hospital said that it would continue to provide the respirator in the light of continuing uncertainty about its legal obligation to provide it. . . .

Discussion

This sad story illustrates the problem of what to do when a family demands medical treatment that the attending physician concludes cannot benefit the patient. Only 600 elderly people are treated with respirators for more than six months in the United States each year.[3] Presumably, most of these people are actually or potentially conscious. It is common practice to discontinue the use of a respirator before death when it can no longer benefit a patient.[4,5]

We do not know Mrs. Wanglie's treatment preferences. A large majority of elderly people prefer not to receive prolonged respirator support for irreversible unconsciousness.[6] Studies show that an older person's designated family proxy overestimates that person's preference for life-sustaining treatment in a hypothetical coma.[7-9] The implications of this research for clinical decision making have not been cogently analyzed.

A patient's request for a treatment does not necessarily oblige a provider or the health care system. Patients may not demand that physicians injure them (for example, by mutilation), or provide plausible but inappropriate therapies (for example, amphetamines for weight reduction), or therapies that have no value (such as laetrile for cancer). Physicians are not obliged to violate their personal moral views on medical care so long as patients' rights are served. Minnesota's Living Will law says that physicians are "legally bound to act consistently within my wishes within limits of reasonable medical practice" in acting on requests and refusals of treatment.[10] Minnesota's Bill of Patients' Rights says that patients "have the right to appropriate medical . . . care based on individual needs . . . [which is] limited where the service is not reimbursable."[11] Mrs. Wanglie also had aortic insufficiency. Had this condition worsened, a surgeon's refusal to perform a life-prolonging valve replacement as medically inappropriate would hardly occasion public controversy. As the Minneapolis *Star Tribune* said in an editorial on the eve of the trial,

> The hospital's plea is born of realism, not hubris. . . . It advances the claim that physicians should not be slaves to technology—any more than patients should be its prisoners. They should be free to deliver, and act on, an honest and time-honored message: "Sorry, there's nothing more we can do."[12]

Disputes between physicians and patients about treatment plans are often handled by transferring patients to the care of other providers. In this case, every provider contacted by the hospital or the family refused to treat this patient with a respirator. These refusals occurred before and after this case became a matter of public controversy and despite the availability of third-party reimbursement. We believe they represent a medical consensus that respirator support is inappropriate in such a case.

The handling of this case is compatible with current practices regarding informed consent, respect for patients' autonomy, and the right to health care. Doctors should inform patients of all medically reasonable treatments, even those available from other providers. Patients can refuse any prescribed treatment or choose among any medical alternatives that physicians are willing to prescribe. Respect for autonomy does not empower patients to oblige physicians to prescribe treatments in ways that are fruitless or inappropriate. Previous "right to die" cases address the different situations of a patient's right to choose to be free of a prescribed therapy. This case is more about the nature of the patient's choice in using that entitlement.

The proposal that this family's preference for this unusual and costly treatment, which is commonly regarded as inappropriate, establishes a right to such treatment is ironic, given that preference does not create a right to other needed, efficacious, and widely desired treatments in the United States. We could not afford a universal health care system based on patients' demands. Such a system would irrationally allocate health care to socially powerful people with strong preferences for immediate treatment to the disadvantage of those with less power or less immediate needs.

After the conclusion was reached that the respirator was not benefiting the patient, the decision to seek a review of the duty to provide it was based on an ethic of "stewardship." Even though the insurer played no part in this case, physicians' discretion to prescribe requires responsible handling of requests for inappropriate treatment. Physicians exercise this stewardship by counseling against or denying such treatment or by submitting such requests to external review. This stewardship is not aimed at protecting the assets of insurance companies but rests on fairness to people who have pooled their resources to insure their collective access to appropriate health care. Several citizens complained to Hennepin County Medical Center that Mrs. Wanglie was receiving expensive treatment paid for by people who had not consented to underwrite a level of medical care whose appropriateness was defined by family demands.

Procedures for addressing this kind of dispute are at an early stage of development. Though the American Medical Association[13] and the Society of Critical Care Medicine[14] also support some decisions to withhold requested treatment, the medical center's reasoning most closely follows the guidelines of the American Thoracic Society.[15] The statements of these professional organizations do not clarify when or how a physician may legally withdraw or withhold demanded life-sustaining treatments. The request for a conservator to review the medical conclusion before considering the medical obligation was often misconstrued as implying that the husband was incompetent or ill motivated. The medical center intended to emphasize the desirability of an independent review of its medical conclusion before its obligation to provide the respirator was reviewed by the court. I believe that the grieving husband was simply mistaken about whether the respirator was benefiting his wife. A direct request to remove the respirator seems to center procedural oversight on the soundness of the medical decision making rather than on the nature of the patient's need. Clearly, the gravity of these decisions merits openness, due process, and meticulous accountability. The relative merits of various procedures need further study.

Ultimately, procedures for addressing requests for futile, marginally effective, or inappropriate therapies require a statutory framework, case law, professional standards, a social consensus, and the exercise of professional responsibility. Appropriate ends for medicine are defined by public and professional consensus. Laws can, and do, say that patients may choose only among medically appropriate options, but legislatures are ill suited to define medical appropriateness. Similarly, health-facility policies on this issue will be difficult to design and will focus on due process rather than on specific clinical situations. Public or private payers will ration according to cost and overall efficacy, a rationing that will become more onerous as therapies are misapplied in individual cases. I believe there is a social consensus that intensive care for a person as "overmastered" by disease as this woman was is inappropriate.

Each case must be evaluated individually. In this case, the husband's request seemed entirely inconsistent with what medical care could do for his wife, the standards of the community, and his fair share of resources that many people pooled for their collective medical care. This case is about limits to what can be achieved at the end of life.

References

1. Tomlinson T, Brody H. Futility and the ethics of resuscitation. JAMA 1990; 264:1276–80.
2. In re Helga Wanglie, Fourth Judicial District (Dist. Ct., Probate Ct. Div.) PX-91-283. Minnesota, Hennepin County.
3. Office of Technology Assessment Task Force. Life-sustaining technologies and the elderly. Washington, D.C.: Government Printing Office, 1987.
4. Smedira NG, Evans BH, Grais LS, et al. Withholding and withdrawal of life support from the critically ill. N Engl J Med 1990; 322:309–15.
5. Lantos JD, Singer PA, Walker RM, et al. The illusion of futility in clinical practice. Am J Med 1989; 87:81–4.
6. Emanuel LL, Barry MJ, Stoeckle JD, Ettelson LM, Emanuel EJ. Advance directives for medical care—a case for greater use. N Engl J Med 1991; 324:889–95.
7. Zweibel NR, Cassel CK. Treatment choices at the end of life: a comparison of decisions by older patients and their physician-selected proxies. Gerontologist 1989; 29:615–21.
8. Tomlinson T, Howe K, Notman M, Rossmiller D. An empirical study of proxy consent for elderly persons. Gerontologist 1990; 30:54–64.
9. Danis M, Southerland LI, Garrett JM, et al. A prospective study of advance directives for life-sustaining care. N Engl J Med 1991; 324:882–8.
10. Minnesota Statutes. Adult Health Care Decisions Act. 145b.04.
11. Minnesota Statutes. Patients and residents of health care facilities: Bill of rights. 144.651:Subd. 6.
12. Helga Wanglie's life. Minneapolis Star Tribune. May 26, 1991:18A.
13. Council on Ethical and Judicial Affairs. American Medical Association. Guidelines for the appropriate use of do-not-resuscitate orders. JAMA 1991; 265:1868–71.
14. Task Force on Ethics of the Society of Critical Care Medicine. Consensus report on the ethics of foregoing life-sustaining treatments in the critically ill. Crit Care Med 1990; 18:1435–9.
15. American Thoracic Society. Withholding and withdrawing life-sustaining therapy. Am Rev Respir Dis (in press).

NO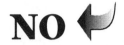

Felicia Ackerman

The Significance of a Wish

The case of Helga Wanglie should be seen in the general context of conflicts that can arise over whether a patient should be maintained on life-support systems. Well-publicized conflicts of this sort usually involve an institution seeking to prolong the life of a patient diagnosed as terminally ill and/or permanently comatose, versus a family that claims, with varying degrees of substantiation, that the patient would not have wanted to be kept alive under these circumstances. But other sorts of conflicts about prolonging life also occur. Patients who have indicated a desire to stay alive may face opposition from family or medical staff who think these patients' lives are not worth prolonging. Such cases can go badly for patients, who may have difficulty getting their preferences even believed, let alone respected.[1]

Helga Wanglie's case is not as clear cut. But in view of the fact that keeping her on a respirator will prolong her life, that there is more reason to believe she would have wanted this than to believe she would not have wanted it, that medical diagnoses of irreversible unconsciousness are not infallible, and that her private health insurance plan has not objected to paying for her respirator support and in fact has publicly taken the position that cost should not be a factor in treatment decisions, I believe HCMC [Hennepin County Medical Center] should continue to maintain Mrs. Wanglie on a respirator. This respirator support is medically and economically feasible, and it serves a recognized medical goal—that of prolonging life and allowing a chance at a possible, albeit highly unlikely, return to consciousness.

The Significance of Medical Expertise

Dr. Steven Miles, ethics consultant at HCMC, has argued that continued respirator support is "medically inappropriate" for Mrs. Wanglie. The argument is based on a criterion of medical appropriateness that allows doctors to prescribe respirators for any of three purposes: to allow healing, to alleviate suffering, and to enable otherwise disabled persons to continue to enjoy life. Since keeping Mrs. Wanglie on a respirator serves none of these ends, it is argued, such treatment is medically inappropriate.

From Felicia Ackerman, "The Significance of a Wish," *Hastings Center Report,* vol. 21, no. 4 (July–August 1991). Copyright © 1991 by The Hastings Center. Reprinted by permission.

But just what does "medically inappropriate" mean here? A clear case of medical inappropriateness would be an attempt to cure cancer with laetrile, since medicine has presumably shown that laetrile cannot cure cancer. Moreover, since laetrile's clinical ineffectiveness is a technical medical fact about which doctors are supposed to have professional expertise, it is professionally appropriate for doctors to refuse to grant a patient's request to have laetrile prescribed for cancer. But HCMC's disagreement with Mrs. Wanglie's family is not a technical dispute about a matter where doctors can be presumed to have greater expertise than laymen. The parties to the dispute do not disagree about whether maintaining Mrs. Wanglie on a respirator is likely to prolong her life; they disagree about whether her life is worth prolonging. This is not a medical question, but a question of values. Hence the term "medically inappropriate," with its implication of the relevance of technical medical expertise, is itself inappropriate in this context. It is as presumptuous and *ethically* inappropriate for doctors to suppose that their professional expertise qualifies them to know what kind of life is worth prolonging as it would be for meteorologists to suppose their professional expertise qualifies them to know what kind of destination is worth a long drive in the rain.

It has also been argued that continued respirator support does not serve Mrs. Wanglie's interests since a permanently unconscious person cannot "enjoy any realization of the quality of life."[2] Yet were this approach to be applied consistently, it would undermine the idea frequently advanced in other life-support cases that it is in the interests of the irreversibly comatose to be "allowed" to die "with dignity." Such people are not suffering or even conscious, so how can death benefit them or serve their interests? The obvious reply in both cases is that there is a sense in which it is in a permanently comatose person's interests to have his or her previous wishes and values respected. And there is some evidence that Mrs. Wanglie would want to be kept alive.

But why suppose doctors are any more obliged to serve this want than they would be to help gratify some nonmedical desire such as a desire to be remembered in a certain way? An obvious answer is that prolonging life is a medical function, as is allowing a possible return to consciousness. Medical diagnoses of irreversible coma are not infallible, as the recent case of Carrie Coons clearly demonstrates. The court order to remove her feeding tube, requested by her family, was rescinded after Mrs. Coons regained consciousness following five and a half months in what was diagnosed as an irreversible vegetative state.[3] Such cases cast additional light on the claim that respirator support is medically inappropriate and not in Mrs. Wanglie's interests. When the alternative is death, the question of whether going for a long-shot chance of recovering consciousness is worth it is quite obviously a question of values, rather than a technical medical question doctors are especially professionally qualified to decide.

The Significance of Quality of Life

Medical ethicists who take into account the possibility that seemingly irreversibly comatose patients might regain consciousness have offered further general arguments against maintaining such patients on life-support systems. One such argument relies on the fact that "the few patients who have recovered consciousness after a prolonged period of unconsciousness were severely disabled,"[4] with disabilities including blindness, inability to speak, permanent distortion of limbs, and paralysis. Since many blind, mute, and/or paralyzed people seem to find their lives well worth living, however, the assumption that disability is a fate worse than death seems highly questionable. Moreover, when the patient's views on the matter are unknown, maintaining him on a respirator to give him a chance to regain consciousness and then decide whether to continue his disabled existence seems preferable to denying him even the possibility of a choice by deciding in advance that he would be better off dead. Keeping alive someone who would want to die and "allowing" to die someone who would want a chance of regained consciousness are not parallel wrongs. While both obviously go against the patient's values, only the latter has the additional flaw of doing this in a way that could actually affect his conscious experience.

The other argument asserts that since long-term treatment imposes emotional and often financial burdens on the comatose patient's family and most patients, before losing consciousness, place a high value on their families' welfare, presumably these patients would rather die than be a burden to their loved ones.[5] Though very popular nowadays, this latter sort of argument is cruel because it attributes extreme self-abnegation to those unable to speak for themselves. It is also biased because it assumes great sacrificial love on the part of the patient, but not the family. Why not argue instead that a loving family will not want to deny a beloved member a last chance at regained consciousness and hence that it is *not* in the interest of the patient's loved ones to withdraw life supports? Mrs. Wanglie's family clearly wants her kept alive.[6]

The Significance of a Gesture

Mrs. Wanglie's family claims that she would want to be kept alive. Yet Dr. Cranford suggests that her family at first denied having previously discussed the matter with her, and that it was only after the HCMC committed itself to going to court that the family claimed Mrs. Wanglie had said she would want to be kept alive. Dr. Miles mentions that during the months when she was on a respirator before becoming unconscious, Mrs. Wanglie at times pulled at her respirator tubing.

I agree that Mrs. Wanglie's views are less than certain. Yet for reasons given above and also because death is irrevocable, there should be a presumption in favor of life when a patient's views are unclear or unknown. Pulling at a respirator tube is obviously insufficient evidence of even a fleeting desire to die; it may simply be a semi-automatic attempt to relieve discomfort, like pulling away in a dentist's chair even when one has an overriding desire that the dental work be performed. Basically, although the circumstances of the family's claim about Mrs. Wanglie's statement of her views make the claim questionable, it is their word against nobody's. No one claims that she ever said she would prefer *not* to be kept alive, despite her months of conscious existence on a respirator.

It has also been argued that we should not allow patients to demand medically inappropriate care when the costs of that care are borne by others who have not consented to do so. I have already discussed the question of medical appropriateness. And a private health plan is paying for Mrs. Wanglie's care, a plan whose officials have publicly stated that cost should not be a factor in treatment decisions. The pool of subscribers to the plan, whose premiums are what indirectly subsidize Mrs. Wanglie's care, have, by being members of this plan, committed themselves to a practice of medicine that does not take cost into account. It would be unfair to make cost a factor in Mrs. Wanglie's treatment decision now. Public statements by health insurance plan officials are expected to be taken into account by consumers selecting health insurance and must not be reneged upon. Mrs. Wanglie's insurer is not seeking to renege. Instead, it is her *doctors* who have decided that her life is not worth prolonging.

Moreover, to say it would be the underlying disease rather than the act of removing the respirator that would cause Helga Wanglie's death is not helpful. If Mrs. Wanglie is, as the HCMC staff claims, irreversibly respirator-dependent, then saying that removing the respirator would cause her death is just as logical as saying that withdrawing a rope from a drowning man would cause his death, even if his death is to be "attributed" to his drowning. If the person in either case has an interest in living, one violates his interest by withdrawing the necessary means. This is what HCMC is seeking court permission to do to Mrs. Wanglie.

References

1. For example, consider the case of seventy-eight-year-old Earl Spring, whose mental deterioration did not prevent him from saying that he did not want to die. The statement of this preference was not considered conclusive reason to keep him on dialysis over his family's objections. Similarly, the *New York Times Magazine* recently described the situation of a severely disabled, elderly woman whose explicit advance directive that she wanted everything possible done to keep her alive was apparently ignored by both her husband and the hospital's ethics committee (K. Bouton, "Painful Decisions: The Role of the Medical Ethicist," 5 August 1990).
2. This argument comes from an unpublished letter from Dr. Steven Miles, made available to me by the *Hastings Center Report* at his request.
3. The Coons case was widely reported in newspapers. For example, see C. DeMare, " 'Hopeless' Hospital Patient, 86, Comes Out of Coma," *Albany Times Union,* 12 April 1989. Additional cases of this sort are cited in President's Commission for the Study of Ethical Problems in Medicine and Biomedical and Behavioral Research, *Deciding to Forego Life-Sustaining Treatment* (Washington, D.C.: U.S. Government Printing Office, 1983).
4. President's Commission, *Deciding to Forego Life-Sustaining Treatment,* p. 182.
5. President's Commission, *Deciding to Forego Life-Sustaining Treatment,* p. 183.
6. I have given this sort of argument in a letter to the *New York Times,* 4 November 1987, as well as in a short story about terminal illness, "The Forecasting Game," in *Prize Stories 1990: The O. Henry Awards,* ed. W. Abrahams (New York: Doubleday, 1990), pp. 315–35, and in an op-ed "No Thanks, I Don't Want to Die with Dignity," *Providence Journal-Bulletin,* 19 April 1990 (reprinted in other newspapers under various different titles).

POSTSCRIPT

Should Doctors Be Able to Refuse Demands for "Futile" Treatment?

Three days after the Minnesota court named Oliver Wanglie as his wife's legal conservator, thus preserving his right to make decisions about her treatment, Helga Wanglie died of multisystem organ failure. Her aggressive treatment had been continued throughout. Mr. Wanglie said, "We felt that when she was ready to go that the good Lord would call her, and I would say that's what happened." Her daughter said that her mother's care had been excellent; "We just had a disagreement on ethics."

A series of cases involving infants has extended the debate on medical futility. The most publicized case is that of "Baby K," who was born in 1992 with most of her brain missing. In most cases of this condition (anencephaly), babies die within a few days. Baby K's mother, however, insisted that Fairfax Hospital in Falls Church, Virginia, provide ventilator support to help the baby breathe, which kept her alive in a nursing home. In February 1994 the hospital's request to stop this treatment was denied by a federal appeals court, which extended to this case a federal law requiring hospitals to treat emergency patients even if they cannot pay. Payment was not an issue here, however, because the mother is a member of a Health Maintenance Organization, which paid the bills. Despite continued treatment, Baby K died in April 1995 at the age of three.

E. Haavi Morreim addresses the issue of how to preserve respect for moral diversity while preventing patients, families, physicians, and society from coercing one another into providing costly ineffective treatments in "Profoundly Diminished Life: The Casualties of Coercion," *Hastings Center Report* (January/February 1994).

John S. Paris and Frank E. Reardon provide a comprehensive overview of the cases in this area in "Physician Refusal of Requests for Futile or Ineffective Treatments," a chapter in *Emerging Issues in Biomedical Policy, vol. 2,* edited by Robert H. Blank and Andrea L. Bonnicksen (Columbia University Press, 1993). They and other authors discuss the Gilgunn case, another futility case, in "Use of a DNB Order Over Family Objections," *Journal of Intensive Care Medicine* (January–February 1999). See also "Futility and Hospital Policy," by Tom Tomlinson and Diane Czlonka, *Hastings Center Report* (May–June 1995); *Wrong Medicine,* by Lawrence J. Schneiderman and Nancy Jecker (Johns Hopkins University Press, 1995); and Marjorie and Howard Zucker, *Medical Futility and the Evaluation of Life-Sustaining Interventions* (Cambridge University Press, 1997).

On the Internet ...

NARAL Online

This is the home page of the National Abortion and Reproductive Rights Action League (NARAL), an organization that works to promote reproductive freedom and dignity for women and their families.

http://www.naral.org

The Ultimate Pro–Life Resource List

The Ultimate Pro-Life Resource List is the most comprehensive listing of right-to-life resources on the Internet.

http://www.prolifeinfo.org

The Lindesmith Center–Drug Policy Foundation

This site offers articles concerning the issue of punishing pregnant drug users as well as articles about the case of *Cornelia Whitner v. State of South Carolina.*

http://www.lindesmith.org/news/nyt30.html

PART 3

Choices in Reproduction

*F*ew bioethical issues could be of greater personal and social significance than questions concerning reproduction. Advances in medical technology, such as in vitro fertilization and egg donation have opened new possibilities for infertile couples, while challenging traditional notions of family. Some advances in genetic manipulation, such as cloning, are still in the experimental stage and raise complex ethical issues. Another type of technological advance, the ability to see images of the developing fetus, has enhanced our understanding of both normal growth and birth defects. This technology has provided evidence of the impact of the mother's behavior on fetal development. While many behaviors of pregnant women expose fetuses to risk, and while fathers' exposure to chemicals and other toxic substances also affect fetuses, attention has focused mainly on the mothers' use of illegal drugs. Preventing risk to fetuses raises troubling questions concerning the role of police and the courts in medical matters and the best way to assist drug-addicted women. In the late 1990s the polarized debate about the morality of abortion found a new focus: late-term abortions and the controversial procedures used at this stage of fetal development. The issues in this section come to grips with some of the most perplexing and fundamental questions that confront medical practitioners, individual women and their partners, and society in general.

- Should Abortions Late in Pregnancy Be Banned?

- Should Pregnant Women Be Punished for Exposing Fetuses to Risk?

ISSUE 7

Should Abortions Late in Pregnancy Be Banned?

YES: M. LeRoy Sprang and Mark G. Neerhof, from "Rationale for Banning Abortions Late in Pregnancy," *Journal of the American Medical Association* (August 26, 1998)

NO: David A. Grimes, from "The Continuing Need for Late Abortions," *Journal of the American Medical Association* (August 26, 1998)

ISSUE SUMMARY

YES: Physician M. LeRoy Sprang and osteopathic physician Mark G. Neerhof assert that late-term abortion is needlessly risky, inhumane, and ethically unacceptable. They state that all abortions of 23 weeks or later should be considered unethical unless the fetus has a lethal condition or the mother's life is endangered.

NO: While acknowledging that early abortion is safer, simpler, and less controversial, physician David A. Grimes contends that late-term abortion is fundamentally important to women's health because some medical conditions of both women and fetuses cannot be diagnosed early in pregnancy and because of the prevalence of incest and rape.

Abortion is the most divisive bioethical issue of our time. The issue has been a persistent one in history, but in the past 30 years or so the debate has polarized. One view—known as "pro-life"—sees abortion as the wanton slaughter of innocent life. The other view—"pro-choice"—considers abortion as an option that must be available to women if they are to control their own reproductive lives. According to the pro-life view, women who have access to "abortion on demand" put their own selfish whims ahead of an unborn child's right to life. According to the pro-choice view, women have the right to choose to have an abortion—especially if there is an overriding reason, such as preventing the birth of a child with a severe genetic defect or one conceived as a result of rape or incest.

Behind these strongly held convictions, as political scientist Mary Segers has pointed out, are widely differing views of what determines value (that is, whether value is inherent in a thing or ascribed to it by human beings), the relation between law and morality, and the use of limits of political solutions to social problems, as well as the value of scientific progress. Those who condemn abortion as immoral generally follow a classical tradition in which abortion is a public matter because it involves our conception of how we should live together in an ideal society. Those who accept the idea of abortion, on the other hand, generally share the liberal, individualistic ethos of contemporary society. They believe that abortion is a private choice, and that public policy should reflect how citizens actually behave, not some unattainable ideal.

While the moral right to an abortion remains an unresolved issue, certain types of abortion arouse more controversy than others. In the past few years the morality of late-term, or partial-birth, abortion has been the focus of heated debate in Congress, state legislatures, and other forums. In June 1995 a Partial-Birth Abortion Ban Act was introduced in Congress. The medical term for such abortions is *intact dilatation and extraction* (D&X), a variation of *dilatation and evacuation* (D&E). In intact D&X the fetus is partially delivered feet first and the contents of the brain partially extracted so that the fetus is born dead but otherwise intact. This is the most commonly used procedure in the second trimester. The number of late-term abortions performed annually, and whether this procedure is necessary, are points of disagreement.

This is what we know about abortion practices in America today: Abortion has been legal since the 1973 Supreme Court decision of *Roe v. Wade* declared that a woman has a constitutional right to privacy, which includes an abortion. According to the National Center on Health Statistics, abortion at eight weeks or less gestation is seven times safer than childbirth, although there are some unknown risks—primarily the effect of repeated abortions on subsequent pregnancies. Abortion is common: Each year about 1.5 million abortions are performed. That is, one out of four pregnancies (and half of all unintended pregnancies) end in abortion. Still, statistics released in 1998 show that the abortion rate in the United States is at its lowest point in 20 years. About 90 percent of all abortions are performed within the first 12 weeks of pregnancy by a method called suction aspiration. Eighty percent of the women who have abortions are unmarried, and nearly 63 percent are between the ages of 15 and 24. (In comparison, however, in 1965 there were between 200,000 and 1.2 million illegal abortions, and 20 percent of all deaths from childbirth or pregnancy were caused by botched abortions.) The national fertility rate reached a peak in 1990 and is somewhat lower today.

The following selections present differing views on the necessity and ethical justification for late-term abortion. M. LeRoy Sprang and Mark G. Neerhof argue that such abortions are unsafe for women, inhumane, and most often performed on fetuses that could survive. David A. Grimes counters that late-term abortion is safe and must be available for the health and well-being of the women most often involved in such procedures. These women are typically young, poor and uneducated, or minorities.

**M. LeRoy Sprang and
Mark G. Neerhof**

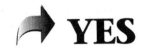 **YES**

Rationale for Banning Abortions
Late in Pregnancy

The abortion issue remains in the public eye and the media headlines largely because of a single late-term abortion procedure referred to in the medical literature as intact dilation and extraction (D&X) and in the common vernacular as partial-birth abortion. This [selection] reviews the medical and ethical aspects of this procedure and of late-term abortions in general. . . .

Ethical considerations.— Intact D&X is most commonly performed between 20 and 24 weeks and thereby raises questions of the potential viability of the fetus. . . .

Beyond the argument of potential viability, many prochoice organizations and individuals assert that a woman should maintain control over that which is part of her own body (ie, the autonomy argument). In this context, the physical position of the fetus with respect to the mother's body becomes relevant. However, once the fetus is outside the woman's body, the autonomy argument is invalid. The intact D&X procedure involves literally delivering the fetus so that only the head remains within the cervix. At this juncture, the fetus is merely inches from being delivered and obtaining full legal rights of personhood under the US Constitution. What happens when, as must occasionally occur during the performance of an intact D&X, the fetal head inadvertently slips out of the mother and a live infant is fully delivered? For this reason, many otherwise prochoice individuals have found intact D&X too close to infanticide to ethically justify its continued use.

Professional, legislative, and public concerns.— An extraordinary medical consensus has emerged that intact D&X is neither necessary nor the safest method for late-term abortion. In addition to American Medical Association (AMA) and ACOG [American College of Obstetricians and Gynecologists] policy statements, Warren Hern, MD, author of *Abortion Practice* has questioned the efficacy of intact D&X. "I have very serious reservations about this procedure. . . . You really can't defend it. . . . I would dispute any statement that this is the safest procedure to use."[1] . . .

From M. LeRoy Sprang and Mark G. Neerhof, "Rationale for Banning Abortions Late in Pregnancy," *Journal of the American Medical Association*, vol. 280, no. 8 (August 26, 1998), pp. 744–747. Copyright © 1998 by The American Medical Association. Reprinted by permission.

Legislative bodies across the United States have decided that intact D&X is not appropriate. In fact, 28 states have approved a ban, and Congress also overwhelmingly voted to ban the procedure with strong bipartisan support.[2] ...

Termination of Late-Term Pregnancies

Many of the medical and ethical issues that pertain to intact D&X also apply to late-term pregnancy terminations, defined for the purposes of this [selection] as termination beyond 20 weeks' gestation. Pregnancy termination at this gestational age can be accomplished either by labor induction or by D&E [dilation and evacuation].

Most clinicians would argue for maintaining the option of late pregnancy termination to save the life of the mother, which is an extraordinarily rare circumstance. Maternal health factors demanding pregnancy termination in the periviable period can almost always be accommodated without sacrificing the fetus and without compromising maternal well-being. The high probability of fetal intact survival beyond the periviable period argues for ending the pregnancy through appropriate delivery. In a similar fashion, the following discussion does not apply to fetuses with anomalies incompatible with prolonged survival. When pregnancy termination is performed for these indications, it should be performed in as humane a fashion as possible. Therefore, intact D&X should not be performed even in these circumstances. ...

Ethical considerations.— The autonomy of the pregnant woman is increasingly counterbalanced by fetal development, the increasing tendency to attribute personhood to the fetus, and the increasing likelihood of independent fetal viability. Fetal development affects maternal autonomy on an inversely sliding scale. As a fetus evolves into an individual capable of survival independent of its mother (and thus personhood), the conditional fetal rights argument gains greater merit.

A second ethical principle concerns beneficence, ie, one individual's obligation to act for the benefit of another. As the fetus matures, the majority of individuals would extend greater and greater beneficence to the fetus. According to Stubblefield, "Inevitably, there must be a gestational age limit for abortion. I would avoid performing abortions after 22 weeks unless the mother's life were endangered or unless the fetus had major malformations so severe as to preclude prolonged survival. ... When termination of pregnancy will be undertaken at or after 23 weeks because of serious risk for maternal health, the fetus should be considered as well."[3]

A third ethical principle concerns justice and denotes balancing the rights of distinct individuals. As the fetus develops, more and more people recognize that there are 2 distinct individuals involved. To take a position that would make the value of the fetus depend solely on private choice and on the individual exercise of power fails to understand the importance of communal safeguards against capricious power over life and death.[4]

Conclusions

Medical professionals have an obligation to thoughtfully consider the medical and ethical issues surrounding pregnancy termination, particularly with respect to intact D&X and late-term abortions. Having done so, we conclude the following: (1) Intact D&X (partial-birth abortion) should not be performed because it is needlessly risky, inhumane, and ethically unacceptable. This procedure is closer to infanticide than it is to abortion. (2) Abortions in the periviable period (currently 23 weeks) and beyond should be considered unethical, unless the fetus has a condition incompatible with prolonged survival or if the mother's life is endangered by the pregnancy. (3) If a maternal medical condition in the periviable period indicates pregnancy termination, the physician should wait, if the medical condition permits, until fetal survival is probable and then proceed with delivery. Such medical decisions must be individualized.

Physicians must preserve their role as healing, compassionate, caring professionals, while recognizing their ethical obligation to care for both the woman and the unborn child. In July 1997, the ACOG Executive Board supplemented its policy on abortion toward this end, stating, "ACOG is opposed to abortion of the healthy fetus that has attained viability in a healthy woman."[5]

We hope that with thoughtful discussions regarding specific issues such as those considered in this [selection], the opposing forces in the ongoing, stagnant abortion debate will find middle ground on which most can agree. The question is often asked, "But who should decide?" Ultimately, at least in the United States, the public will decide. The results of an August 1997 national poll showed public opinion firmly in the camp of "drawing a line" on abortion rights, with 61% believing that abortion should be legal only under certain circumstances, and 22% defending the legality of abortion under any circumstances.[6] Society will not [countenance] infanticide. According to Boston University ethicist and health law professor George Annas, JD, MPH, Americans see "a distinction between first trimester and second trimester abortions. The law doesn't, but people do. And rightfully so."[7] He explained that after approximately 20 weeks, the American public sees a baby. The American public's vision of this may be much clearer than that of some of the physicians involved.

References

1. Gianelli DM. Outlawing abortion method. *American Medical News.* November 20, 1995:3, 70–72.
2. *Status of Bans on "Partial-Birth Abortion" and Other Abortion Methods.* New York, NY: Center for Reproductive Law and Policy; June 29, 1998.
3. Stubblefield PJ. Pregnancy termination. In: Gabbe SG, Niebyl JR, Simpsons JL, eds. *Obstetrics, Normal and Problem Pregnancies.* 3rd ed. New York, NY: Churchill Livingston; 1996:1243–1278.
4. Callahan D. The abortion debate: can this chronic public illness be cured? In: Chervenak FA, McCullough LD, eds. *Clin Obstet Gynecol.* 1992;35:783–791.

5. *ACOG Statement of Policy.* Approved by executive board and published in ACOG newsletter; July 1997.
6. Padawer R. "Partial-birth" battle changing public views. *USA Today.* November 17, 1997:17A.
7. Gianelli DM. Medicine adds to debate on late-term abortion. *American Medical News.* March 3, 1997:3, 54–56.

David A. Grimes 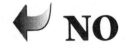 **NO**

The Continuing Need for Late Abortions

Late abortion is the most controversial aspect of the most divisive social issue of our times.[1] The debate has been strident, confusing, and at times, misleading.[2] ...

Epidemiology and Techniques of Late Abortion

For decades, late induced abortions have been uncommon in the United States. From 1972 through 1992, the proportion of all induced abortions that were performed at 21 or more weeks' gestation ranged from 0.8% to 1.7%.[3] The upper gestational age limit varies by state. However, the claim that many women have elective abortions in the third trimester lacks support. Most reports of abortions at 25 or more weeks' gestation are due to reporting errors or to fetal demise. Between 1979 and 1980, only 3 cases of approximately 70,000 reported induced abortions in Georgia took place at 25 weeks or more. Two procedures were performed for fetal anencephaly, and insufficient information was available for the third.[4] This is believed to be the only published [material] on this procedure.

Dilation and evacuation (D&E) is the most frequent method used for late abortion in the United States. In 1992, D&E accounted for 86% of all abortions at 21 or more weeks' gestation, whereas labor induction accounted for 14%....

Morbidity and Mortality of Late Abortions

... Compared with labor induction, D&E is preferable in terms of compassion, cost, comfort, and convenience. Negative reactions to second-trimester abortion are directly related to contact with the fetus. Aborting a fetus can be emotionally difficult for women, especially for those who are alone in a hospital in the middle of the night. In contrast, during D&E abortion women have no contact with the fetus. The operation transfers the emotional burden of abortion from women, who have often suffered greatly, to the staff. Dilation and evacuation abortion obviates the need for costly overnight stays in hospital, as is customary with labor induction. Women having D&E abortions are spared a "maxi-labor" followed by a "mini-delivery." Instead of enduring labor, women receive local or general anesthesia for the brief operation. Finally, because D&E

From David A. Grimes, "The Continuing Need for Late Abortions," *Journal of the American Medical Association,* vol. 280, no. 8 (August 26, 1998), pp. 747–750. Copyright © 1998 by The American Medical Association. Reprinted by permission.

abortion takes place on an outpatient basis, women's lives are less disrupted than with hospitalization for 1 or more nights.

Characteristics of Women Who Have Late Abortions

Women who have late abortions often are disadvantaged. Teenagers, especially those younger than 15 years, and women of minority status disproportionately have late abortions.[3] Many of these patients either do not suspect the pregnancy or attempt to conceal it until the pregnancy becomes evident. Menstrual irregularity is an important risk factor.[5] Women with irregular menses often discover late that they are pregnant. Other risk factors include young age, low educational attainment, having had a sexually transmitted disease, and ambivalence about the decision to abort. Thus, many of the factors associated with late abortions are not easily changed.[6]

Women seeking late abortions are often disadvantaged in other ways, such as lack of knowledge about options, lack of money to pay for the procedure, lack of transportation to a provider, and alcohol or other drug dependence. Some young women are unaware of the availability of late abortions. Since enactment of the Hyde Amendment, the federal government has not paid for indigent women to have abortions, and few states subsidize abortion services. Hence, some women need weeks to raise the money to pay for an abortion, which delays the procedure until the second trimester. Of note, states that fund abortions have significantly lower rates of teen pregnancy, low-birth-weight babies, premature births, and births with late or no prenatal care than do other states.

Geography poses yet another barrier: more than 80% of US counties do not have an abortion provider. Providers of late abortion are even more scarce. In 1993, only 13% of US abortion providers offered abortions at 21 weeks, and the cost averaged more than $1000.[7]

Indications for Late Abortion

Late abortions are fundamentally important to women's reproductive health.[1] Antenatal fetal diagnosis, such as maternal α-fetoprotein screening and amniocentesis, is predicated on the availability of induced abortion. Although techniques such as chorionic villus sampling and early amniocentesis have allowed earlier diagnosis, by the time results of midtrimester amniocentesis or ultrasound are available, a woman may be beyond 20 weeks' gestation.[8]

Ironically, the availability of late abortion is pronatalist. About 98% of women who undergo genetic screening receive reassuring news.[9] Without the availability of prenatal diagnosis with abortion as an option, many of these women would not have become pregnant or would have aborted all pregnancies that occurred.[10] As noted by Cook,[11] "Macroethical reasons favouring legal abortion in such circumstances rest on the potential to do greater good than harm in the community, and reveal the positive, life-affirming aspects of legally available abortion services."

Illnesses of women and fetal anomalies lead to requests for late abortions. Late abortion can be lifesaving for women with medical disorders aggravated by pregnancy.[12] Conditions such as Eisenmenger syndrome carry a high risk of maternal morbidity and mortality in pregnancy, the latter ranging from 20% to 30%.[13] In recent years, I have performed late abortions for a Kampuchean refugee with craniopagus conjoined twins and a 25-year-old woman with a 9 × 15-cm thoracic aortic aneurysm from newly diagnosed Marfan syndrome. Cancer sometimes makes late abortion necessary. For example, either radical hysterectomy or radiation therapy for cervical cancer before fetal viability involves abortion.

Incest and rape are other compelling indications. Pregnancies resulting from incest among young teenagers or among women with mental handicaps may escape detection until the pregnancy is advanced. Approximately 32,000 pregnancies result from rape each year in the United States; about half of rape victims receive no medical attention, and about one third do not discover the pregnancy until the second trimester.[14]

Gestational Age Limit for Abortion

The appropriate upper gestational age limit for abortion remains elusive. Most Americans reject absolutist positions on abortion. Absolutist positions are problematic "because no such account can claim final intellectual or moral authority, given the necessarily disputable nature of all accounts of the independent moral status of the fetus."[15]

Instead, most Americans choose the moderate or gradualist view. This holds that the fetus gains increasing human worth as pregnancy advances. "The main difficulty with moderate views of abortion is that they lack the precision of the liberal and the conservative views. Knowledge of fetal development is constantly increasing and no sharp divisions can be drawn between one stage and the next."[16] Given these ambiguities, compassion, tolerance, and judgment are needed to balance the competing interests of fetus, woman, and society.

Some argue that the gestational age limit for abortion should be the point of viability. This is a shifting target, and physicians cannot predict the probability of extrauterine survival for a given fetus. However, few abortion supporters would consider elective abortion after viability morally acceptable, except in rare circumstances in which the fetus has an anomaly incompatible with life.[17] Others[18] claim that neurological development should define the limit: when the fetus becomes sentient, abortion should be impermissible.

Women ultimately determine the status of the fetus. "Thus, before viability, a pregnant woman is free to withhold, confer, or, having once conferred, withdraw the status of being a patient from the fetus." In other words, "for secular gynecologic ethics, the abortion controversy regarding previable fetuses is resolved for physicians by the autonomous decision of the woman regarding her pregnancy and the dependent moral status of the fetus as a patient."[15]

Attempts to Ban a Late Abortion Method

... If late abortions were restricted or eliminated, the alternatives that would remain for women would include illegal abortion, adoption, and rearing a child initially unwanted. Studies of women denied abortions have provided important insights.[19] Some women denied abortion seek the procedure elsewhere and succeed; the high rates of reported spontaneous abortion among women in these studies are suspicious. Few women (7%–19%) place their children for adoption.

Children born after their mothers are denied abortion face serious challenges. In a classic study from Scandinavia, these children had a more insecure childhood, more delinquency, more psychiatric care, and more early marriages than did children in a comparison group.[19] ... Denying requested abortions has adverse consequences that persist at least into early adulthood.

Conclusions

As noted by Macklin,[20] "The three leading principles of bioethics—respect for persons, beneficence and justice—together provide an ethical mandate for guaranteeing to women throughout the world a legal right to safe abortion." This mandate is especially important for the immature, disadvantaged, and often seriously ill women requesting late abortions in the United States. Regardless of political views on abortion, the scientific evidence is clear and incontrovertible: legal abortion, including late abortion, has been a resounding public health success.

Early abortion is safer, simpler, and less controversial than late abortion. Improving sex education, promoting access to safe and effective contraception, and removing economic and geographic barriers to early abortion can help to reduce the number of late abortions. This is a goal around which there should be broad consensus. Nevertheless, as experience has revealed,[3] the need for late abortion will not disappear. Hence, our continuing responsibility as physicians and as a society is to ensure that these procedures are as safe, comfortable, and compassionate as possible. Women deserve no less from their physicians.

References

1. Rosenfield A. The difficult issue of second-trimester abortion. *N Engl J Med.* 1994;331:324–325.
2. Rich F. Partial-truth abortion. *New York Times.* March 9, 1997:15.
3. Koonin LM, Smith JC, Ramick M, Green CA. Abortion surveillance—United States, 1992. *MMWR Morb Mortal Wkly Rep.* 1996:45 (SS-3):1–36.
4. Spitz AM, Lee NC, Grimes DA, Schoenbucher AK, Lavoie M. Third-trimester induced abortion in Georgia, 1979 and 1980. *Am J Public Health.* 1983;73:594–595.
5. Burr WA, Schulz KF. Delayed abortion in an area of easy accessibility. *JAMA.* 1980;244:44–48.
6. Guilbert E, Marcoux S, Rioux JE. Factors associated with the obtaining of a second-trimester induced abortion. *Can J Public Health.* 1994;85:402–406.
7. Henshaw SK. Factors hindering access to abortion services. *Fam Plann Perspect.* 1995;27:54–59, 87.

8. Timothy J, Harris R. Late terminations of pregnancy following second trimester amniocentesis. *Br J Obstet Gynaecol.* 1986;93:343–347.
9. Farmakides G, Bracero L, Marion R, Fleischer A, Schulman H. Pregnancy termination after detection of fetal chromosomal or metabolic abnormalities. *J Perinatol,* 1988;8:101–104.
10. Hewitt J, Coyle PC. Termination of pregnancy limit: 28, 24, or 18 weeks. *Lancet.* 1988;1:186–187.
11. Cook RJ. Legal abortion: limits and contributions to human life. In: Porter R, O'Connor M, eds. *Abortion: Medical Progress and Social Implications.* London, England: Pitman; 1985:211–227.
12. Bowers CH, Chervenak, JL, Chervenak FA. Late-second-trimester pregnancy termination with dilation and evacuation in critically ill women. *J Reprod Med.* 1989;34:880–883.
13. Gleicher N, Midwall J, Hochberger D, Jaffin H. Eisenmenger's syndrome and pregnancy. *Obstet Gynecol Surv.* 1979;34:721–741.
14. Holmes MM, Resnick HS, Kilpatrick DG, Best CL. Rape-related pregnancy: estimates and descriptive characteristics from a national sample of women. *Am J Obstet Gynecol.* 1996;175:320–324.
15. McCullough LB, Chervenak FA. *Ethics in Obstetrics and Gynecology.* New York, NY: Oxford University Press; 1994:166–195.
16. Campbell AV. Viability and the moral status of the fetus. In: Porter R, O'Connor M, eds. *Abortion: Medical Progress and Social Implications.* London, England: Pitman; 1985:228–243.
17. Chervenak FA, Farley MA, Walters L, Hobbins JC, Mahoney MJ. When is termination of pregnancy during the third trimester morally justifiable? *N Engl J Med.* 1984;310:501–504.
18. Jones DG. Brain birth and personal identity. *J Med Ethics.* 1989;15:173–178.
19. Dagg PKB. The psychological sequelae of therapeutic abortion: denied and completed. *Am J Psychiatry.* 1991;148:578–585.
20. Macklin R. Abortion controversies: ethics, politics and religion. In: Baird DT, Grimes DA, van Look PFA, eds. *Modern Methods of Inducing Abortion.* Oxford, England: Blackwell Science; 1995:170–189.

POSTSCRIPT

Should Abortions Late in Pregnancy Be Banned?

In June 2000, the U.S. Supreme Court struck down a Nebraska law making it a crime to perform a "partial birth abortion." The 5–4 vote was the first abortion rights ruling in eight years. Approximately 30 states have laws similar to the Nebraska statute.

After President Bill Clinton vetoed the first Partial-Birth Abortion Ban Act in April 1996, Senator Rick Santorum (R-Pennsylvania) reintroduced the bill. In the second round, medical organizations, such as the American Medical Association (AMA), which had either taken no position or urged the president to veto the first bill, now supported it. Others, such as the American College of Obstetrics and Gynecologists, found that while intact dilation and extraction did not seem to be the only procedure available in any case, only the woman's physician should make the decision about what procedure to use. The AMA's position, later rescinded, was particularly controversial because it agreed to support the legislation if Senator Santorum added two procedural amendments that served physicians' interests.

Congress passed the bill a second time in 1997, and again President Clinton vetoed it because, he said, it failed to include an exception for abortions that would be performed to prevent "serious harm" to a woman's health. More than two dozen states have passed late-term abortion bans. In Wisconsin abortion clinics shut down for a week after the late-term abortion ban was passed because doctors and staff feared that they would be prosecuted for performing early-term as well as late-term abortions. The abortion clinics remained closed until local district attorneys agreed not to prosecute physicians who performed abortions before 16 weeks' gestation.

In "Partial Birth Abortion, Congress, and the Constitution," *The New England Journal of Medicine* (July 23, 1998), George J. Annas reviews the legislative and judicial history of partial-birth abortion as well as of government regulation of medical procedures. See also "Late-Term Abortion," by Janet E. Gans Epner, Harry S. Jonas, and Daniel L. Seckinger, *Journal of the American Medical Association* (August 26, 1998), which provides background on the issue.

For a history of the political and ethical issues surrounding abortion in the United States, see Eva R. Rubin's *The Abortion Controversy: A Documentary History* (Greenwood, 1994). Abortion technology may change if mifepristone, also known as RU-486, becomes widely used. This drug provides a nonsurgical technique for terminating early pregnancies. Long used in Europe, it was approved for use in the United States by the Food and Drug Administration in 1996.

ISSUE 8

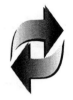

Should Pregnant Women Be Punished for Exposing Fetuses to Risk?

YES: Jean Toal, from Majority Opinion, *Cornelia Whitner, Respondent, v. State of South Carolina, Petitioner* (July 15, 1997)

NO: Alexander Morgan Capron, from "Punishing Mothers," *Hastings Center Report* (January–February 1998)

ISSUE SUMMARY

YES: In a case involving a pregnant woman's use of crack cocaine, a majority of the Supreme Court of South Carolina ruled that a state legislature may impose additional criminal penalties on pregnant drug-using women without violating their constitutional right of privacy.

NO: Law professor Alexander Morgan Capron argues that the Supreme Court of South Carolina's decision may lead society to punish pregnant women who expose fetuses to many different types of risk, including women who have multiple births due to fertility drugs.

At first glance, Cornelia Whitner and Bobbi McCaughey have absolutely nothing in common. Cornelia Whitner gave birth to a baby after using crack cocaine in the last trimester of pregnancy. She was arrested and convicted of child neglect. Bobbi McCaughey gave birth to seven babies in November 1997 to public acclaim and an avalanche of gifts and community support. Yet she too placed her babies at risk, simply by the use of fertility drugs and her decision to continue the multiple pregnancy. Through laws and public attitudes, society views the risks taken by Whitner and McCaughey very differently and punishes or rewards women accordingly.

In 1989, fueled by the specter of an epidemic of drug use resulting in the birth of thousands of "crack babies," the Medical University of South Carolina established a program that required drug-using pregnant women to seek treatment and prenatal care or face criminal prosecution. This program applied only to patients attending the university's obstetric clinic, primarily poor black women, and not to private patients. Patients enrolled in the clinic saw a video and were given written information about the harmful effects of substance abuse during pregnancy. The information warned that the Charleston, South Carolina, police, the court system, and child protective services might become involved if illegal drug use were detected.

Women who met certain criteria were required to undergo periodic urine screening for drugs. A patient who had a positive urine test or who failed to keep scheduled appointments for therapy or prenatal care could be arrested and placed in custody. If a woman delivered a baby who tested positive for drugs, she would be arrested immediately after her medical release and her newborn taken into protective custody. If the drug use was detected within the first 27 weeks of gestation, the patient was charged with possession of an illegal substance; after that date, the charge was possession and distribution of an illegal substance to a minor. If the drug use were detected during delivery, the woman would be charged with unlawful neglect of a child.

This stringent policy was developed as a result of clinicians' concern about the harmful effects of drug use on fetal development and prosecutors' desires to take a strong public stand condemning drug use. Although the stated goal was to get women into treatment, there were few places that women could receive treatment and the necessary support, such as transportation and child care. At the time there was no women-only residential treatment center for substance-abusing pregnant women anywhere in the state.

The program ended because the federal Office of Protection from Research Risks determined that it constituted human experimentation conducted without required institutional review board approval. This determination was based on a published report comparing the outcomes before and after the program. The university's approval as a site that could receive federal funds was placed in jeopardy.

By the time the policy was discontinued in September 1994 as the result of a settlement with the Civil Rights Division of the federal Department of Health and Human Services, 42 pregnant women had been arrested. One of those women was Cornelia Whitner, whose baby was born with cocaine metabolites in his system. Whitner admitted to using crack cocaine during her pregnancy. Charged with criminal child neglect, she pled guilty and was sentenced to eight years in prison. She appealed the decision on the grounds that the law covered children, not fetuses, and her case went to the Supreme Court of South Carolina.

The court's majority decision, written by Justice Jean Toal, found that the state's statute includes a fetus within its definition of "child" and ruled that the state was not violating Whitner's constitutional right of privacy by punishing her for endangering her child through an already illegal activity. Alexander Morgan Capron finds the decision troubling because it can lead to a far greater range of acts for which prosecution is possible. This can include, theoretically, exposing fetuses to risk through multiple-birth pregnancies caused by using fertility drugs. He concludes that medical professionals must do more to help women adopt behaviors that reduce risk to their children.

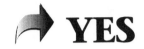 **YES**

Majority Opinion

Whitner *v.* South Carolina ... ,

This case concerns the scope of the child abuse and endangerment statute in the South Carolina Children's Code. We hold the word "child" as used in that statute includes viable fetuses.

Facts

On April 20, 1992, Cornelia Whitner (Whitner) pled guilty to criminal child neglect, S.C.Code Ann. § 20-7-50 (1985), for causing her baby to be born with cocaine metabolites in its system by reason of Whitner's ingestion of crack cocaine during the third trimester of her pregnancy. The circuit court judge sentenced Whitner to eight years in prison. Whitner did not appeal her conviction.

Thereafter, Whitner filed a petition for Post Conviction Relief (PCR), pleading the circuit court's lack of subject matter jurisdiction to accept her guilty plea as well as ineffective assistance of counsel. Her claim of ineffective assistance of counsel was based upon her lawyer's failure to advise her the statute under which she was being prosecuted might not apply to prenatal drug use. The petition was granted on both grounds. The State appeals.

Law/Analysis

... South Carolina law has long recognized that viable fetuses are persons holding certain legal rights and privileges. In 1960, this Court decided Hall v. Murphy, 236 S.C. 257, 113 S.E.2d 790 (1960). That case concerned the application of South Carolina's wrongful death statute to an infant who died four hours after her birth as a result of injuries sustained prenatally during viability. The Appellants argued that a viable fetus was not a person within the purview of the wrongful death statute, because, inter alia, a fetus is thought to have no separate being apart from the mother.

We found such a reason for exclusion from recovery "unsound, illogical and unjust," and concluded there was "no medical or other basis" for the

From *Cornelia Whitner, Respondent, v. State of South Carolina, Petitioner,* 328 S.C. 1, 492 S.E. 2d 777 (1997). Notes and some case citations omitted.

"assumed identity" of mother and viable unborn child. In light of that conclusion, this Court unanimously held: "We have no difficulty in concluding that a fetus having reached that period of prenatal maturity where it is capable of independent life apart from its mother is a person."

Four years later, in Fowler v. Woodward, 244 S.C. 608, 138 S.E.2d 42 (1964), we interpreted Hall as supporting a finding that a viable fetus injured while still in the womb need not be born alive for another to maintain an action for the wrongful death of the fetus.

> Since a viable child is a person before separation from the body of its mother and since prenatal injuries tortiously inflicted on such a child are actionable, it is apparent that the complaint alleges such an "act, neglect or default" by the defendant, to the injury of the child. . . .
>
> Once the concept of the unborn, viable child as a person is accepted, we have no difficulty in holding that a cause of action for tortious injury to such a child arises immediately upon the infliction of the injury. . . .

More recently, [in State v. Horne,] we held the word "person" as used in a criminal statute includes viable fetuses. . . . The defendant in that case stabbed his wife, who was nine months' pregnant, in the neck, arms, and abdomen. Although doctors performed an emergency caesarean section to deliver the child, the child died while still in the womb. The defendant was convicted of voluntary manslaughter and appealed his conviction on the ground South Carolina did not recognize the crime of feticide.

This Court disagreed. In a unanimous decision, we held it would be "grossly inconsistent . . . to construe a viable fetus as a 'person' for the purposes of imposing civil liability while refusing to give it a similar classification in the criminal context." Accordingly, the Court recognized the crime of feticide with respect to viable fetuses.

Similarly, we do not see any rational basis for finding a viable fetus is not a "person" in the present context. Indeed, it would be absurd to recognize the viable fetus as a person for purposes of homicide laws and wrongful death statutes but not for purposes of statutes proscribing child abuse. Our holding in Hall that a viable fetus is a person rested primarily on the plain meaning of the word "person" in light of existing medical knowledge concerning fetal development. We do not believe that the plain and ordinary meaning of the word "person" has changed in any way that would now deny viable fetuses status as persons.

The policies enunciated in the Children's Code also support our plain meaning reading of "person." S.C.Code Ann. § 20-7-20(C) (1985), which describes South Carolina's policy concerning children, expressly states: "It shall be the policy of this State to concentrate on the prevention of children's problems as the most important strategy which can be planned and implemented on behalf of children and their families." (emphasis added) The abuse or neglect of a child at any time during childhood can exact a profound toll on the child herself as well as on society as a whole. However, the consequences of abuse or neglect which takes place after birth often pale in comparison to those resulting from abuse suffered by the viable fetus before birth. This policy of prevention supports a reading of the word "person" to include viable fetuses. Furthermore, the scope of the Children's Code is quite broad. It applies "to all children who have need of services." . . . When coupled with the comprehensive remedial purposes of the Code, this language supports the inference that the legislature intended to include viable fetuses within the scope of the Code's protection.

Whitner advances several arguments against an interpretation of "person" as used in the Children's Code to include viable fetuses. We shall address each of Whitner's major arguments in turn.

Whitner's first argument concerns the number of bills introduced in the South Carolina General Assembly in the past five years addressing substance abuse by pregnant women. Some of these bills would have criminalized substance abuse by pregnant women; others would have addressed the issue through mandatory reporting, treatment, or intervention by social service agencies. Whitner suggests that the introduction of several bills touching the specific issue at hand evinces a belief by legislators that prior legislation had not addressed the issue. Whitner argues the introduction of the bills proves that section 20-7-50 was not intended to encompass abuse or neglect of a viable fetus.

We disagree with Whitner's conclusion about the significance of the proposed legislation. Generally, the legislature's subsequent acts "cast no light on the intent of the legislature which enacted the statute being construed." . . . Rather, this Court will look first to the language of the statute to discern legislative intent, because the language itself is the best guide to legislative intent. . . . Here, we see no reason to look beyond the statutory language. . . . Additionally, our existing case law strongly supports our conclusion about the meaning of the statute's language.

Whitner also argues an interpretation of the statute that includes viable fetuses would lead to absurd results obviously not intended by the legislature. Specifically, she claims if we interpret "child" to include viable fetuses, every action by a pregnant woman that endangers or is likely to endanger a fetus, whether otherwise legal or illegal, would constitute unlawful neglect under the statute. For example, a woman might be prosecuted under section 20-7-50 for smoking or drinking during pregnancy. Whitner asserts these "absurd" results could not have been intended by the legislature and, therefore, the statute should not be construed to include viable fetuses.

We disagree for a number of reasons. First, the same arguments against the statute can be made whether or not the child has been born. After the birth of a child, a parent can be prosecuted under section 20-7-50 for an action that is likely to endanger the child without regard to whether the action is illegal in itself. For example, a parent who drinks excessively could, under certain circumstances, be guilty of child neglect or endangerment even though the underlying act—consuming alcoholic beverages—is itself legal. Obviously, the legislature did not think it "absurd" to allow prosecution of parents for such otherwise legal acts when the acts actually or potentially endanger the "life, health or comfort" of the parents' born children. We see no reason such a result should be rendered absurd by the mere fact the child at issue is a viable fetus.

Moreover, we need not address this potential parade of horribles advanced by Whitner. In this case, which is the only case we are called upon to decide here, certain facts are clear. Whitner admits to having ingested crack cocaine during the third trimester of her pregnancy, which caused her child to be born with cocaine in its system. Although the precise effects of maternal crack use during pregnancy are somewhat unclear, it is well documented and within the realm of public knowledge that such use can cause serious harm to the viable unborn child.... There can be no question here Whitner endangered the life, health, and comfort of her child. We need not decide any cases other than the one before us.

We are well aware of the many decisions from other states' courts throughout the country holding maternal conduct before the birth of the child does not give rise to criminal prosecution under state child abuse/endangerment or drug distribution statutes.... Many of these cases were prosecuted under statutes forbidding delivery or distribution of illicit substances and depended on statutory construction of the terms "delivery" and "distribution." ... Obviously, such cases are inapplicable to the present situation. The cases concerning child endangerment statutes or construing the terms "child" and "person" are also distinguishable, because the states in which these cases were decided have entirely different bodies of case law from South Carolina....

Massachusetts, however, has a body of case law substantially similar to South Carolina's, yet a Massachusetts trial court [in Commonwealth v. Pellegrini,] has held that a mother pregnant with a viable fetus is not criminally liable for transmission of cocaine to the fetus.... Specifically, Massachusetts law allows wrongful death actions on behalf of viable fetuses injured in utero who are not subsequently born alive. Mone v. Greyhound Lines, Inc., 368 Mass. 354, 331 N.E.2d 916 (1975). Similarly, Massachusetts law permits homicide prosecutions of third parties who kill viable fetuses. See Commonwealth v. Cass, 392 Mass. 799, 467 **783 N.E.2d 1324 (1984) (ruling a viable fetus is a person for purposes of vehicular homicide statute); Commonwealth v. Lawrence, 404 Mass. 378, 536 N.E.2d 571 (1989) (viable fetus is a person for purposes of common law crime of murder). Because of the similarity of the case law in Massachusetts to ours, the Pellegrini decision merits examination.

In Pellegrini, the Massachusetts Superior Court found that state's distribution statute does not apply to the distribution of an illegal substance to a viable fetus. The statute at issue forbade distribution of cocaine to persons under the age of eighteen. Rather than construing the word "distribution," however, the superior court found that a viable fetus is not a "person under the age of eighteen" within the meaning of the statute. In so finding, the court had to distinguish [Commonwealth v.] Lawrence and [Commonwealth v.] Cass, both of which held viable fetuses are "persons" for purposes of criminal laws in Massachusetts.

The Massachusetts trial court found Lawrence and Cass "accord legal rights to the unborn only where the mother's or parents' interest in the potentiality of life, not the state's interest, are sought to be vindicated." In other words, a viable fetus should only be accorded the rights of a person for the sake of its mother or both its parents. Under this rationale, the viable fetus lacks rights of its own that deserve vindication. Whitner suggests we should interpret our decisions in Hall, Fowler, and Horne to accord rights to the viable fetus only when doing so protects the special parent-child relationship rather than any individual rights of the fetus or any State interest in potential life. We do not think Hall, Fowler, and Horne can be interpreted so narrowly.

If the Pellegrini decision accurately characterizes the rationale underlying Mone, Lawrence, and Cass, then the reasoning of those cases differs substantially from our reasoning in Hall, Fowler, and Horne. First, Hall, Fowler, and Horne were decided primarily on the basis of the meaning of "person" as understood in the light of existing medical knowledge, rather than based on any policy of protecting the relationship between mother and child. As a homicide case, Horne also rested on the State's—not the mother's—interest in vindicating the life of the viable fetus. Moreover, the United States Supreme Court has repeatedly held that the states have a compelling interest in the life of a viable fetus.... If, as Whitner suggests we should, we read Horne only as a vindication of the mother's interest in the life of her unborn child, there would be no basis for prosecuting a mother who kills her viable fetus by stabbing it, by shooting it, or by other such means, yet a third party could be prosecuted for the very same acts. We decline to read Horne in a way that insulates the mother from all culpability for harm to her viable child. Because the rationale underlying our body of law—protection of the viable fetus—is radically different from that underlying the law of Massachusetts, we decline to follow the decision of the Massachusetts Superior Court in Pellegrini....

Right to Privacy

Whitner argues that prosecuting her for using crack cocaine after her fetus attains viability unconstitutionally burdens her right of privacy, or, more specifically, her right to carry her pregnancy to term. We disagree.

Whitner argues that section 20-7-50 burdens her right of privacy, a right long recognized by the United States Supreme Court.... She cites Cleveland Board of Education v. LaFleur, 414 U.S. 632, 94 S.Ct. 791, 39 L.Ed.2d 52 (1974), as standing for the proposition that the Constitution protects women from measures penalizing them for choosing to carry their pregnancies to term.

In LaFleur, two junior high school teachers challenged their school systems' maternity leave policies. The policies required "every pregnant school teacher to take maternity leave without pay, beginning [four or] five months before the expected birth of her child." A teacher on maternity leave could not return to work "until the beginning of the next regular school semester which follows the date when her child attains the age of three months." The two teachers, both of whom had become pregnant and were required against their wills to comply with the school system's policies, argued that the policies were unconstitutional.

The United States Supreme Court agreed. It found that "[b]y acting to penalize the pregnant teacher for deciding to bear a child, overly restrictive maternity leave regulations can constitute a heavy burden on the exercise of these protected freedoms." The Court then scrutinized the policies to determine whether "the interests advanced in support of" the policy could "justify the particular procedures [the School Boards] ha[d] adopted." Although it found that the purported justification for the policy—continuity of instruction—was a "significant and legitimate educational goal," the Court concluded that the "absolute requirement[ ] of termination at the end of the fourth or fifth month of pregnancy" was not a rational means for achieving continuity of instruction and that such a requirement "may serve to hinder attainment of the very continuity objectives that they are purportedly designed to promote." Finding no rational relationship between the purpose of the maternity leave policy and the means crafted to achieve that end, the Court concluded the policy violated the Due Process Clause of the Fourteenth Amendment.

Whitner argues that the alleged violation here is far more egregious than that in LaFleur. She first suggests that imprisonment is a far greater burden on her exercise of her freedom to carry the fetus to term than was the unpaid maternity leave in LaFleur. Although she is, of course, correct that imprisonment is more severe than unpaid maternity leave, Whitner misapprehends the fundamentally different nature of her own interests and those of the government in this case as compared to those at issue in LaFleur.

First, the State's interest in protecting the life and health of the viable fetus is not merely legitimate. It is compelling. . . .

Even more importantly, however, we do not think any fundamental right of Whitner's—or any right at all, for that matter—is implicated under the present scenario. It strains belief for Whitner to argue that using crack cocaine during pregnancy is encompassed within the constitutionally recognized right of privacy. Use of crack cocaine is illegal, period. No one here argues that laws criminalizing the use of crack cocaine are themselves unconstitutional. If the State wishes to impose additional criminal penalties on pregnant women who engage in this already illegal conduct because of the effect the conduct has on the viable fetus, it may do so. We do not see how the fact of pregnancy elevates the use of crack cocaine to the lofty status of a fundamental right.

Moreover, as a practical matter, we do not see how our interpretation of section 20-7-50 imposes a burden on Whitner's right to carry her child to term. In LaFleur, the Supreme Court found that the mandatory maternity leave policies burdened women's rights to carry their pregnancies to term because the policies prevented pregnant teachers from exercising a freedom they would have enjoyed but for their pregnancies. In contrast, during her pregnancy after the fetus attained viability, Whitner enjoyed the same freedom to use cocaine that she enjoyed earlier in and predating her pregnancy—none whatsoever. Simply put, South Carolina's child abuse and endangerment statute as applied to this case does not restrict Whitner's freedom in any way that it was not already restricted. The State's imposition of an additional penalty when a pregnant woman with a viable fetus engages in the already proscribed behavior does not burden a woman's right to carry her pregnancy to term; rather, the additional penalty simply recognizes that a third party (the viable fetus or newborn child) is harmed by the behavior.

Section 20-7-50 does not burden Whitner's right to carry her pregnancy to term or any other privacy right. Accordingly, we find no violation of the Due Process Clause of the Fourteenth Amendment.

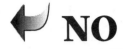

Punishing Mothers

What should society do when a woman, in producing children, exposes them to avoidable risks? That recurring question—which plunges one quickly and deeply into the murky waters of child protection, women's rights, and the far reaches of medical science—has been back on the front pages recently. Two very different stories illustrate how context affects our answer.

Multiple Births

[In the] fall [of 1997] the international media cast the bright, warm glow of an approving spotlight on Carlisle, Iowa, the home of Kenny and Bobbi Mc-Caughey, who gave birth to four boys and three girls on 20 November. The babies, who were born two months premature and ranged from 2.5 to 3.4 pounds, seem to be doing well, making them the first surviving septuplets in the world. With the use of fertility drugs and in vitro fertilization, multiple births are becoming more frequent; for example, fifty-seven quintuplets were born in the United States in 1995. A few months before the McCaugheys' babies, septuplets were born in Saudi Arabia but six died, and in May 1985 an American woman carrying seven fetuses gave birth to six (the seventh was stillborn) but lost three within nineteen days.

Most media coverage was supportive of the McCaugheys, as were friends and neighbors in their small town, the governor of Iowa, and numerous business enterprises, which promised a new house (to replace the two bedroom home the couple had shared with their two-year-old daughter Mikayla), an extra-large van, and life-time supplies of such items as disposable diapers. While parents who had experienced the heavy demands of multiple births warned of everything from sleepless nights to bankruptcy, the general sentiment was summed up by the septuplets' maternal grandfather Robert Hepworth, who termed their births "a miracle."

Still, a few objections were voiced by physicians as well as ethicists. Fertility specialists in Britain, where artificial reproduction (but not the use of fertility drugs) is closely regulated, raised "serious questions about whether such a multiple pregnancy should have been allowed to happen," viewing it less as a triumph of medicine than as a "medical disaster."[1]

From Alexander Morgan Capron, "Punishing Mothers," *Hastings Center Report* (January–February 1998), pp. 31–33. Copyright © 1998 by The Hastings Center. Reprinted by permission.

Though most critics did not go so far as to argue that the McCaugheys should not have used fertility drugs unless they were willing to undergo "selective reduction" early in the pregnancy (in which the number of fetuses would have been reduced from seven to at most two or three), Gregory Pence did suggest they had made an unethical choice. Rather than claiming it was "God's will," the McCaugheys should take responsibility for the choice they made. "They took bad odds and hoped that all seven would be healthy, and in so doing, they took the risk of having seven disabled or dead babies."[2]

More frequently, the criticism focused instead on the physicians involved. Through ultrasound scans and other means of monitoring, fertility specialists can tell when their interventions will lead to the release of a dangerously high number of eggs, so the woman can avoid conceiving that month or can undergo egg harvesting and in vitro fertilization, with only a few of the resulting embryos being transferred to the uterus and the rest frozen for later use if needed. Peter Brinsden, medical director at Bourn Hall in Cambridge where Louise Brown, the first test-tube baby, was born in 1978, chided physicians who do not use their medical powers responsibly. "The aim of fertility treatment should be to give couples one or two children at most."

Besides the stress that multiple births place on parents (and on their marriage) after the children are born, the general experience with such pregnancies is that they are very dangerous for mother and fetuses alike. Overstimulation of the ovaries can lead in rare cases to heart failure, and carrying many fetuses is associated with potentially fatal blood clots and miscarriages.

Even when such fetuses survive their crowded uterine environment, they will almost certainly be born many weeks early and very small, conditions that give rise to a litany of medical and developmental risks, such as chronic lung disease, mental retardation, and blindness. If, like the McCaughey babies, they succeed in weathering the risks of pregnancy, prematurity, and low birth weight, and emerge relatively intact from weeks of vigorous and very expensive care in a neonatal intensive care unit (NICU), such children still face an elevated risk of child abuse.

Addicted Babies

Direct charges of child neglect lay at the heart of another recent motherhood story, as recounted in a decision handed down by the Supreme Court of South Carolina less than a month before the McCaughey septuplets' birth.[3] The spotlight on public attention that shone on Cornelia Whitner after she gave birth in Pickens County several years ago was certainly less intense but also much less warm than that which greeted the birth of the McCaughey septuplets in Des Moines.

Ms. Whitner's baby was born with cocaine metabolites in his system, and she admitted using crack cocaine during the third trimester of her pregnancy. Charged with criminal child neglect under S.C. Code §20-7-50, Ms. Whitner pled guilty and was sentenced to eight years in prison.

Rather than appealing her conviction, Ms. Whitner filed a petition for Post Conviction Relief, arguing that §20-7-50 covered children but not fetuses.

Thus, she claimed, she had received ineffective assistance of her trial counsel, who failed to advise her that the statute might not apply to prenatal drug abuse, and the trial court lacked jurisdiction to accept a guilty plea to a nonexistent offense. After her petition was granted on both grounds, the state appealed to the Supreme Court of South Carolina.

The South Carolina Children's Code provides that "Any person having the legal custody of any child... who shall, without lawful excuse, refuse or neglect to provide... the proper care and attention for such child... so that the life, health or comfort of such child... is endangered or is likely to be endangered, shall be guilty of a misdemeanor." Another provision of the code defines "child" as "a person under the age of eighteen."

Is a fetus a "person" for the purposes of the children's code? Looking to the language of the statute (in light of comparable language in other contexts) as well as to the policy behind the law, the state supreme court answered "yes." It thus reached a different conclusion from other courts in similar prosecutions over the past dozen years around the country.

As the abuse of illegal drugs—particularly but not exclusively crack cocaine—swelled in the late 1980s to epidemic levels, physicians became concerned about the growing number of babies who had been exposed to these drugs prenatally. Though early medical reports—magnified through the lens of the popular media into a picture of NICUs filled with the Charles Mansons of the future—probably overstated the physical and behavioral consequences of prenatal drug exposure, studies have by now established that many babies whose mothers used cocaine and other drugs during pregnancy will have been harmed, in ways that are not always remediable.

Thus, it is hardly surprising that public officials took steps to deter maternal drug abuse and to punish women whose use of drugs exposed their children to harm before birth. Prosecutions took two forms. In some cases, women were charged under statutes forbidding delivery or distribution of illicit substances, in other cases, under statutes that punish child endangerment. Yet in decision after decision in the early 1990s, state courts rejected these prosecutions and held the statutes inapplicable to pregnant women's drug use insofar as the harm alleged occurred before a child's birth.

The *Whitner* Decision

The South Carolina Supreme Court reached a different conclusion in the *Whitner* case. Since the case involved only a child endangerment provision, the court did not need to deal with the issue of how "delivery" of a drug would be established under a statute forbidding drug distribution. And the court found "no question" that "Whitner endangered the life, health, and comfort of her child" when she ingested crack cocaine in the third trimester of the pregnancy.

Nor did the court have much difficulty in interpreting its statute to include a fetus within the meaning of "child" because, unlike most of the other states that had rejected prosecutions for prenatal drug abuse, South Carolina had substantial case law construing "person" to include a viable fetus.

The earlier cases dealt with two situations. Going back to 1960, South Carolina's courts have allowed wrongful death actions arising from injuries sustained prenatally by a viable fetus, whether born alive or (after a 1964 decision) stillborn. The second context first arose in a homicide prosecution of a man who stabbed his nine-months-pregnant wife in the neck, arms, and abdomen. Despite an attempted caesarean delivery, the child died while still in utero, and the defendant was convicted of voluntary manslaughter.[4] Proclaiming a desire to be consistent with its holdings in the civil cases, the state supreme court upheld the conviction and recognized the crime of feticide, at least as to fetuses who were capable of surviving outside the womb.

In light of these earlier holdings, the *Whitner* court felt there was no "rational basis for finding a viable fetus is not a 'person' in the... context" of the child endangerment statute. In this ruling, it departed from the conclusion reached by a Massachusetts court that refused to recognize criminal liability of a pregnant woman for transmitting cocaine to her viable fetus, even though that state, like South Carolina, allows wrongful death actions for viable fetuses injured in utero and homicide prosecutions of third parties who kill viable fetuses. While the Massachusetts court had read its precedents as limited to cases in which the "mother's or parents' interest in the potentiality of life, not the state's interest, are sought to be vindicated,"[5] the South Carolina court held that the state may protect the interests of a viable fetus even from its mother.

Maternal Liability

Since South Carolina is not unusual in vindicating the interests of children for prenatal injuries in torts cases, adoption of the *Whitner* court's reasoning by other courts would have profound implications for state regulation of the behavior of expectant mothers.

First, the implication of the decision—though nowhere directly addressed—is that it is acceptable for the state to monitor the status of pregnant women and of their babies, such as by doing tests for illicit drugs without consent. If toxicology screening requires informed consent, then women who know that such tests will label them child abusers will refuse permission.

Conversely, if such screening is seen as acceptable without consent, under some general public health doctrine, then pregnant addicts may avoid routine prenatal care so as not to be arrested and incarcerated, and they may even seek to deliver their children outside usual medical settings—all to the detriment of their health and that of their child-to-be. Further, some pregnant addicts might seek late-term abortions, rather than deliver a baby with telltale signs of drug usage.[6]

It is also hard to believe that the court's holding in *Whitner* will stay confined to viable fetuses. While the courts may feel constrained to limit feticide prosecutions to cases where the victim is viable, civil damages are awarded for injuries that occur not just before viability but even before conception and are then manifested after birth. A similar reading of the child endangerment statute can be expected, especially in light of the medical evidence that the developing fetus is probably at greater risk of injury from maternal drug abuse in the first few months of gestation than in the final months.

While the *Whitner* court repeatedly emphasized that it was only address-ing the situation before it—a pregnant woman's abuse of an illegal substance —there is nothing in the child protection law that limits the range of acts for which prosecution is possible. The focus of §20-7-30 is on preventing action or inaction that endangers a child's "life, health or comfort." While the statute excepts acts done with "lawful excuse," it is not clear that anything short of necessity would provide such an excuse—certainly not the mere comfort or convenience of an expectant mother.

The conduct that would therefore be most likely to lead to prosecution would be maternal drinking, since the link between fetal harm and prenatal exposure to alcohol is, if anything, even better documented than the link to prenatal exposure to illegal drugs. Alcoholic beverages carry warnings of this risk, and obstetricians routinely warn their patients to refrain from drinking even before their pregnancies are confirmed. Failure to follow such advice, or medical advice either to take or to refrain from taking prescription drugs or fol-lowing other medical regimes, could thus lay the basis for a child endangerment prosecution if shown to have led to serious harm to a child.

Indeed, in the words of the South Carolina court, there does not appear to be "any rational basis" for limiting the wrongful acts that could form the basis for a prosecution, whether the conduct occurred pre-viability or was otherwise legal for a woman who was not pregnant. And, to return to the Iowa septuplets, application of the *Whitner* doctrine would appear to expose to prosecution any woman who decided to initiate a pregnancy following fertility treatment if she was informed about the great risks of multiple births.

Of course, future Bobbi McCaugheys are unlikely to give much thought to such matters, and for good reason, as society regards the decision to proceed with a multiple pregnancy very differently from the abuse of illegal drugs. Yet both are situations in which children are exposed to the risk of death or severe handicaps, and both are situations in which the medical profession needs to do much more to help women (and their partners) to adjust their behavior in ways that offer their children a better start in life.

References

1. Chris Mihill and Sarah Boseley, "Multiple Births: When the Shine Wears Off a Miracle," *The Guardian* (London), 21 November 1997, p. 17.
2. Gregory Pence, "McCaughey Septuplets: God's Will or Human Choice?" *Birming-ham Sunday News*, 30 November 1997, p. C1.
3. Whitner v. State, 1997 W.L. 680091 (S.C.), filed 15 July 1997 and amended and refiled on grant of rehearing 27 October 1997.
4. State v. Horne, 282 S.C. 444, 319 S.E.2d 703 (1984).
5. Commonwealth v. Pellegrini, No. 87970 (Mass. Super. Ct., 15 October 1990), slip op. at 11.
6. The *Whitner* court rejected the argument that the pressure to take this step amounted to a penalty on the decision to carry a pregnancy to term in viola-tion of the woman's right of privacy recognized in Cleveland Board of Education v. LaFleur, 414 U.S. 632 (1974).

POSTSCRIPT

Should Pregnant Women Be Punished for Exposing Fetuses to Risk?

The U.S. Supreme Court agreed in February 2000 to hear the case of *Ferguson v. City of Charleston,* brought by a woman who states that she was wrongfully arrested and jailed while pregnant.

Since 1985 an estimated 200 women in 30 states have been prosecuted for drug use during pregnancy. The article that led the federal government to determine that the Medical University of South Carolina's drug use program constituted research is "Cocaine in Pregnancy: Confronting the Problem," by Edgar O. Horger III, Shirley B. Brown, and Charles Molony Condon, *Journal of the South Carolina Medical Association* (October 1990).

A comprehensive review of the development of the policy and its legal and ethical implications is "The Charleston Policy on Cocaine Use During Pregnancy: Cautionary Tale," by Philip H. Jos, Mary Faith Marshall, and Martin Perlmutter, *Journal of Law, Medicine & Ethics* (Summer 1995).

Deborah Hornstra argues that we should not think of babies as having a right to be born healthy and that proposing such a right destroys the maternal-fetal relationship by casting the fetus and mother as adversaries. See "A Realistic Approach to Maternal-Fetal Conflict," *Hastings Center Report* (September–October 1998).

See also Bonnie Steinbock's *Life Before Birth: The Moral and Legal Status of Embryos and Fetuses* (Oxford University Press, 1992) and Janna C. Merrick and Robert H. Blank, eds., *The Politics of Pregnancy: Policy Dilemmas in the Maternal-Fetal Relationship* (Haworth Press, 1993).

The McCaughey septuplets continue to do well, and despite their early claims that the parents would not capitalize on their births, Kenny McCaughey now appears in television commercials. For an analysis of this issue, see Arlene Judith Kloztako's, "Medical Miracle or Medical Mischief? The Saga of the McCaughey Septuplets," *Hastings Center Report* (May–June 1998). In December 1998 eight babies were born in Texas to Nkem Chukwu and her husband Iyke Louis Idobi through the use of fertility drugs. The smallest of the babies died. The cost of hospital care for the babies is estimated at $250,000 each.

See also Drew Humphries, *Crack Mothers: Pregnancy, Drugs, and the Media* (Ohio State University Press, 1999).

On the Internet ...

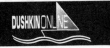

Society for Adolescent Medicine

The Society for Adolescent Medicine is composed of professionals committed to improving the physical and psychosocial health of adolescents. This Web site provides many resources on the topic of adolescent health.

`http://www.adolescenthealth.org/samfinal/mission_goals.ht`

Jehovah's Witnesses and Blood—NEWS

This site presents various newspaper articles and other news items on Jehovah's Witnesses and blood. The articles are from different countries and present more than one view on the issue of refusing medical treatment based on religious grounds.

`http://home.online.no/~jansh/wteng/blood/news.htm`

PART 4

Children and Bioethics

*C*hildren are often the subjects of controversies in biomedical ethics. Too young to make fully autonomous decisions, vulnerable to the pressures and interests of adults (including parents and health care providers), children are nonetheless persons in their own right with clear interests and a need for guidance and protection. Unless proven otherwise, parents are presumed to be the primary decision makers for their children. The common belief is that parents know and love their children, have a family history of values and choices, and can make informed choices about the best interests of their children. Yet this ideal does not always hold true, and in many cases what parents find acceptable, physicians or public health officials see as medical negligence. This section presents some of the most vexing dilemmas in medical ethics.

- Should Adolescents Make Their Own Life-and-Death Decisions?

- Do Parents Harm Their Children When They Refuse Medical Treatment on Religious Grounds?

ISSUE 9

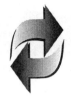

Should Adolescents Make Their Own Life-and-Death Decisions?

YES: Robert F. Weir and Charles Peters, from "Affirming the Decisions Adolescents Make About Life and Death," *Hastings Center Report* (November–December 1997)

NO: Lainie Friedman Ross, from "Health Care Decisionmaking by Children: Is It in Their Best Interest?" *Hastings Center Report* (November–December 1997)

ISSUE SUMMARY

YES: Ethicist Robert F. Weir and pediatrician Charles Peters assert that adolescents with normal cognitive and developmental skills have the capacity to make decisions about their own health care. Advance directives, if used appropriately, can give older pediatric patients a voice in their care.

NO: Pediatrician Lainie Friedman Ross counters that parents should be responsible for making their child's health care decisions. Children need to develop virtues, such as self-control, that will enhance their long-term, not just immediate, autonomy.

Apatient is brought to the emergency room after an accident. The physicians believe that he will die if he does not receive a blood transfusion, but the patient says that he is a Jehovah's Witness and will not accept blood. A cancer patient has undergone months of debilitating therapy with discouraging results; she says that she does not want any more treatment. These patients have the right to refuse treatment because they are adults. What if they were 15 or 16 years old? Would they have the same rights or could their wishes be overruled?

If there is one Golden Rule of contemporary bioethics, it is that competent adults are legally and ethically empowered to make health care decisions for themselves. Competent in this context means able to understand the choices and the consequences of decisions made. People base these decisions on values and preferences, personal experiences, religious beliefs, the availability of alternatives, level of pain and suffering, economic consequences, or any combination of these and other factors.

Except in unusual situations, parents are presumed to be in the best position to make these decisions for their children. Children, especially young children, are assumed to have neither the cognitive skills nor the mature judgment to make complex choices that may have far-reaching health consequences. Parents share the consequences of the decision so they make it with the best interests of their children and themselves in mind.

But adolescents are neither children nor fully mature adults. Where do they fit in this scheme? There are differences of opinion of how to define adolescence. Depending on the definition, adolescence may begin as young as 10 and end as late as 21. Legally the age of 18 defines the end of adolescence. However, that may not be an appropriate boundary for health care decision making. Those who support the idea that young people of a certain age should make their own health care decisions tend to call them "adolescents"; those who are critical of this view tend to call them "children" or "minors." In general adolescents have achieved a degree of emotional and intellectual maturity that surpasses that of young children. Still, they may be unable to appreciate long-term consequences of their actions.

In making health care decisions for children and adolescents, an alliance among the patient, parents, and physicians sometimes develops. Together they choose among alternative plans for treatment or, in the case of terminal illness, palliative care instead of aggressive treatment. However, parents, adolescents, and physicians do not always agree.

The selections that follow present two opposing views on whether adolescents should make their own life-and-death decisions. Robert F. Weir and Charles Peters argue for adolescent capacity and autonomy. They summarize an expanding body of professional literature to indicate that, with a few exceptions, adolescents are capable of making major health decisions and giving informed consent. Lainie Friedman Ross argues against the 1995 American Academy of Pediatrics recommendations that give children a greater voice in their care. She contends that it is the parents' right and responsibility to make decisions that enhance their children's long-term autonomy.

Robert F. Weir and Charles Peters

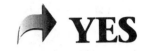 **YES**

Affirming the Decisions Adolescents Make About Life and Death

Some Illustrative Cases

Scott Rose was a talented adolescent who loved poetry, music, writing, and acting. Unfortunately, he had Nezelof syndrome, a cellular immunodeficiency disease similar to the condition of the famous "bubble boy" in Houston. Scott refused to remain in a similar enclosure, preferring to live as normal a life as his condition permitted. At the age of fourteen, with his lungs deteriorating and his suffering increasing, Scott decided that he could accept no more life-sustaining treatment. Against his physician's wishes but with tacit approval from his family, Scott died by disconnecting himself from the ventilator that was keeping him alive in a community hospital in Oklahoma.

C.G. was a fifteen-year-old with end-stage cystic fibrosis. During the last year of his life, he was hospitalized four times in a critical care unit for pneumonia and respiratory distress. He repeatedly expressed fear that his life would end in a slow, agonizing death. He realized that he was dying and stated that he did not want to "smother" or die on a ventilator. On his last admission, he experienced increasing respiratory distress and became disoriented as his carbon dioxide rose. However, his parents were adamant, insisting to the attending physician that "everything possible" be done to keep C.G. alive, including prolonged intubation and mechanical ventilation.

Benito Agrela was born with an enlarged liver and spleen. He received a liver transplant when he was eight years old, had a second liver transplant when he was fourteen, and then stopped taking his medication several months after the second transplant because he could not tolerate its side effects. When the Florida Department of Social Services discovered that he was not taking his antirejection medications, they forcibly removed him from his parents' home and admitted him to a transplant floor of a Miami hospital. After he refused further treatment, his case was taken to court; the circuit court judge spent several hours with Benito and his physicians, then ruled that Benito had a legal right to refuse the medications and return home. Before his death at the age of

From Robert F. Weir and Charles Peters, "Affirming the Decisions Adolescents Make About Life and Death," *Hastings Center Report,* vol. 27, no. 6 (November–December 1997). Copyright © 1997 by The Hastings Center. Reprinted by permission.

fifteen, Benito said: "I should have the right to make my own decision. I know the consequences, I know the problems."

M.C. was ten years old when she was diagnosed with acute lymphoblastic leukemia. During two years of chemotherapy, she maintained excellent grades, joined a swim team, and demonstrated, according to her teachers, "a particularly mature and far-reaching perspective on her life." Then the leukemia relapsed. Following discussions with a health care team and her parents, she decided that a partially matched, related donor bone marrow transplant was her best chance for continued life. Before she received the transplant, at the age of thirteen, she told her parents and others that she did not want to "grow up to be a vegetable," did not want to be supported on "a lot of machines," and did not want to be a psychological or financial burden on the family. Two months after the transplant, she was diagnosed as having an Epstein Barr virus-associated lymphoproliferative disorder. Despite aggressive treatment efforts in a pediatric ICU, her condition did not improve. Four days later the ventilator sustaining her life was withdrawn, at the request of her family and in keeping with her previously expressed wishes.

B.C. was a sixteen-year-old adolescent who was diagnosed with cystic fibrosis shortly after birth. Over the years, both his medical condition and his relationship with his parents deteriorated. He watched several friends with cystic fibrosis die, and mentioned on several occasions that he did not want to be placed on a ventilator. Nevertheless, even as his pulmonary tests deteriorated rapidly, his parents refused to discuss death with him, or any decisions that might need to be made about limiting life-sustaining treatment, the possibility of do-not-resuscitate status, or his preferences about treatment options. When he was soon thereafter admitted, unresponsive, following an unsuccessful suicide attempt, his parents requested that no life-sustaining measures be employed. They forbade the medical staff from discussing this matter with B.C., even when he became sufficiently alert to communicate.

Our reason for presenting these cases is simple. Every day, in hospitals throughout this country, adolescent patients cope with chronic conditions, struggle to survive with life-threatening illnesses, and think about the burdens of continued existence compared with the prospect of death. Sometimes, as indicated by Scott Rose and Benito Agrela, these adolescent patients conclude that death is preferable to the suffering they are experiencing, decide to refuse further life-sustaining interventions, and carry out that decision in spite of opposition from physicians and/or parents. Other times, as in the case of M.C., parents and physicians carry out the decision to abate life-sustaining treatment, knowing it to be consistent with the adolescent patient's wishes. Yet other times, as in the cases of C.G. and B.C., parents request, and physicians carry out, a plan of care that has not been discussed with the adolescent patient and may be completely contrary to his or her expressed wishes.

Such cases reflect the considerable uncertainty that sometimes surrounds the medical management of these patients. Do most adolescents have the capacity to make major decisions about their lives and health, even when they are hospitalized? Do only *some* adolescents have this decisionmaking capacity and, if so, what kinds of lines need to be drawn in terms of adolescent decisional abilities? Do adolescents have the right not only to *assent*, but also to *consent*—and to refuse to consent—to recommended medical treatment or participation in research studies?...

Adolescents as Capable Decisionmakers

An expanding body of professional literature indicates that adolescents, with some exceptions, are capable of making major health decisions and giving informed consent, whether in a clinical or research setting. An increasing number of professionals in developmental psychology, pediatrics, biomedical ethics, and health law agree that a fundamental reorientation toward adolescents—in clinical medicine, in research settings, and in the law—is necessary to increase adult acceptance of the important decisions that many adolescents now seem capable of making for themselves.

Numerous studies can be cited to make the basic point. Almost twenty years ago, a comprehensive analysis of the literature in developmental psychology by Thomas Grisso and Linda Vierling indicated that "generally minors below the ages of 11–13 do not possess many of the cognitive capacities one would associate with the psychological elements of 'intelligent' consent."[1] By contrast, the authors stated that there "is little evidence that minors of age 15 and above as a group are any less competent to provide consent than are adults." On the basis of their literature analysis, they concluded that "minors are entitled to have some form of consent or dissent regarding the things that happen to them in the name of assessment, treatment, or other professional activities that have generally been determined unilaterally by adults in the minor's interest." Similar conclusions came from an empirical study reported by Lois Weithron and Susan Campbell.[2]

In the pediatric literature, Sanford Leikin surveyed the findings of developmental psychologists, mainly those of Jean Piaget, and applied them to the issue of minors' assent or dissent to medical treatment. He observed that while cognitive development cannot always be equated with chronological age, good evidence exists "that, by age 14 years, many minors attain the cognitive developmental stage associated with the psychological elements of rational consent." As to other adolescent ages, he concluded that "minors between 11 and 14 years of age appear to be in a transition period... [and] there appear to be no psychological grounds for the general assumption that minors 15 years of age or older cannot provide competent consent."[3]

In a subsequent publication Leikin addressed the question of how parents and physicians should respond to the decisions made by adolescents to withhold or withdraw life-sustaining treatment. In large part, he argued, it depends on the psychological development of the adolescent in question and that person's ability to make "authentic choices" guided by logical thought patterns, a physiologic understanding of illness, and a willingness to make decisions independent of authority figures (a willingness, he pointed out, not usually found in adolescents less than fourteen or fifteen years of age).[4] Other writers agree.[5]...

Legal Developments

Even if most adolescents between age fourteen and seventeen increasingly are regarded as having the capacity to make health decisions for themselves, and even if leading pediatric groups have for over twenty years called for an expansion of adolescent rights in health care settings, important questions about the law remain. . . .

Traditionally, state laws reflected the view that adolescents and other legal minors under the age of twenty-one were incapable of understanding, deliberating about, and making decisions regarding important health care choices. The power to make such decisions was vested in parents, legal guardians, or someone standing in *loco parentis* to a child. Any physician who might have provided nonemergency medical care to a legal minor without parental consent risked being charged with civil battery (performing treatment without consent), even if there was no charge of malpractice.[6]

Legal minors and personal health decisions.   During the past three decades, this view of legal minors has changed in a number of ways. One important change involves the age of majority. Until 1971, the standard age of majority was twenty-one, with a perennial debate focusing on the differences in age required for voting compared with the age required for being drafted into the military. That debate stopped with the passage of the 26th amendment to the Constitution in 1971, thereby permitting persons aged between eighteen and twenty to vote in federal elections. Most state legislatures subsequently lowered the age of majority to eighteen, thus granting legal adulthood to millions of persons who previously could not vote, make contractual obligations, or consent to medical treatment apart from their parents.[7]

Another change in the law involves the creation of exceptional legal categories for some adolescents to make personal health decisions. Two such categories are common among the states. Some adolescents, depending on the state, are legally recognized as *emancipated minors* on the basis of marriage, parenthood, military service, consent of parents (for example, adolescents who are "thrown away" by parents after family conflicts), judicial order of emancipation, or financial independence. Some state statutes (such as in Arizona, Idaho, Massachusetts, Montana, Nevada, North Carolina, Oregon, and Texas) specifically grant emancipated minors the right to consent to medical treatment.

Other adolescents are legally recognized in some jurisdictions as *mature minors* for the purpose of making health decisions because of their individual ability to understand the nature and purposes of recommended medical treatment. The "mature minor rule" recognizes that some adolescents are sufficiently mature to make their own decisions about recommended medical treatment and, when necessary, to go against their parents' views regarding the treatment. Physicians who carry out these decisions seem to run little legal risk, since there are no reported judicial decisions over the past twenty-five years in which parents have recovered damages for the medical treatment of an adolescent over the age of fifteen without parental consent.[8]

A third change in the law pertains to *minor treatment statutes* according to which states permit legal minors to consent to certain types of medical care. These statutes usually specify certain health problems for which legal minors can seek medical treatment without parental consent, precisely because the nature of the health problems is such that some adolescents would probably choose to go without medical treatment rather than seek their parents' consent for the treatment. Such statutes are typically limited to treatment for sexually transmitted diseases, pregnancy and pregnancy prevention (including abortion in some states, but not sterilization), alcohol and other drug abuse, and in some states, psychiatric problems.

Legal minors, end-of-life decisions, and state legislatures.   Despite these changes, most state legislatures have not addressed the issue of treatment refusal by adolescents, especially in circumstances in which a refusal of life-sustaining treatment is likely to result in the adolescent's death. Thus, even though forty-seven states have living will statutes (the exceptions are Massachusetts, Michigan, and New York) and forty-eight states have surrogate decisionmaking statutes that include end-of-life decisions (the exceptions are Alabama and Alaska), the legislative statutes in thirty-eight states and the District of Columbia do not specifically address end-of-life decisions made by legal minors.[9]

Most state legislatures seem to think that adolescents either do not die in clinical settings, or are incapable of making informed consent or informed refusal decisions about treatment options, must be protected from their own lack of judgment, or simply should not be permitted to give legally binding advance directions regarding life-sustaining treatments and surrogate decision-makers. If a given adolescent does not qualify for emancipation under state law, does not live in one of the three states (Alaska, Arkansas, and Mississippi) having a mature-minor statute, and is unable or unwilling for some reason to go through a judicial hearing to be designated a mature minor, he or she is left with only three options: (1) persuading parents and physicians to act according to the adolescent's expressed views on life-sustaining treatment, (2) persuading parents to execute an advance directive on the patient's behalf (in the seven states having this legal option), or (3) acquiescing to the views of legal adults (namely, parents and physicians) regarding the medical circumstances under which the remaining portion of life is to be lived....

Advance Directives and Moral Persuasion

Most adolescents who want to participate in the decisionmaking process connected with their medical conditions, especially in regard to decisions about life-sustaining medical interventions, have chronic conditions that often deteriorate over time: certain kinds of cancer, cystic fibrosis, AIDS, complicated types of heart disease, and so on. Having experienced years of physical and psychological suffering, gone through multiple hospitalizations and numerous treatments, probably experienced depression, and probably observed the suffering and dying of several hospitalized friends with similar medical problems, these adolescent patients are frequently mature beyond their chronological years. They have had, at the very least, multiple opportunities to think about the inescapable suffering that characterizes their lives, the features of life that make it worth continuing, the benefits and burdens that accompany medical treatment, and the prospect of death. At least some of these adolescents want to give voice to their values, provide directions for parents, physicians, and nurses regarding end-of-life care, and be assured that their wishes and preferences will be respected and carried out should their medical conditions deteriorate to the point that they will no longer be able to communicate their deeply felt views.

How parents, physicians, nurses, and other health professionals respond to these adolescents' desires for control and self-determination at the end of life is vitally important. These adults, individually and collectively, may simply *choose not to* listen. Alternatively, parents, physicians, and other adults involved in these cases may think that these personal life-and-death decisions are *primarily matters of law*, quite apart from the wishes and preferences expressed by individual patients. If so, the attending physician will likely check with hospital legal counsel, who will report on relevant statutory and case law and give legal advice that, understandably, will be protective of the hospital's legal interests....

There is a third alternative. Parents, physicians, and other adults involved in these cases may regard the thoughtful comments, the verbalized reflections on the meaning of life and death, and the communicated choices regarding treatment options by *at least some* (perhaps most) adolescents with life-threatening conditions as *efforts of moral persuasion*, quite apart from what the law may or may not say.[10] Parents may reluctantly conclude that their son or daughter has suffered enough, seen enough, and communicated enough to convince them that however much they may want their child to live, he or she has the moral right to make end-of-life decisions that, when carried out, will result in death. Physicians, nurses, and other health care professionals also may be convinced.

Advance directives can help meet this goal, especially if the use of such directives becomes an acceptable part of the informed consent process in pediatric medicine. Enabling at least some adolescent patients—patients with chronic, life-threatening conditions—to communicate their decisions about treatment options through oral or written advance directives would also provide a measure of legal protection for physicians. Pediatricians, family practice physicians, and other physicians having such cases would be more able to document the specific end-of-life treatment decisions made by these patients, the maturity and decisionmaking capacity of individual patients, and the conversations about consenting to or refusing life-sustaining treatment that had taken place with the patients and their parents.

References

1. Thomas Grisso and Linda Vierling, "Minors' Consent to Treatment: A Developmental Perspective," *Professional Psychology* 9 (August 1978): 412–427; at 420.

2. Lois A. Weithorn and Susan B. Campbell, "The Competency of Children and Adolescents to Make Informed Treatment Decisions," *Child Development* 53 (1982): 1589–98.
3. Sanford L. Leikin, "Minors' Assent or Dissent to Medical Treatment," *Journal of Pediatrics* 102 (1983): 173.
4. Sanford L. Leikin, "A Proposal Concerning Decisions to Forgo Life-Sustaining Treatment for Young People," *Journal of Pediatrics* 108 (1989): 17–22, at 20; Leikin, "The Role of Adolescents in Decisions Concerning Their Cancer Therapy," *Cancer Supplement* 71 (15 May 1993): 3342–46.
5. For example, C. E. Lewis, "A Comparison of Minors' and Adults' Pregnancy Decisions," *American Journal of Orthopsychiatry* 50 (1980): 446–53; Richard H. Nicholson, ed., *Medical Research with Children* (Oxford: Oxford University Press, 1986), p. 140–52; Angela Holder, *Legal Issues in Pediatrics and Adolescent Medicine,* 2d ed. (New Haven: Yale University Press, 1985), p. 133.
6. Sarah D. Cohn, "The Evolving Law of Adolescent Health Care," *Clinical Issues* 2 (1991): 201–7, at 201; Angela R. Holder, "Disclosure and Consent Problems in Pediatrics," *Law, Medicine & Health Care* 16 (1988): 219–28; Steven M. Selbst, "Treating Minors Without Their Parents," *Pediatric Emergency Care* 1 (1985): 168–73.
7. Richard A. Leiter, ed., *National Survey of State Laws* (Detroit: Gale Research Inc., 1993), pp. 279–91.
8. Angela R. Holder, "Children and Adolescents: Their Right to Decide about Their Own Health Care," in *Children and Health Care: Moral and Social Issues,* ed. Loretta Kopelman and John C. Moskop (Boston: Kluwer Academic Publishers, 1989), p. 163.
9. Information from Choice in Dying, New York, 1995.
10. Robert F. Weir, "Advance Directives as Instruments of Moral Persuasion," in *Medicine Unbound,* ed. Robert H. Blank and Andrea L. Bonnicksen (New York: Columbia University Press, 1994), pp. 171–87.

NO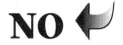

Lainie Friedman Ross

Health Care Decisionmaking by Children

In pediatrics, the doctor-patient relationship traditionally has included three parties: the physician, the child, and his or her parents. Parents were not merely surrogate decisionmakers on the grounds of child incompetence, but rather, parents were believed to have both a right and a responsibility to partake in their child's medical decisions.[1] In this [selection] I will examine the evolving position regarding the role of the child in the decisionmaking process as advocated by the American Academy of Pediatrics (AAP). I will offer both moral and pragmatic arguments why I believe this position is misguided.

Recommendations of the American Academy of Pediatrics

In 1995, the AAP published its recommendations for the role of children in health care decisionmaking. The AAP recommended that the child's voice be given greater weight as the child matured. The AAP categorized children as (1) those who lack decisionmaking capacity; (2) those with a developing capacity; and (3) those who have decisionmaking capacity for health care decisions.[2]

For children who lack decisionmaking capacity, the AAP recommended that their parents should make decisions unless their decisions are abusive or neglectful. When children have developing decisionmaking capacity, the physician should seek parental permission and the child's assent. In many cases, the child's dissent should be binding, or at minimum, the physician should seek third-party mediation for parent-child disagreement. Although the child who dissents to life-saving care can be overruled, attempts should be made to persuade the child to assent for "coercion in diagnosis or treatment is a last resort." When children have decisionmaking capacity, the AAP concluded that the children should give informed consent for themselves and their parents should be viewed as consultants.

A major problem with the AAP recommendations is that it assumes decisionmaking capacity can be defined and measured, although the AAP offers no guidance as to what this definition is or how to test for it. Instead, the AAP recommends individual assessment of decisionmaking capacity in each case.

From Lainie Friedman Ross, "Health Care Decisionmaking by Children: Is It in Their Best Interest?" *Hastings Center Report*, vol. 27, no. 6 (November–December 1997). Copyright © 1997 by The Hastings Center. Reprinted by permission.

However, since there are no criteria on which to base maturity or decisionmaking capacity, the decision of whether to respect a child's decision is dependent upon the judgment of the particular pediatrician—a judgment he or she has no training to make.

My main concern with the AAP recommendations, however, is what should be done when parents and children disagree on health care decisions: according to the AAP, if there is parental-child disagreement and the child is judged to have decisionmaking authority, the child's decision should be binding. If the child has developing capacity, various mechanisms to resolve the conflict should be attempted. They propose:

> short term counseling or psychiatric consultation for patient and/or family, "case management" or similar multidisiplinary conference(s), and/or consultation with individuals trained in clinical ethics or a hospital based ethics committee. In rare cases of refractory disagreement, formal legal adjudication may be necessary.

I will ignore the difficulties in determining whether a minor has decisionmaking capacity and assume that some minors are competent to make at least some health care decisions. If autonomy is based solely on competency, then competent children should have decisionmaking autonomy in the health care setting. It is my view, however, that even if children are competent, there is a morally significant difference between competent minors and adults. Competency is a necessary but not a sufficient condition on which to base respect for a minor's health care decisionmaking autonomy.

Competency of Children

The psychological literature divides the process of giving informed consent into three components: the patient's consent is informed (made knowingly), is competent (made intelligently), and is voluntary.[3] Although a survey of the literature reveals scant empirical data, existing data suggest that most health care decisions made by adults and children do not fulfill these three components.[4] The data also suggest that adults and older children do not significantly differ in their consent skills.[5] If competency is the only criterion on which respect for autonomy in health care is based, then this difference in treatment cannot be justified.

No test has been developed that uniformly distinguishes all competent individuals from incompetent individuals. Given that competency is context-specific, it is doubtful whether such a test could be developed. And even if a nonculturally biased, objective test could be devised, individual testing of every potential patient would exact a high price in terms of efficiency, privacy, and respect for autonomy. Instead, adults have traditionally been presumed competent and children have been presumed incompetent. That is, respect for autonomy in health care uses both a threshold concept of competency and an age-standard.

To some extent the age-standard is arbitrary as there are individuals above the line (older than the legal age of emancipation) who are incompetent and individuals below the line (younger than the legal age of emancipation) who are competent. But the statutes are not capricious: in general, individuals above the line are more likely to be competent than individuals below it.

Autonomy of Children

One reason to limit the child's present-day autonomy is based on the argument that parents and other authorities need to promote the child's life-time autonomy. Given the value that is placed on self-determination, it makes sense to grant adults autonomy provided that they have some threshold level of competency. Respect is shown by respecting their present project pursuits. But respect for a threshold of competency in children places the emphasis on present-day autonomy rather than on a child's life-time autonomy. Children need a protected period in which to develop "enabling virtues"—habits, including the habit of self-control, which advance their life-time autonomy and opportunities. Although many adults would also benefit from developing their potentials and improving their skills and self-control, at some point (and it is reasonable to use the age of emancipation as the proper cut-off), the advantages of self-determination outweigh the benefits of further guidance and its potential to improve life-time autonomy.

A second reason to limit the child's present-day autonomy is the fact that the child's decisions are based on limited world experience and so her decisions are not part of a well-conceived life plan. Again, many adults have limited world experience, but children have a greater potential for improving their knowledge base and for improving their skills of critical reflection and self-control.... By protecting the child from his own impetuosity, his parents help him obtain the background knowledge of the world and the capacities that will allow him to make decisions that better promote his life plans. His parents' attempt to help him flourish may not be achieved, but that does not invalidate their attempt.

A third reason childhood competency should not necessarily entail respect for a child's autonomy is the significant role that intimate families play in our lives. Elsewhere, I have argued that when the family is intimate, parents should have wide discretion in pursuing family goals, goals which may compete and conflict with the goals of particular members.[6] In general, parental autonomy promotes the interests and goals of both children and parents. It serves the needs and interests of the child to have autonomous parents who will help him become an autonomous individual capable of devising and implementing his own life plan. It serves the adults' interest in having and raising a family according to their own vision of the good life. These interests do not abruptly cease when the child becomes competent. If anything, now parents have the opportunity to inculcate their beliefs through rational discourse, instead of through example, bribery, or force.

There are also pragmatic reasons to permit parents to override the present-day autonomy of competent children. First, one can argue for a determination of competency that allows unusually mature children to be emancipated. The problem, as I have already mentioned, is that no such test exists. Second, one can acknowledge that it is best if parents recognize their child's maturity and treat them accordingly, but deny that this justifies granting competent children legal emancipation. Many parents respect their mature child's decisions voluntarily. Laura Purdy remarks: "It is plausible to think that children's maturity is not completely unrelated to parental good sense."[7] Child liberationists may object because a voluntary approach only encourages parents to respect their children's autonomy, but it does not legally enforce it. However, the voluntary approach is more consistent with a policy to limit the state's role in intrafamilial decisions, which is important for the family's ability to flourish.

Health Care Rights in Context

A final argument against respecting the health care decisions of minors is based on placing the notion of health care rights in context. Most individuals who support health care decisionmaking for children view it as an exception and do not seek to emancipate children in other spheres. But why should a child who is competent to make major health care decisions not have the right to make other types of decisions? That is, if a fourteen-year-old is competent to make life-and-death decisions, then why can't this fourteen-year-old buy and smoke cigarettes? Participate in interscholastic football without his parents' consent? Or even drop out of school? ...

What would it mean to endorse equal rights for children? It is a radical proposal with wide repercussions.[8] It would mean that children could make binding contracts, and that there would be the dissolution of child labor laws, mandatory education, statutory rape laws, and child neglect statutes. As such, it would give children rights for which they are ill-prepared and deny them the protection they need from predatory adults. It would leave children even more vulnerable than they presently are.

Endorsement of child liberation would make a child's membership in a family voluntary. For example, Howard Cohen argues that children should be allowed to change families, either because the child's parents are abusive, or because a neighbor or wealthy stranger offers him a better deal.[9] Such freedom ignores the important role that continuity and permanence play in the parent-child relationship—a significance the child may not yet appreciate.[10] ...

The Family as the Locus of Decisionmaking

One of my major concerns with the AAP's recommendations is their willingness to involve third-parties in the decisionmaking process. My concern is that these decisions undermine the family. Physicians provide only for the child's transient medical needs; his parents provide for all of his needs and are responsible for raising the child in such a way that he becomes an autonomous responsible adult. Goldstein and colleagues at Yale University's Child Study Center expressed their concern that health care professionals sometimes forget where their professional responsibilities end, and described the harm that we do when we think we can replace parents.[11] By deciding that the child's decision should be respected over the parents' decision, physicians are replacing the parents' judgment that the decision should be overridden with their judgment that the child's decision should be respected. To do so makes this less an issue of respecting the child's autonomy, and more about deciding who knows what is best for the child. In general, parents are the better judge as they have a more vested interest in their child's well-being and are responsible for the day-to-day decisions of child-rearing. It behooves physicians to be humble as they are neither able nor willing to take over this daily function.

I do not mean to suggest that children, particularly mature children, should be ignored in the decisionmaking process. Diagnostic tests and treatment plans should be explained to children to help them understand what is being done to them and to garner, when possible, their cooperation. Parents should include their children in the decisionmaking process both to get their active support and to help them learn how to make such decisions. However, when there is parental-child disagreement, the child's decision should not be decisive nor should health care providers, as I have argued, seek third-party mediation. Rather, as I have already argued, there are both moral and pragmatic reasons why the parents should have final decisionmaking authority.

References

1. Allen Buchanan and Dan Brock, *Deciding for Others: The Ethics of Surrogate Decision Making* (New York: Cambridge University Press, 1989).
2. American Academy of Pediatrics, Committee on Bioethics, "Informed Consent, Parental Permission, and Assent in Pediatric Practice," *Pediatrics* 95 (1995): 314-17.
3. Thomas Grisso and Linda Vierling, "Minor's Consent to Treatment: A Developmental Perspective," *Professional Psychology* 9, no. 3 (1978): 412-27.
4. Paul S. Appelbaum, Charles W. Lidz, and Alan Meisel, *Informed Consent: Legal Theory and Clinical Practice* (New York: Oxford University Press, 1987); Stanley Milgram, *Obedience to Authority: An Experimental View* (New York: Harper and Row, 1974).
5. Grisso and Vierling, "Minor's Consent to Treatment."
6. Lainie Friedman Ross, *Health Care Decision Making for Children,* unpublished manuscript, 1996.
7. Laura M. Purdy, *In Their Best Interest? The Case Against Equal Rights for Children* (New York: Cornell University Press, 1992).
8. Richard Farson, "A Child's Bill of Rights," in *Justice: Selected Readings,* ed. Joel Feinberg and Hyman Gross (Belmont, Calif.: Dickenson Publishing Co. 1977).
9. Howard Cohen, *Equal Rights for Children* (Totowa, N.J.: Rowman and Littlefield, 1980); John Harris, "The Political Status of Children," in *Contemporary Political Philosophy,* ed. Keith Graham (Cambridge, Mass.: Cambridge University Press, 1982), pp. 35-55.
10. Joseph Goldstein, Anna Freud, and Albert J. Solnit, *Before the Best Interests of the Child* (New York: The Free Press, 1979).
11. Joseph Goldstein et al., *In the Best Interest of the Child* (New York: The Free Press, 1986).

POSTSCRIPT

Should Adolescents Make Their Own Life-and-Death Decisions?

In 1994 three cases of adolescents refusing medical treatment were featured in the news. The first case concerns Benito Agrela and is discussed in the selection by Weir and Peters. The second case concerns Billy Best, a sixteen-year-old from Massachusetts who refused chemotherapy for Hodgkin's disease, a form of cancer. Because he felt that his parents and his physician would not understand his reasons, Best ran away from home. After he was assured that he did not have to undergo chemotherapy, he returned home, began a course of alternative therapies, and his cancer went into remission. The third case concerns Lee Lor, a fifteen-year-old who was diagnosed with ovarian cancer. Her family is from the Hmong community of Asian refugees. They disagreed with the diagnosis and wanted herbal treatment instead of surgery. After Lee was forcibly removed from her parent's home to undergo chemotherapy, she ran away. She too came home when assured that she would not have to undergo treatment. She is still alive, according to the most recent reports.

These three cases are discussed in Isabel Traugott and Ann Alpers, "In Their Own Hands: Adolescents' Refusals of Medical Treatment," *Archives of Pediatric and Adolescent Medicine* (September 1, 1997). Although published in 1985, *Legal Issues in Pediatrics and Adolescent Medicine* by Angela Roddey Holder (Yale University Press) is still a classic text. She supports the right of competent adolescents to make treatment decisions. Other documents supporting this position are the 1995 statement of the American Academy of Pediatrics (cited in the selection by Ross) and "Health Care Decision Making Guidelines for Minors," (Midwest Bioethics Center, 1995). Hillary Rodham Clinton also supports children's rights in several articles, including "Children's Rights: A Legal Perspective," *Children's Rights: Contemporary Perspectives*, edited by Patricia A. Vardin and Ilene N. Brody (Teachers College Press, 1979). Among those critical of the movement to grant children and adolescents more decision-making authority is Laura M. Purdy, *In Their Best Interests? The Case Against Equal Rights for Children* (Cornell University Press, 1992). In "Minor Rights and Wrongs," *Journal of Law, Medicine & Ethics* (Summer 1996), Michelle Oberman urges particular concern about cases in which adolescents refuse life-sustaining treatment.

In *The Adolescent "Alone": Decision Making in Health Care in the United States* (Cambridge University Press, 1999), Jeffrey Blustein, Nancy N. Dubler, and Carol Levine present a series of papers and case studies concerning adolescents who do not have a parent or surrogate in their lives to help them make health care decisions.

ISSUE 10

Do Parents Harm Their Children When They Refuse Medical Treatment on Religious Grounds?

YES: American Academy of Pediatrics, from "Religious Objections to Medical Care," *Pediatrics* (February 1997)

NO: Mark Sheldon, from "Ethical Issues in the Forced Transfusion of Jehovah's Witness Children," *The Journal of Emergency Medicine* (vol. 14, no. 2, 1996)

ISSUE SUMMARY

YES: The Committee on Bioethics of the American Academy of Pediatrics states that all children deserve medical treatment that is likely to prevent substantial harm, suffering, or death, regardless of the parents' religious objections to treatment.

NO: Professor of philosophy Mark Sheldon assesses the case of Jehovah's Witness parents who refuse to allow their children to undergo blood transfusions and concludes that they cannot be said to be truly harming or neglecting their children. Rather, they are placing their children's spiritual interests above worldly ones.

On May 6, 1989, an 11-year-old Minnesota boy named Ian Lundman complained of stomach pains. Acting in accordance with her beliefs as a lifelong Christian Scientist, his mother, Katherine McKown, prayed for Ian but did not call a doctor. When the boy had not improved the following day, Ms. McKown sought the healing prayers of two Christian Science practitioners. Three days later, Ian was dead.

Christian Scientists believe that healing through prayer is scientific and effective and that if a patient dies, it is because the prayers had not been strong enough. Based on a state law that allows parents to rely on spiritual treatment for their children, Minnesota courts dismissed manslaughter charges against Ian's mother, stepfather, and the Christian Science practitioners. In 1993 Ian's father, Douglass Lundman, filed a civil suit against the four people that were involved in his son's death. A doctor testified that Ian had diabetes that could easily have been treated with insulin, while representatives of the First Church of Christ, Scientist (the official name of the church) testified that many people have been healed through prayer. The jury awarded Mr. Lundman $1.5 million in damages and assessed the Christian Science Church $9 million. An appeals court upheld the judgment against the four defendants but dismissed the punitive damages against the Church. In January 1996 the U.S. Supreme Court turned down a petition to restore the punitive damages, leaving the $1.5 million award intact.

Although few such cases reach the Supreme Court, they occur with troubling frequency and place some of the most cherished values in American society into conflict. Religious freedom and family privacy are pitted against society's obligation, through the medical profession and the courts, to protect the health and welfare of all children. In the most extreme cases, such as Ian's, honoring one value inevitably means violating the other.

Some of the debate turns on what constitutes child abuse and neglect. The legal picture is neither clear nor consistent. The federal Child Abuse Prevention and Treatment Act of 1974 defines abuse and neglect as "the physical and mental injury, negligent treatment, or maltreatment of a child under the age of 18 by a person who is responsible for the child's welfare under circumstances which indicate that the child's health and welfare is harmed or threatened thereby." However, state interpretations of the federal definition vary.

Cultural and religious differences clearly influence the interpretation of abuse and neglect statutes, especially where medical neglect is involved. Christian Scientists have been leaders in convincing many state legislatures to exclude religiously based refusals of medical treatment from child abuse and neglect statutes, and more than 40 states have passed laws recognizing spiritual treatment as an acceptable form of health care for children. In the past decade, however, some states have revoked these laws.

In general, the perspective of Jehovah's Witnesses differs from those of Christian Science and other religions that offer alternatives to modern medical care. Jehovah's Witnesses refuse only one intervention: the transfusion of whole blood and blood products. This refusal reflects a core belief in their religion. Jehovah's Witnesses take biblical bans on "eating" blood literally. Blood transfusion is held to violate this ban, and those who accept blood in this manner face loss of eternal life. Because blood transfusion is a common procedure in surgery and in the treatment of some diseases, cases involving refusal by Jehovah's Witnesses arise relatively frequently.

The following selections probe these dilemmas. The Committee on Bioethics of the American Academy of Pediatrics argues that parents harm children when they deny them the benefits of medical care because of religious beliefs. They advocate the repeal of laws that allow religious exemptions and support additional efforts to educate the public about children's medical needs. Mark Sheldon asserts that the concept of harm is not appropriately applied to cases involving Jehovah's Witnesses because parents are sincerely acting in what they believe to be the child's higher interests—protecting the possibility of eternal life.

American Academy of Pediatrics 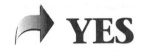 **YES**

Religious Objections to Medical Care

The Problem

The American Academy of Pediatrics (AAP) recognizes that religion plays a major role in the lives of many children and adults in the United States and is aware that some in the United States believe prayer and other spiritual practices can substitute for medical treatment of ill or injured children. Through legislative activity at the federal and state levels, some religious groups have sought, and in many cases attained, government recognition in the form of approved payment for this "nonmedical therapy" and exemption from child abuse and neglect laws when children do not receive needed medical care. The AAP opposes such payments and exemptions as harmful to children and advocates that children, regardless of parental religious beliefs, deserve effective medical treatment when such treatment is likely to prevent substantial harm or suffering or death.

The US Constitution requires that government not interfere with religious practices or endorse particular religions. However, these constitutional principles do not stand alone and may, at times, conflict with the independent government interest in protecting children.[1] Government obligation arises from that interest when parental religious practices subject minor children to possible loss of life or to substantial risk of harm. [2,3] Constitutional guarantees of freedom of religion do not permit children to be harmed through religious practices, nor do they allow religion to be a valid legal defense when an individual harms or neglects a child.[4]

Acute Illness or Injury

The AAP asserts that every child should have the opportunity to grow and develop free from preventable illness or injury.[5] Children also have the right to appropriate medical evaluation when it is likely that a serious illness, injury, or other medical condition endangers their lives or threatens substantial harm or suffering. Under such circumstances, parents and other guardians have a responsibility to seek medical treatment, regardless of their religious beliefs and

From American Academy of Pediatrics, Committee on Bioethics, "Religious Objections to Medical Care," *Pediatrics,* vol. 99, no. 2 (February 1997), pp. 279–280. Copyright © 1997 by The American Academy of Pediatrics. Reprinted by permission.

preferences. Unfortunately, certain groups have obtained exemptions from legal sanctions and state child abuse and neglect reporting laws based on the child's "treatment" by spiritual means, such as prayer.[6] The overall effect has been to limit the government's ability to protect children from abuse or neglect.

The AAP is concerned about religious doctrines that urge parents to avoid seeking medical help when their children are seriously ill. Each year, some parents' religious views lead them to eschew appropriate medical care for their children, resulting in substantial harm or suffering or death due to treatable conditions such as meningitis, bowel obstruction, diabetes mellitus, or pneumonia (*Boston Globe*. August 12, 1993:1; *Pittsburgh Post-Gazette*. March 16, 1991:B1).[4,7] The AAP considers failure to seek medical care in such cases to be child neglect, regardless of the motivation. The basic moral principle of justice requires that children be protected uniformly by laws and regulations at the local, state, and federal levels. Parents and others who deny a child necessary medical care on religious grounds should not be exempt from civil or criminal action that otherwise would be appropriate. State legislatures and regulatory agencies should remove religious exemption clauses from statutes and regulations to ensure that all parents understand that they should seek appropriate medical care for their children.

Preventive Care

Some religious tenets hold that members should not seek or receive medical care for any condition, including pregnancy. These beliefs can result in increased perinatal and maternal mortality.[8] Some religious groups deny children the benefits of routine preventive care. For example, some parents, acting in accord with state laws, refuse to have their children immunized because of religious beliefs. The AAP does not support the stringent application of medical neglect laws when children do not receive recommended immunizations. Although the risk to unimmunized individuals is relatively low, serious adverse reactions to vaccination are rare and the AAP strongly endorses universal immunization. Recent outbreaks of vaccine-preventable infectious diseases, with consequent serious complications and deaths, have been linked to groups that refused immunization for religious reasons.[9–12]

The AAP therefore supports the use of appropriate public health measures, such as mandatory mass vaccinations in epidemic situations, when necessary to protect communities and their unimmunized members. In addition, the AAP is concerned that children unimmunized for any reason may expose young children, not yet old enough to be protected, to infections such as pertussis or invasive *Haemophilus influenzae* disease. The risk is especially high in child care facilities. In such situations, all parents of children in the facility should be informed of the hazards.

Mature Minors

The weight given to parental religious beliefs in decisions affecting their children's well-being declines with the child's increasing age and development. That is, as minors mature, their interest in and capacity for participating in health care decisions affecting themselves increases, as does their ability to make decisions regarding their parents' religious views. The law and AAP policy recognize the doctrine of the "mature minor."[13] This concept acknowledges that many children, usually beginning in adolescence, can contribute to or make medical decisions, including those about life-sustaining treatment. Thus, in selected cases, disputes may be avoided when a minor has the capacity to make an independent decision in light of religious values and recommended medical therapy.

Need for Care and Respect

The AAP wishes to underscore its recognition of the important role of religion in the personal, spiritual, and social lives of many individuals and cautions physicians and other health care professionals to avoid unnecessary polarization when conflict over religious practices arises. Pediatricians should seek to make collaborative decisions with families whenever possible and should take great care when considering seeking authority to override parental preferences. Nevertheless, physicians who believe that parental religious convictions interfere with appropriate medical care that is likely to prevent substantial harm or suffering or death should request court authorization to override parental authority or, under circumstances involving an imminent threat to a child's life, intervene over parental objections. When caring for children whose prognoses are grave even with treatment, physicians should use restraint in pursuing a court order to initiate or continue treatment when parents object to it. In such situations, physicians should work with the parents and children to ensure provision of appropriate palliative care. Threatening or seeking state intervention should be the last resort, undertaken only when treatment is likely to prevent substantial harm or suffering or death. Even under these circumstances, physicians should respect parental religious beliefs and the role of parents in rearing their children. Of course, a physician may withdraw from these cases, after securing acceptable alternative medical care, when continuing in the doctor-patient-family relationship would violate the physician's own moral precepts.

The AAP emphasizes that all children who need medical care that is likely to prevent substantial harm or suffering or death should receive that treatment. The AAP opposes religious doctrines that advocate opposition to medical attention for sick children. Adherence to such views precludes appropriate assessment and intervention to protect the children. The AAP believes that laws should not encourage or tolerate parental action that prevents implementing appropriate medical treatment, nor should laws exempt parents from criminal or civil liability in the name of religion.

References

1. *Planned Parenthood of Central Missouri v Danforth*, 428 US 52, 74(1976)
2. *Prince v Commonwealth of Massachusetts*, 321 US 158, 170(1944)
3. *Jehovah's Witnesses v King County Hospital Unit No. 1*, 278 F Supp 488 (WD Wash 1967), affirmed per curiam 390 US 598(1968)

4. *Walker v Superior Court,* 763 P2d 852, 860 (Calif 1988), *cert denied,* 491 US 905(1989)
5. *UN Convention on the Rights of the Child.* New York, NY: United Nations; 1989
6. Skolnick A. Religious exemptions to child neglect laws still being passed despite convictions of parents. *JAMA.* 1990; 264:1226, 1229, 1233
7. *State of Minnesota v McKown,* 475 NW2d 63 (Minn 1991), *cert denied,* 112 S Ct 882(1992)
8. Kaunitz AM, Spence C, Danielson TS, Rochat RW, Grimes DA. Perinatal and maternal mortality in a religious group avoiding obstetric care. *Am J Obstet Gynecol.* 1984;150:826–831
9. Rodgers DV, Gindler JS, Atkinson WL, Markowitz LE. High attack rates and case fatality during a measles outbreak in groups with religious exemption to vaccination. *Pediatr Infect Dis J.* 1993;12:288–292
10. Etkind P, Lett SM, Macdonald PD, Silva E, Peppe J. Pertussis outbreaks in groups claiming religious exemptions to vaccinations. *AJDC.* 1992;146:173–176
11. Novotny T, Jennings CE, Doran M, et al. Measles outbreaks in religious groups exempt from immunization laws. *Public Health Rep.* 1988;103:49–54
12. Centers for Disease Control. Outbreak of measles among Christian Science students—Missouri and Illinois, 1994. *MMWR.* 1994;43:463–465
13. Committee on Bioethics, American Academy of Pediatrics. Informed consent, parental permission, and assent in pediatric practice. *Pediatrics.* 1995;95:314–317

Mark Sheldon

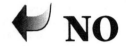 **NO**

Ethical Issues in the Forced Transfusion of Jehovah's Witness Children

Beliefs of Jehovah's Witnesses

Jehovah's Witnesses are Christians who believe the Bible is the Word of God in its entirety. Their name is taken from a statement that appears in the book of Isaiah: "Ye are my witnesses, saith Jehovah" (Isa. 43:10).... Presently, there are estimated to be approximately 2.2 million Jehovah's Witnesses in more than 200 countries around the world, with about 554,000 Witnesses in the United States (1).

As a group, Jehovah's Witnesses have faced numerous challenges. In the 1930s and 1940s, when their right to make home visitations was challenged, the courts affirmed their right to freedom of speech. Jehovah's Witnesses comply with most modern medical and surgical procedures, and a number of Witnesses are physicians and surgeons (2). They do not smoke, use recreational drugs, or have abortions. They view life as sacred. Why, then, do Witnesses appear to contradict this commitment to the idea that life is sacred, and reject blood transfusions at critical moments when it is a matter of life and death? In their pamphlet, *Jehovah's Witnesses and the Question of Blood* (3), they make the following statement:

> The issues of blood for Jehovah's Witnesses ... involves the most fundamental principles on which they as Christians base their lives. Their relationship with their creator and God is at stake.

The seriousness of the question of blood for Witnesses can be compared to the seriousness of idolatry for Jews....

It is the Acts of Apostles, in particular, which serves most centrally as the basis for the rejection of blood transfusions. After listing those things from which believers should abstain, it reads: " ... from which if ye keep yourselves, ye shall do well" (Acts 15:28-29).

Therefore, Jehovah's Witnesses take literally the numerous passages which proscribe the consumption of blood. They believe that the violation of this proscription will result in loss of eternal life. Witnesses do not reject this world. To

From Mark Sheldon, "Ethical Issues in the Forced Transfusion of Jehovah's Witness Children," *The Journal of Emergency Medicine*, vol. 14, no. 2 (1996), pp. 251–257. Copyright © 1996 by Elsevier Science, Inc. Reprinted by permission.

the contrary, they value and seek bodily health. Still, they do not think "physical life is limited to this present, temporal existence" (4). They believe that it is wrong to contrast "physical life" with "eternal life." Rather, Witnesses believe that God will, in the future, destroy life on earth, ending both personal life and conscious spiritual life. Eventually, they believe, God will resurrect the bodies of the faithful, and a limited number "will reign with God in heaven, while the remainder will live a life without end on a renewed earth" (4). They believe that life in the future, therefore, will be physical, earthly, and eternal.....

The Legal Framework

... When adults are concerned, the courts generally have determined that the competent adult Jehovah's Witness, who has no dependent minor children, has a right to refuse blood transfusion (5). When children are concerned, however, the situation is very different. Interestingly enough, the decision that appears to have set the major precedent, *Prince v. Massachusetts* (1944), was not a case dealing with medical treatment, but with child labor laws (5). An aunt, who was the legal custodian of a 9-year-old, had the child on the street with her selling Jehovah's Witness magazines. Although this was in violation of child labor laws, the defense claimed that Jehovah's Witnesses were required by their religion to spread the gospel. The little girl indicated that she wanted to sell the magazines to avoid eternal damnation. Defense, therefore, claimed that this was a violation of her right to freedom of religious belief. In response, the Supreme Court ruled that the state has authority as *parens patriae* to act in the interest of the child's well being, and that, on this basis, parental control can be restricted. While this particular decision had nothing to do with transfusion, the court (6) reached this conclusion:

> Neither the rights of religion nor the rights of parenthood are beyond limitation.... Parents may be free to make martyrs of themselves, but they are not free to make martyrs of their children before they have reached the age when they can make that choice for themselves.

A series of court decisions followed upholding *Prince,* but also dealing with the legitimacy of state intervention in matters that do or do not involve life-or-death situations. Again, it is interesting to note that *Prince* did not involve a life-and-death situation (5).

Witnesses' Views Regarding Children

In their pamphlet, *Jehovah's Witnesses and the Question of Blood* (3), the Witnesses make the following statement:

> Jehovah's Witnesses are sure that obeying the directions from their Creator is for their lasting good....

.The Witnesses then make the point that their refusal of blood transfusion cannot rightfully be construed either as suicide or as an exercise of the right to die, but it must be seen as respect for God's word (3).

In addressing the issue of children, Witnesses (3) make the following argument:

> Likely the aspect of this matter that is most highly charged with emotion involves the treating of children. All of us realize that children need care and protection. God-fearing parents particularly appreciate this. They deeply love their children and keenly feel their God-given responsibility to care for them and make decisions for their lasting welfare.—Ephesians 6:14.
>
> Society, too, recognizes parental responsibility, acknowledging that parents are the ones primarily authorized to provide for and decide for their children. Logically, religious beliefs in the family have a bearing on this. Children are certainly benefited if their parents' religion stresses the need to care for them. That is so with Jehovah's Witnesses, who in no way want to neglect their children. They recognize it as their God-given obligation to provide food, clothing, shelter and health care for them. Moreover, a genuine appreciation of the need to provide for one's children also requires inculcating in them morality and regard for what is right. . . .
>
> Parents who are Jehovah's Witnesses show great love for their children as well as their God by using the Bible to become moral persons. Thus, when these children are old enough to know what the Bible says about blood, they themselves support their parents decision to abstain from blood.—Acts 15:29.

. . . Witnesses indicate that they are fully aware of the significance of their refusal of blood transfusion for their children. However, they state that they do this out of devotion to God and out of love for their children. They claim that they cherish their children and are concerned for their children's future welfare. They do not believe that their actions should be construed as neglect. Rather, they believe that they probably are better parents than many parents in the larger society. They point to society's toleration for loose parenting, which leads to children growing up without respect for life, morality, or themselves. They hold up as examples the early Christian families who died at the hands of the Romans as models. Further, Witnesses claim to have evidence that as their children grow, they made the same choices that their parents previously made for them.

The aspect of the quote that should be emphasized is that Jehovah's Witness parents perceive themselves as acting in their children's best interest. They do not want their children to be "cut off" from the possibility of obtaining eternal life. They do not believe that it is in any way appropriate to describe their actions as involving neglect or disregard for their children. It is true, of course, that their belief that they may be better parents than others does not provide support for their right to deny blood transfusion to their children. Also, it is not clear what evidence they have to support their claim that their children will, when grown, reach the same decision as they have. But it seems clear that to describe their actions as neglectful is problematic. . . .

The Ethics Literature

Uniformly, the ethics literature expresses the view that it is right for the state to take temporary custody of a child to force it to undergo a blood transfusion in cases 1) when the lack of transfusion will lead to the child's death and 2) when the child is too young to give assent. However, I also believe that the basis upon which the state takes such action is not well defended in the existing ethics literature. This section consists of a review of representative arguments supporting state intervention, along with criticism of these arguments.

In 1977, Ruth Macklin (7) wrote, in an article still much referred to and often anthologized, the following:

> It might be argued that Jehovah's Witness parents, in refusing permission for blood to be given to their child, are acting in accordance with their perceived duty to God, as dictated by their religion, and that this duty to God overrides whatever secular duties they may have to preserve the life and health of their child.

Macklin (7) criticized this belief:

> Here it can only be replied that when an action done in accordance with perceived duties to God results in the likelihood of harm or death to another person (whether child or adult), then the duties to preserve life here on earth take precedence. The duties of a physician are to preserve and prolong life and to alleviate suffering. ... Freedom of religion does not include the right to act in a manner that will result in harm or death to another.

A few points in response to Macklin's argument are in order. The first and fundamental question is: from whose perspective is "harm" being defined? Second, she identifies "harm" with "death." These are not necessarily the same. She (7) states:

> If the parents refuse to grant permission for blood to be given to their child when failure to give blood will result in death or severe harm . . . , their prima facie right to retain control over their child no longer exists. . . . the case [at this point] sufficiently resembles that of child neglect [in respect to harm to the child]. . . . in the absence of fulfillment of their duties, it is morally justifiable to take control of the child away from the parent.

From Macklin's point of view, the act "sufficiently resembles child neglect." However, on what basis is this determined to be child neglect? This is only possible to claim if the religious perspective of the parents is set aside. What makes this move acceptable? The vague comment "sufficiently resembles child neglect" does not seem to provide such a basis.

Another interesting discussion of this issue appears in a 1983 article (8) that appeared in *Hospital Progress*. The article states: "The basic ethical principle involved is beneficence: One is obliged to do whatever good one reasonably can for another person" (8). The argument is different from Macklin's in that duty is seen positively (doing good) rather than negatively (avoiding harm). The article indicates a certain concern for the family and recognizes that it is "especially dangerous today, when society tends increasingly to allow the state to take over parents' functions" (8). However, it makes the following point (8):

> When the person is a minor, the obligation of beneficence falls primarily on the parents. When the parents for whatever reasons, even sincerely held religious beliefs, fail in this regard, then society, usually through its legal processes, must step in and provide for the child's good. Certain members of society, such as physicians or hospital administrators, are in a position to detect parental failure in these matters and therefore have a moral obligation to call the child's plight to civil authorities attention.

Two comments are necessary. The first is that the use of the language "parental failure" is heavily condemnatory, and not clearly appropriate. Second, while there may not be a problem, as there was above, in defining "harm," there is the problem of defining "good."

Another document that addresses the issue of state intervention is "Religious Exemptions From Child Abuse Statutes," produced by the Committee on Bioethics of the American Academy of Pediatrics in 1988 (9). This document is essentially a recommendation to change child abuse and neglect statutes that exempt parents on the basis of religious freedom....

Again, as in the Macklin article, the problem exists concerning the fact that whether harm is present depends on the perspective from which it is identified. Also, what truly constitutes the "welfare" of the child is a matter of perspective.

Another representative approach in the ethics literature appears in an article by Gary Benfield, MD, published in *Legal Aspects of Medical Practice* (10). He attempts, he points out, to address the human side of the issue, and he does, one can argue, make a sincere effort to try to understand the feelings of the Jehovah's Witness parents. He describes one of his cases that involved a young Rh-positive mother who gave birth to an Rh-positive male. He quotes (10) the mother:

> Three days after the birth of our son, we were told that on the very day of his birth he was taken from us, by a simple dial of the phone, and given blood.... You have touched the very depth of my being. The pain I felt is the same pain had I been told of my son's death.... I realize it is difficult to understand how two people claiming to love their child are willing to let that child die. We as Jehovah's Witnesses believe in that promised kingdom of God's as a real ruling power, and when that kingdom that we all pray for does come to this earth, our son will be given back to us. We would just have to wait a little longer to watch him grow and to give him all the love we stored up for him in our hearts over the last few months.... Jehovah's Witnesses do not reject blood for their children due to lack of love.... If we violate God's law on blood and the child dies, we have endangered his opportunity for everlasting life in God's new world.

Benfield's comments, in response to the mother's statement, are interesting and revealing. He remarks that after he considered all the options, he chose the one that "would best benefit my innocent patient" (10), a description which seems to impute something negative and possibly exploitative to the mother's relationship with the child. Second, he explains the basis for his choice. This consists of him asking himself, "Can I live with this decision?" (10). His answer is, "Yes." One can argue, however, that there is a problem in resolving an ethical dilemma on this basis. Such a criterion allows for anything that human beings "can live with." It is probably the case that Benfield is a sensitive and caring person, but this is a dangerous way to proceed. Presumably (this comment is not meant to reflect on Benfield but on the methodology he employs to resolve ethical dilemmas), Nazi doctors could "live with" their decisions.

Benfield (10) continues:

> The parents felt that, by giving blood, I would compromise their son's chances for everlasting life. I disagreed. I felt that Jehovah, a loving God, would welcome their child in "God's new world" were he to die having received blood or not. Who was right?

In this passage, Benfield ventures beyond the basis justifying intervention expressed in the ethics literature quoted above. He does not focus on the issue of "harm" or "good" or "welfare." Instead, he is engaged in theological debate. This, of course, prompts a question concerning the expertise a physician must have in order to engage in such commentary, to make a judgment concerning the validity of another's religious belief. The question is not what Benfield does, but why. What legitimately entitles him to force a transfusion on the child? A claim to possess a more valid religious insight than the mother is not available to him simply by virtue of being a physician. Nothing about being a physician provides a basis for his conviction that he understands better than the mother does how God works. In addition, she does not make a decision on the basis of what she "can live with." She acts on the basis of scripture. For her, this is not a matter of speculation or theological debate. She acts in a way that is prescribed for her by her religious tradition.

Observations and Conclusions

The following observations and conclusions should be viewed as preliminary thoughts in response to the issues raised in this article. They are preliminary in the sense that more discussion is warranted....

- The criticism of the ethics literature, contained in this paper, does not imply that there is no basis for the existence of statutes concerned with child abuse and neglect. This is a different question. The state, on this issue, appropriately takes guidance from scientists (psychiatrists and psychologists) who do studies, determine consequences, and measure pain and adverse reaction related to abuse and neglect. The state can develop expertise in this area and can claim knowledge of what constitutes child welfare, benefit, best interest, and harm. But where the issue is ultimately spiritual and where obtaining eternal life is the objective, it is clear that the state can make no claim to any sort of knowledge. Undergoing a blood transfusion may, in fact, cut off one from obtaining eternal life, and the state simply does not have the expertise and knowledge that would enable it to judge the merits of such a claim.

- Given this lack of expertise in such ultimate questions, the state, it seems to me, must accede that all talk of harm, benefit, best interest, and martyrdom amounts to what appears to be rhetoric and not argument. Jehovah's Witness parents, in refusing blood transfusion, cannot be said to be truly harming or neglecting their children. It is simply not the case that knowledge, which would make such a judgment legitimate, is available. That refusing a transfusion is harmful can certainly be believed, and one can argue that such is the case, but it cannot be known. Therefore, the state, in taking temporary guardianship to transfuse the child, cannot be said, with certainty, to be doing this for the child's welfare. It is simply not known whether this is the case.

What, therefore, makes it legitimate to order transfusions for the children of Jehovah's Witness? The most defensible argument is that the state's weakness is also its strength. That is, while the state does not know truly what is in the child's best interest, neither does anyone else. What the parents believe is in the child's best interest may be mistaken. Given that no one knows what is in the child's best interest, the role of the state is to ensure that children ultimately become adults, able to decide, independently, what is in their own best interest. It is not even that the state assumes that it knows it to be in the child's best interest to become an adult. It may not be. It is simply that no one knows what is in the child's best interest, and the responsibility of the state is to make certain that persons who make decisions which are irrevocable do so when they are competent. A source of disquiet is that many people believe, with good reason, that parents know what is in their child's best interest. This is a belief that is not easily dismissed. And, in fact, it is not dismissed here. Ideally, the family is a very significant moral institution. More than any other institution in society, the family, properly focused, values human beings simply because they *are*, not because of any use to which they can be put. And, for this reason, it is probably in a child's best interest (and society's best interest, as well) that the family be maintained to the extent that it is, as a unit, consistent with this objective of such nurturance.

References

1. Mead FS. Handbook of denominations in the United States. Nashville: Abingdon Press; 1980:148.
2. Dixon JL, Smalley MG. Jehovah's Witnesses: the surgical/ethical challenge. JAMA. 1981;246(27): 2471–2.
3. Jehovah's Witnesses and the question of blood. Brooklyn, NY: Watchtower Bible and Tract Society; 1977.
4. Studdard PA, Greene JY. Jehovah's Witnesses and blood transfusion: toward the resolution of a conflict of conscience. Ala J Med Sci. 1986;23(4):455.
5. Hirsh HL, Phifer H. The interface of medicine, religion, and the law: religious objections to medical treatment. Med Law. 1985;4(2):121–39.
6. *Prince v. Massachusetts.*
7. Macklin R. Consent, coercion and conflict of rights. Perspect Biol Med. 1977;20(365):365–6.

8. Editorial. May a Catholic hospital allow bloodless surgery for children? Hosp Prog. 1983;64(9): 58, 60.

9. Committee on Bioethics of the American Academy of Pediatrics. Religious exemptions from child abuse statutes. Pediatrics. 1988;81(1): 169–71.

10. Benfield DG. Giving blood to the critically ill newborn of Jehovah's Witness parents: the human side of the issue. Leg Aspects Med Pract. 1978;6(6):19–22.

POSTSCRIPT

Do Parents Harm Their Children When They Refuse Medical Treatment on Religious Grounds?

One solution to the problem posed by the refusal of Jehovah's Witnesses to undergo blood transfusions is to use alternative treatment methods, such as nonblood replacement fluids and surgical techniques that reduce the need for blood. Under many circumstances, these management alternatives allow even major surgery to be performed without additional risk. Another way to circumvent the religious prohibition is to choose medical, rather than surgical, treatment. In "Accommodating Jehovah's Witnesses' Choice of Nonblood Management," *Perspectives in Health Care Management* (Winter 1990), Donald Ridley, an attorney, argues that the sometimes inappropriate or unproven use of blood transfusions—as well as the lingering danger of transfusion-related infectious diseases, such as hepatitis—means that it may be reasonable to view Jehovah's Witnesses as "people making an informed choice between alternative courses of management." See also J. K. Vinicky et al., "The Jehovah's Witness and Blood: New Perspectives on an Old Dilemma," *Journal of Clinical Ethics* (Spring 1990).

Some of the most difficult situations arise when the patient is an adolescent. Determining whether or not an adolescent has the capacity to refuse blood transfusions is fraught with hazards. Some states have a provision for declaring an adolescent a "mature minor," that is, a person under the legal age of consent who has the capacity to make medical and other decisions. In 1994 a court of appeals in New Brunswick, Canada, set aside the order of a lower court that a 15-year-old Jehovah's Witness with leukemia be made a ward of the Crown in order that he may be given blood transfusions, if necessary. In that case, two doctors testified that the boy understood the consequences of his refusal. In a 1990 Texas case, however, the court ruled against a 16-year-old Jehovah's Witness who refused blood transfusions after he was hit by a train and severely injured. His doctor claimed that he would need transfusions during surgery to save his arm. The lower court supported the doctor and made the county child protective agency a temporary managing conservator. The Texas Court of Appeals upheld the decision, declaring that the parents' right to religious freedom did not include exposing their child to ill health or death. Moreover, because Texas law (like federal law) does not recognize the "mature minor" standard, the appeals court said that the district court was within its discretion in appointing the agency as conservator.

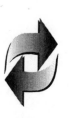

On the Internet ...

National Bioethics Advisory Commission: Publications

The full text of the National Bioethics Advisory Commission report *Cloning Human Beings* is available on this site.

> http://www.bioethics.gov/pubs.html

CNN Interactive: Genetic Testing and Insurance

This site contains an article on genetic testing and insurance along with an interactive section for posting opinions on the subject.

http://cnn.com/HEALTH/bioethics/9808/genetics.part2/template.html

Human Genome Project Information

This site contains articles concerning ethical, legal, and social issues raised by the availablity of genetic information.

> http://www.ornl.gov/hgmis/elsi/elsi.html

PART 5

Genetics

*T*he explosion of technology for unraveling the mysteries of human genetics has created enormous possibilities for the future in terms of understanding heredity and its influence on disease, of identifying people who are at risk for genetic diseases, and eventually of treating at-risk people. The completion of the human genome map raises questions of property rights to genes and the best way to address human cloning. All scientific and technical breakthroughs bring unresolved problems. Earlier abuses of genetic information (much of it misinformation) haunt efforts today to use this information wisely and compassionately. Also, although genetic information is intensely private, many people and institutions want to know, for their own reasons, whether or not a person has a genetic profile for a future disease. What impact will this knowledge have on individuals' lives and futures? These are some of the challenging issues raised in this section.

- Should Genes for Human Diseases Be Patented?

- Should Human Cloning Be Banned?

- Should Information From Genetic Testing Be Available to Employers and Insurers?

- Should Parents Always Be Told of Genetic-Testing Availability?

Should Genes for Human Diseases Be Patented?

YES: Glenn McGee, from "Gene Patents Can Be Ethical," *Cambridge Quarterly of Healthcare Ethics* (Fall 1998)

NO: Jon F. Merz and Mildred K. Cho, from "Disease Genes Are Not Patentable: A Rebuttal of McGee," *Cambridge Quarterly of Healthcare Ethics* (Fall 1998)

ISSUE SUMMARY

YES: Bioethicist Glenn McGee argues that disease gene patents are not patents on products of nature but on scientific innovations. He asserts that correctly framed and issued disease-related gene patents will not preclude access to genetic material for educational and scientific uses.

NO: Bioethicists Jon F. Merz and Mildred K. Cho counter that disease genes are not patentable because they are indeed products of nature that exist independent of the ingenuity, innovation, and manufacture of humans.

T he race to complete mapping of the human genome, the master set of genetic instructions that determines human biology, ended its first phase in May 2000. The task will not be fully completed until every letter of the human genetic code is put into its proper place. Nevertheless, even a "rough draft" is a monumental scientific accomplishment.

Two competitors crossed the finish line together. One was the publicly funded Human Genome Research Institute, headed by Dr. Francis Collins. The other was Celera Genomics Corporation, a private, for-profit company, headed by Dr. Craig Venter. The federal project began in 1990 and cost an estimated $2 billion. Begun in 1998, the Celera effort moved quickly and developed new technology to "sequence" (describe the structure of) genes.

The origins of this vast undertaking span the twentieth century. In 1900 botanists and biologists resurrected the earlier work of Gregor Mendel in explaining the scientific laws of heredity. In 1953 James Watson and Francis Crick discovered the double-helix structure of deoxyribonucleic acid (DNA), the long molecule that is the building block of human life. In 1973 the technology of recombinant DNA made it possible to take a fragment of DNA from one genome and splice it (recombine it) with another. Using recombinant DNA, scientists began to isolate single genes and discover their function. Proposals to characterize the entire human genome began in the 1980s.

To comprehend the scale of what has been accomplished, consider these numbers: Each human cell is made up of 23 chromosome pairs (rod-like structures composed of proteins and cellular DNA). The chromosomes are believed to contain 100,000 or more genes (the fundamental units of heredity). The human genome contains about 3 billion base pairs (subunits of genes). According to Walter Gilbert, a molecular biologist, the amount of information contained in these base pairs is equal to a thousand thousand-page telephone books.

The potential uses for this genetic map are enormous. Some geneticists and physicians believe that the human genome map is an unprecedented resource that will aid in understanding the genes involved in human biology and eventually in diagnosing and treating some of the approximately 4,000 known human genetic diseases as well as others that may have genetic factors. Some skeptics, on the other hand, point out that only a minor percentage of DNA, perhaps less than 10 percent, represent genes and their regulatory sequences. The rest are repetitive or have an unknown function. In this view, the map is incredibly detailed but is not much of a guide to major landmarks.

While the ultimate use of this information remains to be seen, the immediate future is clouded by an ethical debate about its ownership. U.S. patent law dates back to 1790, and a patent clause is part of the Constitution. A patent is a monopoly right granted to an inventor, giving him or her exclusive right to use the invention for a specific time period. The patent holder can license others to use the patent, usually for a fee. In a 1980 landmark case, *Diamond v. Chakrabaty* 447 U.S. 303, the Supreme Court ruled that living things (in this case, hybridized bacteria) can be patented.

In the case of the human genome, the federal government's position is that the information should be made freely available to scientists. Celera, on the other hand, is not releasing its data and has filed more than 6,000 of the 10,000 gene patents now pending. The U.S. Patent and Trademark Office still has not decided how many patents should be granted and what standards to use in their decisions.

The following two selections present opposing views of the patent debate. Glenn McGee asserts that, with some precautions, the government should continue granting patent protection to investigators who generate disease diagnostic information. Jon F. Merz and Mildred K. Cho counter that disease genes, like other products of nature or scientific observations, are not patentable.

Glenn McGee

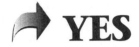 **YES**

Gene Patents Can Be Ethical

W hen one examines the emerging debate about genetic patenting, it becomes clear that those who oppose so-called "gene patents" misunderstand genetics or apply inappropriate moral and jurisprudential theory. In this brief essay I examine some arguments against gene patents of the "methods for detection" variety, and conclude that patents on methods for detecting the presence of a genetic correlation with disease-related (and other) phenotypes can be appropriate, and that with several precautions the U.S. Patent and Trademark Office should continue granting patent protection to investigators who generate genetic disease diagnostic innovations.

There are two arguments against gene patents. The first is that genetic information is a part of nature, and one ought not, indeed cannot, patent nature. Patents allow long-term control of new and innovative processes to be secured by inventors.[1] You have to figure out how to do something in order to receive a patent, and the process you create must have utility. Critics charge that finding a gene is not innovative. Arthur Caplan and Jon Merz, for example, compare the identification of disease genes to the land rush.[2] The basic tools utilized in the multimillion dollar laboratories that identify genes, they point out, are themselves covered by patent protection, and render the search for genes similar to using conventional means to find new territory. Caplan and Merz contend that although the scientists who identified some forms of a gene that correlate with breast cancer are entitled to claim their discovery, discovering new land is not the same thing as owning a process. Put another way, the telescope is indeed an innovative instrument, and someone can indeed patent the technologies involved in telescopes, but it is another thing entirely to point your innovative telescope up at the heavens and begin claiming each new star as a product of technological innovation, thus protecting the process of looking at each new star.[3] The point is well taken. The discoverer of Pluto has not invented a process, no matter how much utility might be claimed from finding and using the discovery of Pluto. If we follow this line of analysis with genes, locating new genes is a matter of sailing into new territory with old boats, so the correct mode of protection for the "finders" of new genes would be something other than patents, akin to land use or water rights laws.

From Glenn McGee, "Gene Patents Can Be Ethical," *Cambridge Quarterly of Healthcare Ethics*, vol. 7, no. 4 (Fall 1998). Copyright © 1998 by Cambridge University Press. Reprinted by permission.

However, it seems to me that opponents of the patenting of disease genes erroneously assume that the U.S. Patent and Trademark Office, and the courts that enforce patent claims, can be a final arbiter for some arcane, metaphysical distinction between "discoveries of nature" and useful technologies made by humans. Opponents of patents for "methods of detecting" a relationship between genes and disease assert that such patents are improper because they involve no "reworking" of a gene from its "natural form," and are thus attempts to patent nature. Opponents of disease-related gene patents argue that genes are natural phenomena discovered using previously patented devices. Merz, Cho, Robertson, and Leonard, for example, write that "the discovery that a particular DNA sequence at a specific locus or that different forms of a gene are associated with a disease does not qualify that scientific knowledge as patentable subject matter because no human alteration of an existing organism or naturally occurring entity is involved... [and] because it is merely an observation of a state of nature or 'nature's handiwork.' "[4] But is it so clear? It seems to me that while disease genes are in one sense discoverable by conventional means, their utility and indeed their meaning as a commercial object is not discovered but rather invented. Investigators who patent alleles [gene pairs] for, or even a gene *for* susceptibility to cancer can legitimately claim a patent for "methods for detecting" a relationship between a particular bit of DNA and some phenotype. The job of the U.S. Patent and Trademark Office is to evaluate whether the patent claims a novel method for detecting a particular relationship between the DNA of a person and some phenotype for a particular purpose (e.g., diagnosing the presence of possibility of future disease states). Methods patents do not patent disease genes per se, but instead the process of making use of that DNA in diagnosis.

There is a subtle distinction to be made between "observing DNA" and constructing a DNA-based product for diagnosis of some disease or phenotype, much too subtle to be captured in any obvious way by the blunt rules about patentable subject matter, let alone by the intent of our Constitutional founders. Nonetheless, the distinction is real, and goes right to the heart of what patents are supposed to do. Disease gene patents are more an innovation of scientists than a discovery. That we sometimes tend to believe otherwise is to some extent a product of *genetic essentialism,* our cultural belief that genes are a simple, self-evident library of data present in everyone and responsible for all aspects of human embodiment and disease. If we begin with the idea that genes are a simple code to be read or stumbled upon, we miss the immensely difficult epidemiological task of clarifying otherwise diffuse relationships between particular environments and genes, and between particular groups and genes. If I find a strange tree in the Vermont forest, take a clipping back to my lab, discover that eating the tree cures a disease, and file a patent application for the tree itself, or for very broad uses of the tree, the U.S. Patent and Trademark Office is likely to reject my application. However, if I take a clipping and purify, package, intensify, or in other ways make a product *derived* from that clipping, the U.S. Patent and Trademark Office may grant me a patent alongside the thousands of other medical device or pharmaceutical patents. It was obvious to the Office that cDNA, express sequence tags (ESTs), and RNA that has been "purified" in some way merited patent issuance. What must be answered is whether the process of describing disease-related genes is like examining a "natural form" (like the regular clipping from the tree), or like changing nature to serve a novel purpose (like making a special tea from my clipping).

There is little hope of demonstrating that a disease-related gene mutation is natural, out there to be discovered and possessed of a priori identity. Disease genes are identified in the application by their phenotypic products, when some bits of DNA can be put to explanatory use for some diagnostic purpose. But this is true also of Nebraska. Nebraska is a state only when we say it is. Its geography, climate, and flora are identifiable only after we establish the boundaries for some other purpose. We do not patent Nebraska. Patents for disease-related gene mutations and genes are by contrast useful when the innovation involved in creating some genetic diagnosis product is useful, novel, and nonobvious. While finding a new gene requires no new or novel piece of equipment, and involves no "purification" by probes or other "artificial" tools, the work of identifying the group of people possessed of a phenotype, the specific methods by which mutations are associated with a particular phenotype, and the methods for putting the epidemiological evidence to specific work in making a diagnosis, are clearly synthetic and novel and are not themselves natural phenomena. Having a phenotype, like having a disease, is in part a matter of social and scientific convention about which states of human life possess relevant or important differences meriting medical intervention or classification. We sometimes forget that even when a gene is highly correlated with a particular disease, that doesn't make the disease "genetic." Finding DNA is a discovery. Correlating it with human life for the purpose of creating a diagnostic process is innovation.

Thus not to allow disease-related gene work patent protection seems misguided. If making an extract of my tree clipping can be classed as innovative and patentable, why should we allow genetic essentialism to persuade us that the line between discovering nature and making technology is unblurred for work involving genetic diagnosis? It is in fact a blurry line, and the best we can hope for is to limit the use of patenting to cases where it clearly protects the making of particular diagnostic tests and elements of viral vectors for gene therapy. The U.S. Patent and Trademark Office does not have special access to the heavens, and to expect that they will treat all disease-related gene mutations and genes as "purely natural" phenomena is to ask them to buy in to a particularly intractable element of genetic essentialism: the claim that genes are natural things, things "in themselves." So far the patent office has wisely refused to endorse this analysis, opting instead to patent genes or alleles when they are employed in a novel product even if that product is tied directly to embodied human biology.

Think about the matter in intellectual rather than simple physical terms and things seem clearer. When the anthropologist begins to observe a new community, her work is quite clearly that of the observer, and her work products are most clearly associated with existing and well-recognized anthropological methods. She may publish initial findings about the community but she will not yet be doing synthetic work. She is pointing a telescope into the heavens, cataloguing a new star. As her work proceeds, though, she will increasingly develop new ways of understanding the community and new modes for gathering data. Much of her new data will take on new forms and be published in different ways, e.g., as personal reports from her slow, partial assimilation into the culture. Let us imagine that she is now approached by a U.S. soft drink company for advice in understanding this new market. Using her synthetic work, she may develop for them a scheme for interpreting the wishes of the community, using an instrument that will tell who will want to buy soda on the basis of signs and signals otherwise uninterpretable. The U.S. Patent and Trademark Office will be receptive to her intellectual patent application for the methods for detecting such receptiveness, even though she began with simple and well-understood methods for gathering knowledge. Her late turn to identify a way of thinking about the community for the purpose of "diagnosing" its interest in soda is novel and patentable. My point by analogy is that the teams working on genetic diagnosis are entitled to the same protection for whatever diagnostic utility they derive. However Faustian is the anthropologist's appropriation of her early project, it would be essentialism to insist that she is merely patenting a priori natural facts. She, and the patent applicants for gene patents, should be able to request patent protection for innovative scholarly work that mutates and culminates in novel products.

It seems to me no one would care much about the preceding debate were it not for the second argument against gene patents, which holds that gene patents create a "toll bridge" barring research using patented genes. Opponents of gene patents hold that a researcher who wants to study some chromosome may not be able to look at human genetic information without paying the people who "found" it. This argument is more important because it suggests that genetic patents will clog up the works of genetic research, creating an anticompetitive environment in which genetic tests will not be developed if researchers in the early stages of work on common diseases will not be able to afford to pay the tolls necessary for start-up research.

However, correctly framed and issued disease-related gene patents will in no way preclude access to genetic material by the thousands of laboratories in high schools, colleges, and of course medical sciences departments that are conducting research in molecular and cellular engineering without using the device actually patented by the patentee. Infringement of the patent occurs when other organizations put the innovation per se to use, and the actual innovation is put to use only when the method for detecting the allele's or gene's correlation with the particular phenotype is applied to a patient. The critical issue is that the patent office be very clear about what it is that the patent claims about the disease or phenotype being diagnosed. A clear patent application is a good one if and only if it identifies a well-studied body of epidemiological data about the effectiveness of use of particular genetic information in finding disposition to, or physiologic evidence of, some phenotype. Companies should not be able to throw up a flag as they identify each new chunk of the genome: there must be utility, and only that useful device is patentable.

In the final analysis, none of us wants to sell Yellowstone, the stars in the sky, or our bodies. The effort to diagnose genetic correlation with disease creates new kinds of information for particular purposes. It is not, as some opponents of genetic patenting would have it, an effort to own the "code of codes" or to lock up investigation of genetic disease.

Notes

1. U.S. Constitution, Article 1, § 8, cl 8; U.S. Code Title 35, § 101, 102 (1982).
2. Caplan A.L., Merz J. Patenting gene sequences. *British Medical Journal* 1996; 312:926; see also Halewood P. Law's bodies: disembodiment and the structure of liberal property rights. *Iowa Law Review* 1996; 81(5): 133–93; Kimbrell A. *The Human Body Shop: The Engineering and Marketing of Life.* New York: Free Press 1993; Barrad C. Genetic information and property theory. *Northwestern University Law Review* 1993; 87(3): 1037–86.
3. Merz J., Cho M., Robertson M., Leonard D. Disease gene patenting is a bad innovation. *Molecular Diagnosis* 1997: 2(4): 299–304.
4. See note 4, Merz et al. 1997: 401.

NO 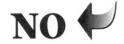　　　Jon F. Merz and Mildred K. Cho

Disease Genes Are Not Patentable:
A Rebuttal of McGee

Dr. McGee presents a cogent argument for the patentability of the diagnosis of gene forms that are found to be associated with disease or other phenotypic manifestations. We're convinced he's wrong. An analogy will help explain why.

Some years ago, in the Black Forest, people hunted down the elusive truffle, that culinary delight, with pigs learned in the art of rooting around in, you guessed it, tree roots. People and pigs had been collaborating in the search for truffles for thousands of years. Among the truffles collected in the forest, none was as highly prized—or as rare—as the White Truffle. It would reward its finder with 10 times the price of other truffles at market. But the White Truffle was much more elusive than other truffles, and a day in the forest would yield an average 1 White Truffle for every 100 regular truffles.

After 20 years of truffle trifles (and meticulous notekeeping), one Franz Statistiner did make an interesting (and, as we shall see, valuable) observation: 9 of every 10 White Truffles that he had gathered over the years were found on the roots of red oak trees, and, overall, 20% of truffles found on red oaks were White!

Franz contemplated keeping his finding secret and simply targeting his pigs on their daily jaunts to search only red oaks, thereby increasing his yield of White Truffles. He was worried, however, that other truffle hunters would soon note his success in the market and figure out his secret. Instead, he went to a patent lawyer.

A good patent lawyer. She wrote and got an imaginary patent with the following claims:

I Claim:

> 1. A method of detecting an increased chance of having White Truffles under a tree comprising directly or indirectly:
>
>> detecting whether or not a tree is a Red Oak Tree;
>> and
>> observing whether or not the tree is more likely to
>> have White Truffles growing under it, wherein Red Oak

From Jon F. Merz and Mildred K. Cho, "Disease Genes Are Not Patentable: A Rebuttal of McGee," *Cambridge Quarterly of Healthcare Ethics*, vol. 7, no. 4 (Fall 1998). Copyright © 1998 by Cambridge University Press. Reprinted by permission.

> Trees have an increased likelihood of having White
> Truffles thereunder.
>
> 2. The method of claim 1, wherein said detecting step comprises look-
>   ing for trees having at least one Red Oak Tree Leaf growing thereon.

Franz then was able to collect royalties from all other hunters who focused their search on red oak trees, making him wildly wealthy. Franz bought the forest.

Sound reasonable? Dr. McGee apparently agrees with us: neither the discovery nor the act of looking at red oak trees for the purpose of diagnosing the increased likelihood of finding White Truffles is patentable subject matter. What has been discovered is a mere phenomenon of nature, an (as yet unexplained) association between an observation of a particular type of tree in the forest and the empirical fact that such trees have a "natural" propensity for White Truffles. It is no more than an observation of a thing and the mental step of understanding the informational value of that thing.

The truffle patent is not only analogous to a disease gene patent, but has been craftily drafted directly from U.S. Patent No. 5,508,167, entitled Methods of Screening for Alzheimer's Disease, which reads:

> What is claimed is:
>
> 1. A method of detecting if a subject is at increased risk of devel-
>   oping late onset Alzheimer's disease (AD) comprising directly or
>   indirectly:
>
>> detecting the presence or absence of an apolipoprotein
>> E type 4 isoform (ApoE4) in the subject;
>>   and
>> observing whether or not the subject is at increased
>> risk of developing late onset AD by observing if the
>> presence of ApoE4 is or is not detected, wherein the
>> presence of ApoE4 indicates said subject is at increased
>> risk of developing late onset AD.

This invention, Dr. McGee and the U.S. Patent and Trademark Office agree, is patentable. What differs? The act of "detecting" in the truffle patent requires one's eyes and knowledge of any unique characteristics of the red oak tree, such as the leaf specified in claim 2. Detecting in the AD patent requires use of PCR, Southern analysis, sequencing, or one of numerous other previously established means of looking at the chemical structure known as DNA. Each entails steps that are obvious to anyone skilled in the pertinent art. The act of looking at trees or genes, respectively, comprises normal knowledge and skill of those trained in their respective arts. Any one device or method for looking might itself be a patentable innovation (such as a microscope, telescope, or PCR), but the special protections afforded by patenting should not be extended to all specific acts of looking.

What else differs? The "invention" underlying the truffle patent is the association of red oak trees with an increased chance of finding White Truffles thereunder. The "invention" underlying the AD patent is the association of a particular allele with an increased chance of disease occurrence. Both are empirical observations; both are simply epidemiologic discoveries about (albeit within our current understanding of) naturally occurring phenomena.

Dr. McGee's argument is based on two false premises. The first is that the difficulty and effort involved in making a discovery, the "immensely difficult epidemiological task of purifying otherwise diffuse relationships between particular environments and genes, and between particular groups and genes," make the discovery patentable.

Everyone agrees that a basic scientific or statistical discovery, regardless of how difficult it was to make or how much effort and money went into it, is not patentable subject matter. As the U.S. Supreme Court stated in a case in which it invalidated claims for a mixture of bacteria, "[P]atents cannot issue for the discovery of the phenomena of nature.... The qualities of these bacteria, like the heat of the sun, electricity, or the qualities of metals, are part of the storehouse of knowledge of all men. They are manifestations of laws of nature, free to all men and reserved exclusively to none."[1] The Supreme Court more recently reiterated that "[t]he laws of nature, physical phenomena, and abstract ideas have been held not patentable.... Thus a new mineral discovered in the earth or a new plant found in the wild is not patentable subject matter. Likewise, Einstein could not patent his celebrated law that $E = mc^2$; nor could Newton have patented the law of gravity."[2] The work Einstein and Newton put into these discoveries was synthetic and novel, but their genius and remarkable efforts do not make their observations of associations between physical entities patentable.

Furthermore, the fact that several research groups independently clone and sequence genes associated with diseases, often within weeks of each other, suggests that the effort is not that innovative to those skilled in the arts. If the entire coding sequence of the human genome is sequenced at the end of the Human Genome Project, it will become even less of an effort to correlate the presence of sequences with disease. At some point, by Dr. McGee's argument, associations between genes and diseases will not be patentable because of the ease—a simple computer search—of finding these (as well as far more complex multigene and gene-environment) relationships. To say that these associations are patentable is "genetic exceptionalism": allowing oneself to be unduly dazzled, nay, mesmerized, by the novelty of biotechnology compared to other technologies. It is genetic exceptionalism to say that finding associations between red oak trees and White Truffles using the well-established method of shoveling is not patentable, but that finding associations between a gene and a disease using well-established methods of mapping, cloning, and sequencing genes, and of identifying people with mutations is patentable.

Dr. McGee's second false premise is that he predicates patentability on the usefulness of the discovery. However, market potential is not a necessary, much less a satisfactory, condition to determining whether something comprises patentable subject matter. It is simply irrelevant. Gold and diamonds, while valuable, are not patentable subject matter, regardless of who first discovered them or how difficult those discoveries were. McGee's arguments show how easy it is to segue from an inquiry about whether something is patentable subject matter to questions about whether that something satisfies the tests for patentability; that is, it must be new, useful, and nonobvious. Under U.S. patent law, however, these are separate issues, and confounding them muddles the underlying question.

Arguing that correlating discoveries with "human life for the purpose of creating a diagnostic process is innovation" as does McGee sets us on a slippery slope that would wreak havoc with healthcare. By this argument, tests used in performing physical examinations (including asking patents questions, feeling their thyroid glands, and listening to their lungs and heart with stethoscopes) as methods of detecting abnormalities should be patentable. Many of the methods used in routine physicals took years of clinical observations and effort, resulted from a synthetic and creative process, and are undoubtedly useful. Yet are they patentable?

At bottom, the "detection" involved in the truffle and disease gene patents itself is not patentable. Everyone is free to look at those things—be they trees or genes—that exist independent of the ingenuity, innovation, and manufacture of humans. The fact that someone discovers a reason for looking does not change that basic premise. The scientific reason itself is not patentable, and it does not render the act of looking in the specific case patentable.

Independent of the foregoing, we believe there are substantive arguments against disease gene patenting based not on patentability of the subject matter but on public policy and ethics. As we have asserted elsewhere, the risks to patient health and access to care, to physician-patient relations, and to the biomedical research enterprise far outweigh the possible benefits that could be attributed to disease gene patents.[3] While we believe the courts should invalidate these broad diagnosis methods patents under the product of nature doctrine, we firmly believe that the unethical patenting practices reflected in these patents should be more firmly enjoined by the medical profession and by healthcare institutions. Unfortunately, the ethical proscriptions have been emasculated by financial pressures, by increasing commercialism of academic medicine, and by profiteering. The profession must clean up its act, or Congress may intervene.

Because of perceived abuse of patents of surgical methods, Congress enacted a law in late 1996 that holds physicians not liable for infringement of "pure process" patents.[4] That law does not apply to "biotechnology patents" (perhaps reflecting Congress's love affair with things biotechnic, and perhaps reflecting the acknowledged assistance of the biotechnology industry in drafting the law),[5] and does not protect laboratories approved under the Clinical Laboratories Improvement Act.[6] That law was a stopgap against more drastic legislation prohibiting medical process patents; if methods patenting continues to burgeon (and diagnostics comprises the largest share of biotechnology patents being issued),[7] Congress should expand the law's protections. Already, the human chorionic gonadotropin patent, a similarly broad diagnostic patent, has led to the abandonment of prenatal testing that had been the standard of care.[8] This is simply unacceptable. These patents are contrary to good medical practice, and must be prohibited.

Notes

1. Funk Brothers Seed Co. v. Kalo Inoculant Co., 333 U.S. 127, 130 (1948).
2. Diamond v. Chakrabarty, 447 U.S. 303, 308–9 (1980).
3. Merz JF, Cho MK, Robertson MJ, Leonard, DGB. Disease gene patenting is a bad innovation. *Molecular Diagnosis* 1997; 2(4): 299–304.
4. Public Law 104-208, § 101(a), 110 Stat 3009-67, 104th Congress, 2nd term, 1996, codified at U.S. Code Title 35 § 287(c) (1997).
5. Congressional Record S12023-4 (30 September 1996).
6. Clinical Laboratories Improvement Act, codified at U.S. Code Title 42 § 263a (1997).
7. Thomas SM, Birtwistle NJ, Brady M, Burke JF. Public-sector patents on human DNA. *Nature* 1997; 388:709.
8. Eichenwald K. Push for royalties threatens use of Down Syndrome test. *New York Times* 1997; May 23: A1.

POSTSCRIPT

Should Genes for Human Diseases Be Patented?

In July 2000 the U.S. House Judiciary Subcommittee on Courts and Intellectual Property held hearings on disease gene patenting. Industry spokesmen pointed to the need to maintain economic incentives in the form of patents for the potential of the human genome map to be realized. Others expressed concern that patent holders, most of whom used federally funded research to develop their products, are restricting access and preventing some physicians from performing genetic tests. The director of the U.S. Patent and Trademark Office responded that the patent laws have worked well, and that the question of whether an invention is patentable should be separated from the question of access to it.

Human gene patenting is also controversial in other countries. For international perspectives, see Patricia Baird, "Patenting and Human Genes," *Perspectives in Biology and Medicine* (Spring 1998), pp. 391–408. Baird points out that developing countries have historically been exploited by scientists who use their populations for study but do not give them access to the resulting inventions. If scientists from poor countries have to pay royalties to use gene sequences, their abilities to apply research findings would be limited.

Mark Sagoff argues that intellectual property can be protected without any implication that anyone has invented or now owns a product of nature. In his view, industry does not want to "upstage the Creator" but wants to enjoy legal protection that encourages investments. See "Patented Genes," in *Issues in Science and Technology* (Spring 1998), pp. 37–41.

The American College of Medical Genetics issued a statement in August 1999 that unequivocally condemns gene patents. Its position is that "genes and their mutations are naturally occurring substances that should not be patented," and that patents on genes with clinical implications must be very broadly licensed. Furthermore, the College states that licensing agreements "should not limit access through excessive royalties and other unreasonable terms."

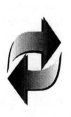

ISSUE 12

Should Human Cloning Be Banned?

YES: George J. Annas, from "Why We Should Ban Human Cloning," *The New England Journal of Medicine* (July 9, 1998)

NO: John A. Robertson, from "Human Cloning and the Challenge of Regulation," *The New England Journal of Medicine* (July 9, 1998)

ISSUE SUMMARY

YES: Law professor George J. Annas contends that human cloning devalues people by depriving them of their uniqueness and would radically alter what it means to be human.

NO: Law professor John A. Robertson asserts that regulatory policy should avoid a ban on cloning, but should ensure that it is performed in a responsible manner.

On February 23, 1997, Ian Wilmut, a Scottish animal husbandry scientist, introduced a lamb named Dolly to the world. In one sense Dolly was unique—the first mammal to be born from a technique that involved transplanting the genetic material of an adult sheep into an egg from which the nucleus had been removed. In another sense, Dolly's distinction was that she was not unique; she was a clone, an exact genetic copy of the donating sheep.

The implications for human cloning were immediately apparent. The question of whether it would be ethical to clone a human has troubled scientists, religious leaders, and ethicists for decades. However, most earlier debates had faded because the prospects seemed remote. Dolly brought about a new and vigorous debate.

Immediately after Wilmut's announcement, President Bill Clinton announced a ban on federal funding for cloning research and asked private researchers to comply voluntarily. He asked the National Bioethics Advisory Commission (NBAC) to study the legal and ethical issues associated with the use of this technology and to make recommendations within 90 days.

The NBAC's report, submitted in June 1997, concludes that "at this time it is morally unacceptable for anyone in the public or private sector, whether in a research or clinical setting, to attempt to create a child using somatic cell nuclear transfer cloning [the technical name for Wilmut's technique]." The

NBAC reached this conclusion because of concerns about the safety of using these techniques in humans, which, they say, "are likely to involve unacceptable risks to the fetus and/or potential child." Although the NBAC does not determine that cloning violates any fundamental ethical principle, it identifies many serious ethical concerns, such as the possibility of psychological harm, confusion over family roles, and potential damage to important social values.

The NBAC's recommendations include, a continuation of the ban on the use of federal funding, a request to private researchers and firms to comply voluntarily with the intent of the ban, and enactment of federal legislation that will prohibit anyone from attempting to create a child through this technique. This legislative ban will, however, be reviewed after three to five years to see whether it should be continued. Further, the NBAC recommends widespread and continuing deliberation on the issues raised by cloning.

The NBAC's report did not please everyone. Some are concerned about attempts to interfere with scientific progress. Also, cloning is argued to provide potential benefits to infertile parents and others who might have a reason to create a genetic duplicate, for example, to provide a bone marrow transplant to a dying child. Others assert that the NBAC, by appealing to safety concerns, has failed to grapple with the central issues. Following the report, the U.S. Senate passed a bill banning cloning. While many scientists and medical organizations support the ban, they worry that the legislation will apply to other, noncontroversial forms of reproductive research. An alternate bill was introduced to meet these concerns, but neither bill was enacted into law. The debate continues.

The following selections illustrate two differing points of view. George J. Annas criticizes the NBAC report and states that cloning will radically alter what it means to be human by replicating a living or dead human with a single genetic parent. John A. Robertson sees potential good rather than evil in cloning humans. Rather than seeking to prohibit all uses of human cloning, we should focus attention on ensuring that cloning is done responsibly.

George J. Annas

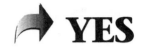 **YES**

Why We Should Ban Human Cloning

In February [1998] the U.S. Senate voted 54 to 42 against bringing an anti-cloning bill directly to the floor for a vote.[1] During the debate, more than 16 scientific and medical organizations, including the American Society of Reproductive Medicine and the Federation of American Societies for Experimental Biology, and 27 Nobel prize–winning scientists, agreed that there should be a moratorium on the creation of a human being by somatic nuclear transplants. What the groups objected to was legislation that went beyond this prohibition to include cloning human cells, genes, and tissues. An alternative proposal was introduced by Senator Edward M. Kennedy (D-Mass.) and Senator Dianne Feinstein (D-Calif.) and modeled on a 1997 proposal by President Bill Clinton and his National Bioethics Advisory Commission. It would, in line with the views of all of these scientific groups, outlaw attempts to produce a child but permit all other forms of cloning research.[2,3] Because the issue is intimately involved with research with embryos and abortion politics, in many ways the congressional debates over human cloning are a replay of past debates on fetal-tissue transplants[4] and research using human embryos.[5] Nonetheless, the virtually unanimous scientific consensus on the advisability of a legislative ban or voluntary moratorium on the attempt to create a human child by cloning justifies deeper discussion of the issue than it has received so far.

It has been more than a year since embryologist Ian Wilmut and his colleagues announced to the world that they had cloned a sheep.[6] No one has yet duplicated their work, raising serious questions about whether Dolly the sheep was cloned from a stem cell or a fetal cell, rather than a fully differentiated cell.[7] For my purpose, the success or failure of Wilmut's experiment is not the issue. Public attention to somatic-cell nuclear cloning presents an opportunity to consider the broader issues of public regulation of human research and the meaning of human reproduction.

Cloning and Imagination

In the 1970s, human cloning was a centerpiece issue in bioethical debates in the United States.[8,9] In 1978, a House committee held a hearing on human cloning in response to the publication of David Rorvik's *In His Image: The Cloning of a*

From George J. Annas, "Why We Should Ban Human Cloning," *The New England Journal of Medicine,* vol. 339, no. 2 (July 9, 1998), pp. 122–125. Copyright © 1998 by The Massachusetts Medical Society. All rights reserved. Reprinted by permission.

Man.[10] All the scientists who testified assured the committee that the supposed account of the cloning of a human being was fictional and that the techniques described in the book could not work. The chief point the scientists wanted to make, however, was that they did not want any laws enacted that might affect their research. In the words of one, "there is no need for any form of regulation, and it could only in the long run have a harmful effect."[11] The book was an elaborate fable, but it presented a valuable opportunity to discuss the ethical implications of cloning. The failure to see it as a fable was a failure of imagination. We normally do not look to novels for scientific knowledge, but they provide more: insights into life itself.[12]

This failure of imagination has been witnessed repeatedly, most recently in 1997, when President Clinton asked the National Bioethics Advisory Commission to make recommendations about human cloning. Although acknowledging in their report that human cloning has always seemed the stuff of science fiction rather than science, the group did not commission any background papers on how fiction informs the debate. Even a cursory reading of books like Aldous Huxley's *Brave New World,* Ira Levin's *The Boys from Brazil,* and Fay Weldon's *The Cloning of Joanna May,* for example, would have saved much time and needless debate. Literary treatments of cloning inform us that cloning is an evolutionary dead end that can only replicate what already exists but cannot improve it; that exact replication of a human is not possible; that cloning is not inherently about infertile couples or twins, but about a technique that can produce an indefinite number of genetic duplicates; that clones must be accorded the same human rights as persons that we grant any other human; and that personal identity, human dignity, and parental responsibility are at the core of the debate about human cloning.

We might also have gained a better appreciation of our responsibilities to our children had we examined fiction more closely. The reporter who described Wilmut as "Dolly's laboratory father,"[13] for example, probably could not have done a better job of conjuring up images of Mary Shelley's *Frankenstein* if he had tried. Frankenstein was also his creature's father and god; the creature told him, "I ought to be thy Adam." As in the case of Dolly, the "spark of life" was infused into the creature by an electric current. Shelley's great novel explores virtually all the noncommercial elements of today's debate.

The naming of the world's first cloned mammal also has great significance. The sole survivor of 277 cloned embryos (or "fused couplets"), the clone could have been named after its sequence in this group (for example, C-137), but this would only have emphasized its character as a laboratory product. In stark contrast, the name Dolly (provided for the public and not used in the scientific report in *Nature,* in which she is identified as 6LL3) suggests a unique individual. Victor Frankenstein, of course, never named his creature, thereby repudiating any parental responsibility. The creature himself evolved into a monster when he was rejected not only by Frankenstein, but by society as well. Naming the world's first mammal clone Dolly was meant to distance her from the Frankenstein myth both by making her something she is not (a doll) and by accepting "parental" responsibility for her.

Unlike Shelley's world, the future envisioned in Huxley's *Brave New World,* in which all humans are created by cloning through embryo splitting and conditioned to join a specified worker group, was always unlikely. There are much more efficient ways of creating killers or terrorists (or even soldiers and workers) than through cloning. Physical and psychological conditioning can turn teenagers into terrorists in a matter of months, so there is no need to wait 18 to 20 years for the clones to grow up and be trained themselves. Cloning has no real military or paramilitary uses. Even clones of Adolf Hitler would have been very different people because they would have grown up in a radically altered world environment.

Cloning and Reproduction

Even though virtually all scientists oppose it, a minority of free-marketers and bioethicists have suggested that there might nonetheless be some good reasons to clone a human. But virtually all these suggestions themselves expose the central problem of cloning: the devaluing of persons by depriving them of their uniqueness. One common example suggested is cloning a dying or recently deceased child if this is what the grieving parents want. A fictional cover story in the March 1998 issue of *Wired,* for example, tells the story of the world's first clone.[14] She is cloned from the DNA of a dead two-week-old infant, who died from a mitochondrial defect that is later "cured" by cloning with an enucleated donor egg. The closer one gets to the embryo stage, the more cloning a child looks like the much less problematic method of cloning by "twinning" or embryo splitting. And proponents of cloning tend to want to "naturalize" and "normalize" asexual replication by arguing that it is just like having "natural" twins.

Embryo splitting might be justified if only a few embryos could be produced by an infertile couple and all were implanted at the same time (since this does not involve replicating an existing and known genome). But scenarios of cloning by nuclear transfer have involved older children, and the only reason to clone an existing human is to create a genetic replica. Using the bodies of children to replicate them encourages all of us to devalue children and treat them as interchangeable commodities. For example, thanks to cloning, the death of a child need no longer be a singular human tragedy but, rather, can be an opportunity to try to replicate the no longer priceless (or irreplaceable) dead child. No one should have such dominion over a child (even a dead or dying child) as to use his or her genes to create the child's child.

Cloning would also radically alter what it means to be human by replicating a living or dead human being asexually to produce a person with a single genetic parent. The danger is that through human cloning we will lose something vital to our humanity, the uniqueness (and therefore the value and dignity) of every human. Cloning represents the height of genetic reductionism and genetic determinism.

Population geneticist R.C. Lewontin has challenged my position that the first human clone would also be the first human with a single genetic parent by arguing that, instead, "a child by cloning has a full set of chromosomes like anyone else, half of which were derived from a mother and half from a father. It happens that these chromosomes were passed through another individual, the cloning donor, on the way to the child. That donor is certainly not the child's 'parent' in any biological sense, but simply an earlier offspring of the original parents."[15] Lewontin takes genetic reductionism to perhaps its logical extreme. People become no more than containers of their parents' genes, and their parents have the right to treat them not as individual human beings, but rather as human embryos—entities that can be split and replicated at their whim without any consideration of the child's choice or welfare. Children (even adult children), according to Lewontin's view, have no say in whether they are replicated or not, because it is their parents, not they, who are reproducing. This radical redefinition of reproduction and parenthood, and the denial of the choice to procreate or not, turns out to be an even stronger argument against cloning children than its biologic novelty. Of course, we could require the consent of adults to be cloned—but why should we, if they are not becoming parents?

Related human rights and human dignity would also prohibit using cloned children as organ sources for their father or mother original. Nor is there any constitutional right to be cloned in the United States that is triggered by marriage to someone with whom an adult cannot reproduce sexually, because there is no tradition of asexual replication and because permitting asexual replication is not necessary to safeguard any existing concept of ordered liberty (rights fundamental to ordered liberty are the rights the Supreme Court sees as essential to individual liberty in our society).

Although it is possible to imagine some scenarios in which cloning could be used for the treatment of infertility, the use of cloning simply provides parents another choice for choice's sake, not out of necessity. Moreover, in a fundamental sense, cloning cannot be a treatment for infertility. This replication technique changes the very concept of infertility itself, since all humans have somatic cells that could be used for asexual replication and therefore no one would be unable to replicate himself or herself asexually. In vitro fertilization, on the other hand, simply provides a technological way for otherwise infertile humans to reproduce sexually.

John Robertson argues that adults have a right to procreate in any way they can, and that the interests of the children cannot be taken into account because the resulting children cannot be harmed (since without cloning the children would not exist at all).[16] But this argument amounts to a tautology. It applies equally to everyone alive; none of us would exist had it not been for the precise and unpredictable time when the father's sperm and the mother's egg met. This biologic fact, however, does not justify a conclusion that our parents had no obligations to us as their future children. If it did, it would be equally acceptable, from the child's perspective, to be gestated in a great ape, or even a cow, or to be composed of a mixture of ape genes and human genes.

The primary reason for banning the cloning of living or dead humans was articulated by the philosopher Hans Jonas in the early 1970s. He correctly noted that it does not matter that creating an exact duplicate of an existing person is impossible. What matters is that the person is chosen to be cloned because of some characteristic or characteristics he or she possesses (which, it is hoped, would also be possessed by the genetic copy or clone). Jonas argued that cloning is always a crime against the clone, the crime of depriving the clone of his or her "existential right to certain subjective terms of being"—particularly, the "right to ignorance" of facts about his or her origin that are likely to be "paralyzing for the spontaneity of becoming himself" or herself.[17] This advance knowledge of what another has or has not accomplished with the clone's genome destroys the clone's "condition for authentic growth" in seeking to answer the fundamental question of all beings, "Who am I?" Jonas continues: "The ethical command here entering the enlarged stage of our powers is: never to violate the right to that ignorance which is a condition of authentic action; or: to respect the right of each human life to find its own way and be a surprise to itself."[17]

Jonas is correct. His rationale, of course, applies only to a "delayed genetic twin" or "serial twin" created from an existing human, not to genetically identical twins born at the same time, including those created by cloning with use of embryo splitting. Even if one does not agree with him, however, it is hypocritical to argue that a cloning technique that limits the liberty and choices of the resulting child or children can be justified on the grounds that cloning expands the liberty and choices of would-be cloners.[18]

Moratoriums and Bans on Human Cloning

Members of the National Bioethics Advisory Commission could not agree on much, but they did conclude that any current attempt to clone a human being should be prohibited by basic ethical principles that ban putting human subjects at substantial risk without their informed consent. But danger itself will not prevent scientists and physicians from performing first-of-their-kind experiments—from implanting a baboon's heart in a human baby to using a permanent artificial heart in an adult—and cloning techniques may be both safer and more efficient in the future. We must identify a mechanism that can both prevent premature experimentation and permit reasonable experimentation when the facts change.

The mechanism I favor is a broad-based regulatory agency to oversee human experimentation in the areas of genetic engineering, research with human embryos, xenografts, artificial organs, and other potentially dangerous boundary-crossing experiments.[19] Any such national regulatory agency must be composed almost exclusively of nonresearchers and nonphysicians so it can reflect public values, not parochial concerns. Currently, the operative American ethic seems to be that if any possible case can be imagined in which a new technology might be useful, it should not be prohibited, no matter what harm might result. One of the most important procedural steps Congress should take in setting up a federal agency to regulate human experimentation would be to put the burden of proof on those who propose to undertake novel experiments (including cloning) that risk harm and call deeply held social values into question.

This shift in the burden of proof is critical if society is to have an influence over science.[20] Without it, social control is not possible. This model applies the precautionary principle of international environmental law to cloning and other potentially harmful biomedical experiments involving humans. The principle requires governments to protect the public health and the environment from realistic threats of irreversible harm or catastrophic consequences even in the absence of clear evid.nce of harm.[21] Under this principle, proponents of human cloning would have the burden of proving that there was some compelling contravailing need to benefit either current or future generations before such an experiment was permitted (for example, if the entire species were to become sterile). Thus, regulators would not have the burden of proving that there was some compelling reason not to approve it. This regulatory scheme would depend on at least a de facto, if not a de jure, ban or moratorium on such experiments and a mechanism such as my proposed regulatory agency that could lift the ban. The suggestion that the Food and Drug Administration (FDA) can substitute for such an agency is fanciful. The FDA has no jurisdiction over either the practice of medicine or human replication and is far too narrowly constituted to represent the public in this area. Some see human cloning as inevitable and uncontrollable.[22,23] Control will be difficult, and it will ultimately require close international cooperation. But this is no reason not to try—any more than a recognition that controlling terrorism or biologic weapons is difficult and uncertain justifies making no attempt at control.

On the recommendation of the National Bioethics Advisory Commission, the White House sent proposed anticloning legislation to Congress in June 1997. The Clinton proposal receded into obscurity until early 1998, when a Chicago physicist, Richard Seed, made national news by announcing that he intended to raise funds to clone a human. Because Seed acted like a prototypical "mad scientist," his proposal was greeted with almost universal condemnation.[24] Like the 1978 Rorvik hoax, however, it provided another opportunity for public discussion of cloning and prompted a more refined version of the Clinton proposal: the Feinstein–Kennedy bill. We can (and should) take advantage of this opportunity to distinguish the cloning of cells and tissues from the cloning of human beings by somatic nuclear transplantation[25] and to permit the former while prohibiting the latter. We should also take the opportunity to fill in the regulatory lacuna that permits any individual scientist to act first and consider the human consequences later, and we should use the controversy over cloning as an opportunity to begin an international dialogue on human experimentation.

References

1. U.S. Senate. 144 Cong. Rec. S561–S580, S607–S608 (1998).
2. S. 1611 (Feinstein–Kennedy Prohibition on Cloning of Human Beings Act of 1998).
3. Cloning human beings: report and recommendations of the National Bioethics Advisory Commission. Rockville, Md.: National Bioethics Advisory Commission, June 1997.
4. Annas GJ, Elias S. The politics of transplantation of human fetal tissue. N Engl J Med 1989;320:1079–82.
5. Annas GJ, Caplan A, Elias S. The politics of human embryo research—avoiding ethical gridlock. N Engl J Med 1996;334:1329–32.

6. Wilmut I, Schnieke AE, McWhir J, Kind AJ, Campbell KH. Viable offspring derived from fetal and adult mammalian cells. Nature 1997;385:810–3.

7. Butler D. Dolly researcher plans further experiments after challenges. Nature 1998;391:825–6.

8. Lederberg J. Experimental genetics and human evolution. Am Naturalist 1966;100:519–31.

9. Watson JD. Moving toward the clonal man. Atlantic Monthly. May 1971:50–3.

10. Rorvik DM. In his image: the cloning of a man. Philadelphia: J.B. Lippincott, 1978.

11. Development in cell biology and genetics, cloning. Hearings before the Subcommittee on Health and the Environment of the Committee on Interstate and Foreign Commerce of the U.S. House of Representatives, 95th Congress, 2d Session, May 31, 1978.

12. Chomsky N. Language and problems of knowledge: the Managua lectures. Cambridge, Mass.: MIT Press, 1988.

13. Montalbano W. Cloned sheep is star, but not sole project, at institute. Los Angeles Times. February 25, 1997:A7.

14. Kadrey R. Carbon copy: meet the first human clone. Wired. March 1998:146–50.

15. Lewontin RC. Confusion over cloning. New York Review of Books. October 23, 1997:20–3.

16. Robertson JA. Children of choice: freedom and the new reproductive technologies. Princeton, N.J.: Princeton University Press, 1994:169.

17. Jonas H. Philosophical essays: From ancient creed to technological man. Englewood Cliffs, N.J.: Prentice-Hall, 1974:162–3.

18. Annas GJ. Some choice: law, medicine and the market. New York: Oxford University Press, 1998:14–5.

19. Annas GJ. Regulatory models for human embryo cloning: the free market, professional guidelines, and government restrictions. Kennedy Inst Ethics J 1994;4:235–49.

20. Hearings before the U.S. Senate Subcommittee on Public Health and Safety, 105th Congress, 1st Session, March 12, 1997. (Or see: http://www-busph.bu.edu/depts/lw/clonetest.htm.)

21. Cross FB. Paradoxical perils of the precautionary principle. Washington Lee Law Rev 1996;53:851–925.

22. Kolata GB. Clone: the road to Dolly, and the path ahead. New York: W. Morrow, 1998.

23. Silver LM. Remaking Eden: cloning and beyond in a brave new world. New York: Avon Books, 1997.

24. Knox RA. A Chicagoan plans to offer cloning of humans. Boston Globe. January 7, 1998:A3.

25. Kassirer JP, Rosenthal NA. Should human cloning research be off limits? N Engl J Med 1998;338:905–6.

NO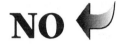

John A. Robertson

Human Cloning and the Challenge of Regulation

The birth of Dolly, the sheep cloned from a mammary cell of an adult ewe, has initiated a public debate about human cloning. Although cloning of humans may never be clinically feasible, discussion of the ethical, legal, and social issues raised is important. Cloning is just one of several techniques potentially available to select, control, or alter the genome of offspring.[1-3] The development of such technology poses an important social challenge: how to ensure that the technology is used to enhance, rather than limit, individual freedom and welfare.

A key ethical question is whether a responsible couple, interested in rearing healthy offspring biologically related to them, might ethically choose to use cloning (or other genetic-selection techniques) for that purpose. The answer should take into account the benefits sought through the use of the techniques and any potential harm to offspring or to other interests.

The most likely uses of cloning would be far removed from the bizarre or horrific scenarios that initially dominated media coverage.[4] Theoretically, cloning would enable rich or powerful persons to clone themselves several times over, and commercial entrepreneurs might hire women to bear clones of sports or entertainment celebrities to be sold to others to rear. But current reproductive techniques can also be abused, and existing laws against selling children would apply to those created by cloning.

There is no reason to think that the ability to clone humans will cause many people to turn to cloning when other methods of reproduction would enable them to have healthy children. Cloning a human being by somatic-cell nuclear transfer, for example, would require a consenting person as a source of DNA, eggs to be enucleated and then fused with the DNA, a woman who would carry and deliver the child, and a person or couple to raise the child. Given this reality, cloning is most likely to be sought by couples who, because of infertility, a high risk of severe genetic disease, or other factors, cannot or do not wish to conceive a child.

From John A. Robertson, "Human Cloning and the Challenge of Regulation," *The New England Journal of Medicine,* vol. 339, no. 2 (July 9, 1998), pp. 119–122. Copyright © 1998 by The Massachusetts Medical Society. All rights reserved. Reprinted by permission.

Several plausible scenarios can be imagined. Rather than use sperm, egg, or embryo from anonymous donors, couples who are infertile as a result of gametic insufficiency might choose to clone one of the partners. If the husband were the source of the DNA and the wife provided the egg that received the nuclear transfer and then gestated the fetus, they would have a child biologically related to each of them and would not need to rely on anonymous gamete or embryo donation. Of course, many infertile couples might still prefer gamete or embryo donation or adoption. But there is nothing inherently wrong in wishing to be biologically related to one's children, even when this goal cannot be achieved through sexual reproduction.

A second plausible application would be for a couple at high risk of having offspring with a genetic disease.[5] Couples in this situation must now choose whether to risk the birth of an affected child, to undergo prenatal or preimplantation diagnosis and abortion or the discarding of embryos, to accept gamete donation, to seek adoption, or to remain childless. If cloning were available, however, some couples, in line with prevailing concepts of kinship, family, and parenting, might strongly prefer to clone one of themselves or another family member. Alternatively, if they already had a healthy child, they might choose to use cloning to create a later-born twin of that child. In the more distant future, it is even possible that the child whose DNA was replicated would not have been born healthy but would have been made healthy by gene therapy after birth.

A third application relates to obtaining tissue or organs for transplantation. A child who needed an organ or tissue transplant might lack a medically suitable donor. Couples in this situation have sometimes conceived a child coitally in the hope that he or she would have the correct tissue type to serve, for example, as a bone marrow donor for an older sibling.[6,7] If the child's disease was not genetic, a couple might prefer to clone the affected child to be sure that the tissue would match.

It might eventually be possible to procure suitable tissue or organs by cloning the source DNA only to the point at which stem cells or other material might be obtained for transplantation, thus avoiding the need to bring a child into the world for the sake of obtaining tissue.[8] Cloning a person's cells up to the embryo stage might provide a source of stem cells or tissue for the person cloned. Cloning might also be used to enable a couple to clone a dead or dying child so as to have that child live on in some closely related form, to obtain sufficient numbers of embryos for transfer and pregnancy, or to eliminate mitochondrial disease.[5]

Most, if not all, of the potential uses of cloning are controversial, usually because of the explicit copying of the genome. As the National Bioethics Advisory Commission noted, in addition to concern about physical safety and eugenics, somatic-cell cloning raises issues of the individuality, autonomy, objectification, and kinship of the resulting children.[5] In other instances, such as the production of embryos to serve as tissue banks, the ethical issue is the sacrifice of embryos created solely for that purpose.

Given the wide leeway now granted couples to use assisted reproduction and prenatal genetic selection in forming families, cloning should not be rejected in all circumstances as unethical or illegitimate. The manipulation of embryos and the use of gamete donors and surrogates are increasingly common. Most fetuses conceived in the United States and Western Europe are now screened for genetic or chromosomal anomalies. Before conception, screening to identify carriers of genetic diseases is widespread.[9] Such practices also deviate from conventional notions of reproduction, kinship, and medical treatment of infertility, yet they are widely accepted.

Despite the similarity of cloning to current practices, however, the dissimilarities should not be overlooked. The aim of most other forms of assisted reproduction is the birth of a child who is a descendant of at least one member of the couple, not an identical twin. Most genetic selection acts negatively to identify and screen out unwanted traits such as genetic disease, not positively to choose or replicate the genome as in somatic-cell cloning.[3] It is not clear, however, why a child's relation to his or her rearing parents must always be that of sexually reproduced descendant when such a relationship is not possible because of infertility or other factors. Indeed, in gamete donation and adoption, although sexual reproduction is involved, a full descendant relation between the child and both rearing parents is lacking. Nor should the difference between negative and positive means of selecting children determine the ethical or social acceptability of cloning or other techniques. In both situations, a deliberate choice is made so that a child is born with one genome rather than another or is not born at all.

Is cloning sufficiently similar to current assisted-reproduction and genetic-selection practices to be treated similarly as a presumptively protected exercise of family or reproductive liberty?[10] Couples who request cloning in the situations I have described are seeking to rear healthy children with whom they will have a genetic or biologic tie, just as couples who conceive their children sexually do. Whether described as "replication" or as "reproduction," the resort to cloning is similar enough in purpose and effects to other reproduction and genetic-selection practices that it should be treated similarly. Therefore, a couple should be free to choose cloning unless there are compelling reasons for thinking that this would create harm that the other procedures would not cause.[10]

The concern of the National Bioethics Advisory Commission about the welfare of the clone reflects two types of fear. The first is that a child with the same nuclear DNA as another person, who is thus that person's later-born identical twin, will be so severely harmed by the identity of nuclear DNA between them that it is morally preferable, if not obligatory, that the child not be born at all.[5] In this case the fear is that the later-born twin will lack individuality or the freedom to create his or her own identity because of confusion or expectations caused by having the same DNA as another person.[5,11]

This claim does not withstand the close scrutiny that should precede interference with a couple's freedom to bear and rear biologically related children.[10] Having the same genome as another person is not in itself harmful, as widespread experience with monozygotic twins shows. Being a twin does not deny either twin his or her individuality or freedom, and twins often have a special intimacy or closeness that few non-twin siblings can experience.[12]

There is no reason to think that being a later-born identical twin resulting from cloning would change the overall assessment of being a twin.

Differences in mitochondria and the uterine and childhood environment will undercut problems of similarity and minimize the risk of overidentification with the first twin. A clone of Smith may look like Smith, but he or she will not be Smith and will lack many of Smith's phenotypic characteristics. The effects of having similar DNA will also depend on the length of time before the second twin is born, on whether the twins are raised together, on whether they are informed that they are genetic twins, on whether other people are so informed, on the beliefs that the rearing parents have about genetic influence on behavior, and on other factors. Having a previously born twin might in some circumstances also prove to be a source of support or intimacy for the later-born child.

The risk that parents or the child will overly identify the child with the DNA source also seems surmountable. Would the child invariably be expected to match the phenotypic characteristics of the DNA source, thus denying the second twin an "open future" and the freedom to develop his or her own identity?[5,11,13] In response to this question, one must ask whether couples who choose to clone offspring are more likely to want a child who is a mere replica of the DNA source or a child who is unique and valued for more than his or her genes. Couples may use cloning in order to ensure that the biologic child they rear is healthy, to maintain a family connection in the face of gametic infertility, or to obtain matched tissue for transplantation and yet still be responsibly committed to the welfare of their child, including his or her separate identity and interests and right to develop as he or she chooses.

The second type of fear is that parents who choose their child's genome through somatic-cell cloning will view the child as a commodity or an object to serve their own ends.[5] We do not view children born through coital or assisted reproduction as "mere means" just because people reproduce in order to have company in old age, to fulfill what they see as God's will, to prove their virility, to have heirs, to save a relationship, or to serve other selfish purposes.[14] What counts is how a child is treated after birth. Self-interested motives for having children do not prevent parents from loving children for themselves once they are born.

The use of cloning to form families in the situations I have described, though closely related to current assisted-reproduction and genetic-selection practices, does offer unique variations. The novelty of the relation—cloning in lieu of sperm donation, for example, produces a later-born identical twin raised by the older twin and his spouse—will create special psychological and social challenges. Can these challenges be successfully met, so that cloning produces net good for families and society? Given the largely positive experience with assisted-reproduction techniques that initially appeared frightening, cautious optimism is justified. We should be able to develop procedures and guidelines for cloning that will allow us to obtain its benefits while minimizing its problems and dangers.

In the light of these considerations, I would argue that a ban on privately funded cloning research is unjustified and likely to hamper important types of research.[8] A permanent ban on the cloning of human beings, as advocated by the Council of Europe and proposed in Congress, is also unjustified.[15,16] A more limited ban—whether for 5 years, as proposed by the National Bioethics Advisory Commission and enacted in California, or for 10 years, as in the bill of Senator Dianne Feinstein (D-Calif.) and Senator Edward M. Kennedy (D-Mass.) that is now before Congress—is also open to question.[5,17,18] Given the early state of cloning science and the widely shared view that the transfer of cloned embryos to the uterus before the safety and efficacy of the procedure has been established is unethical, few responsible physicians are likely to offer human cloning in the near future.[5] Nor are profit-motivated entrepreneurs, such as Richard Seed, likely to have many customers for their cloning services until the safety of the procedure is demonstrated.[19] A ban on human cloning for a limited period would thus serve largely symbolic purposes. Symbolic legislation, however, often has substantial costs.[20,21] A government-imposed prohibition on privately funded cloning, even for a limited period, should not be enacted unless there is a compelling need. Such a need has not been demonstrated.

Rather than seek to prohibit all uses of human cloning, we should focus our attention on ensuring that cloning is done well. No physician or couple should embark on cloning without careful thought about the novel relational issues and child-rearing responsibilities that will ensue. We need regulations or guidelines to ensure safety and efficacy, fully informed consent and counseling for the couple, the consent of any person who may provide DNA, guarantees of parental rights and duties, and a limit on the number of clones from any single source.[10] It may also be important to restrict cloning to situations where there is a strong likelihood that the couple or individual initiating the procedure will also rear the resulting child. This principle will encourage a stable parenting situation and minimize the chance that cloning entrepreneurs will create clones to be sold to others.[22] As our experience grows, some restrictions on who may serve as a source of DNA for cloning (for example, a ban on cloning one's parents) may also be defensible.[10]

Cloning is important because it is the first of several positive means of genetic selection that may be sought by families seeking to have and rear healthy, biologically related offspring. In the future, mitochondrial transplantation, germ-line gene therapy, genetic enhancement, and other forms of prenatal genetic alteration may be possible.[3,23,24] With each new technique, as with cloning, the key question will be whether it serves important health, reproductive, or family needs and whether its benefits outweigh any likely harm. Cloning illustrates the principle that when legitimate uses of a technique are likely, regulatory policy should avoid prohibition and focus on ensuring that the technique is used responsibly for the good of those directly involved. As genetic knowledge continues to grow, the challenge of regulation will occupy us for some time to come.

References

1. Silver LM. Remaking Eden: cloning and beyond in a brave new world. New York: Avon Books, 1997.

2. Walters L, Palmer JG. The ethics of human gene therapy. New York: Oxford University Press, 1997.
3. Robertson JA. Genetic selection of offspring characteristics. Boston Univ Law Rev 1996;76:421-82.
4. Begley S. Can we clone humans? Newsweek. March 10, 1997:53-60.
5. Cloning human beings: report and recommendations of the National Bioethics Advisory Commission. Rockville, Md.: National Bioethics Advisory Commission, June 1997.
6. Robertson JA. Children of choice: freedom and the new reproductive technologies. Princeton, N.J.: Princeton University Press, 1994.
7. Kearney W, Caplan AL. Parity for the donation of bone marrow: ethical and policy considerations. In: Blank RH, Bonnicksen AL, eds. Emerging issues in biomedical policy: an annual review. Vol. 1. New York: Columbia University Press, 1992:262-85.
8. Kassirer JP, Rosenthal NA. Should human cloning research be off limits? N Engl J Med 1998;338:905-6.
9. Holtzman NA. Proceed with caution: predicting genetic risks in the recombinant DNA era. Baltimore: Johns Hopkins University Press, 1989.
10. Robertson JA. Liberty, identity, and human cloning. Texas Law Rev 1998;77:1371-456.
11. Davis DS. What's wrong with cloning? Jurimetrics 1997;38:83-9.
12. Segal NL. Behavioral aspects of intergenerational human cloning: what twins tell us. Jurimetrics 1997;38:57-68.
13. Jonas H. Philosophical essays: from ancient creed to technological man. Englewood Cliffs, N.J.: Prentice-Hall, 1974:161.
14. Heyd D. Genethics: moral issues in the creation of people. Berkeley: University of California Press, 1992.
15. Council of Europe. Draft additional protocol to the Convention on Human Rights and Biomedicine on the prohibition of cloning human beings with explanatory report and Parliamentary Assembly opinion (adopted September 22, 1997). XXXVI International Legal Materials 1415 (1997).
16. Human Cloning Prohibition Act, H.R. 923, S.1601 (March 5, 1997).
17. Act of Oct. 4, 1997, ch. 688, 1997 Cal. Legis. Serv. 3790 (West, WESTLAW through 1997 Sess.).
18. Prohibition on Cloning of Human Beings Act, S. 1602, 105th Cong. (1998).
19. Stolberg SG. A small spark ignites debate on laws on cloning humans. New York Times. January 19, 1998:A1.
20. Gusfield J. Symbolic crusade: status politics and the American temperance movement. Urbana: University of Illinois Press, 1963.
21. Wolf SM. Ban cloning? Why NBAC is wrong. Hastings Cent Rep 1997;27(5):12.
22. Wilson JQ. The paradox of cloning. The Weekly Standard. May 26, 1997:23-7.
23. Zhang J, Grifo J, Blaszczyk A, et al. In vitro maturation of human preovulatory oocytes reconstructed by germinal vesicle transfer. Fertil Steril 1997;68:Suppl:S1. abstract.
24. Bonnicksen AL. Transplanting nuclei between human eggs: implications for germline genetics. Politics and the Life Sciences. March 1998:3-10.

POSTSCRIPT

Should Human Cloning Be Banned?

Several scientists have reported advances in the technology of cloning. In July 1998 a group of Hawaiian scientists reported that they had cloned 22 adult mice, 7 of which are clones of clones from the cells of a single mouse. In December 1998 a group of Japanese scientists reported the birth of eight calves, cloned from a single cow. Four of the calves died during birth. Later the same month Korean researchers reported combining a human egg and a cell to produce the first stages of a human embryo. Because of ethical considerations, they said, they stopped the experiment and did not continue to attempt to create a human clone. Human cloning, while still not a reality, seems to be moving forward.

Meanwhile, scientific critics of Wilmut's research question whether Dolly is a true clone and whether the technique that created her is applicable. Only one Dolly was produced from 277 tries because the other embryos died at various stages of development. Wilmut responded to these criticisms with what he maintains is definitive DNA fingerprinting to prove that Dolly was produced from the original cell.

In a series of articles collectively entitled "Cloning Human Beings: Responding to the National Bioethics Advisory Commission's Report," *Hastings Center Report* (September–October 1997), five scholars write about their opinions of the NBAC report. Richard Lewontin critiques the NBAC report in "The Confusion Over Cloning," *New York Review of Books* (October 23, 1997). A special issue of *The Sciences* (September/October 1997) is devoted to "The Promise and Peril of Cloning." It contains several articles on the science and ethics of cloning, including "Whose Self Is It, Anyway?" In this article, Philip Kitcher observes that even genetic clones would not be exactly the same as the original because "the traits people value most come about through a complex interaction between genotypes and environments."

In "Should Human Cloning Research Be Off Limits?" *The New England Journal of Medicine* (March 26, 1998), Jerome P. Kassirer and Nadia A. Rosenthal oppose restrictive legislative bans on cloning while encouraging a wide public debate based on full knowledge of the scientific facts. Patrick D. Hopkins analyzes public information in "How Popular Media Represent Cloning as an Ethical Problem," *Hastings Center Report* (March–April 1998). Gina Kolata, *Clone: The Road to Dolly and the Path Ahead* (William Morrow, 1998), is a journalistic account of the science and implications of cloning. See also Glenn McGee, ed., *The Human Cloning Debate*, 2d ed. (Berkeley Hills Books, 2000).

ISSUE 13

Should Information From Genetic Testing Be Available to Employers and Insurers?

YES: Andrew Sullivan, from "Promotion of the Fittest," *The New York Times Magazine* (July 23, 2000)

NO: Thomas H. Murray, from "Genetics and the Moral Mission of Health Insurance," *Hastings Center Report* (November–December 1992)

ISSUE SUMMARY

YES: Columnist Andrew Sullivan sees no ethical difference between using genetic information to predict future workplace performance and using other means to do so. Sullivan argues that genetic information is more reliable and less discriminatory than other types of information.

NO: Thomas H. Murray, a professor of biomedical ethics, contends that actuarial fairness—the insurance industry's standard—fails to accomplish the social goals of health insurance and that genetic tests should not be used to deny people access to health insurance.

G enetic diseases and predisposition to disease are not uncommon. An estimated 4,000 to 5,000 genetic diseases have already been identified. Some of these diseases are detectable prenatally, such as Down's syndrome, a form of mental retardation, and sickle-cell anemia, a blood disorder. Others are detected at birth, such as phenylketonuria (PKU), a metabolic disorder. Still others become manifest only in adults, such as Huntington's disease, a lethal neurological disorder.

Approximately 1,100 genes that cause disease have been identified, many because of the work of the Human Genome Project and the existence of newer DNA-based technologies. In 1994–1995, for example, two defective genes, labeled BRCA-1 and BRCA-2, were found to be present in Jewish women from Eastern Europe. These genes might explain the high rate of breast cancer in that population. Genetic disorders come in several varieties. Inherited disorders are passed on from parent to child. Acquired disorders appear later in life as a result of genetic alteration, perhaps due to chemical or environmental toxicities. In addition to diseases directly related to a single gene or a pair of genes, a number of common illnesses—such as most breast cancers, Alzheimer's disease, which causes mental and physical deterioration, and coronary artery disease—are most likely caused by a combination of genetics and environment.

Once a disease-causing gene is identified, a test to determine whether or not a particular individual carries that gene is often developed. The ability to test for such genes has benefits and burdens. The most common use is in prenatal screening, in which a fetus can be tested for a number of chromosomal abnormalities. Premarital screening is also used—particularly among ethnic groups predisposed to certain diseases—so that couples can make informed reproductive choices. The knowledge that one is prone to develop a certain disease can lead to preventive measures such as changes in diet, exercise, and early treatment. The knowledge that these tests provide can be reassuring, or it can force difficult choices—such as whether to marry, conceive a child, or abort pregnancy.

Choices become more problematic in diseases where children may be affected later in life. For example, should a child be tested for Huntington's disease? If the child is tested and found to be carrying the gene, should he or she be told? How would a young person weigh the concern of becoming demented in adult life against the importance of having that information for his or her future mate and potential children?

Whatever the personal decisions made in these cases, nearly everyone concerned about genetic testing worries about its impact on insurance. As the number of genetic tests increases, and as they become routine in medical practice, more and more diseases and predispositions will be identified and entered into a person's medical record. Who will have access to that information? For what purposes? Medical information of all kinds is now transmitted routinely to insurance companies who use it to validate claims, accept or deny applications for insurance, and to set actuarial standards (making estimates of future claims).

The following selections present different points of view about the use of genetic tests for insurance. Andrew Sullivan asserts that genetic discrimination in employment and insurance is both rational and inevitable. Although speculative, genetic information is still more reliable than other means conventionally used to predict future performance. Using information from genetic tests, Sullivan argues, is simply a further elaboration of the basic principle of insurance —estimating risk. Thomas H. Murray, on the other hand, contends that insurance has a social purpose of protecting those in need. This purpose would be undermined by allowing genetic tests to determine insurability.

Andrew Sullivan 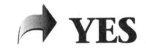 **YES**

Promotion of the Fittest

When you first think about it, it's a no-brainer. When the final stages of mapping the human genome were hyped [in June 2000], both President Bill Clinton and [British] Prime Minister Tony Blair called for a swift, extensive ban on using genetic information to discriminate in employment or insurance. Clinton had already signed an executive order back in February, banning such discrimination for federal employees. True to form, both politicians had polling data to support them. A 1998 survey of 1,000 randomly selected Americans found that 63 percent of them balked at any genetic testing if an employer or health insurer could have access to the data. So a ban on genetic discrimination not only secures privacy and fairness; it also protects good research by reassuring study volunteers that the information they provide is in completely safe hands.

What's not to like? Well, quite a lot, actually. Like most notions that command almost universal assent, the proposed ban on genetic discrimination makes far less sense the more you think about it. A few brave souls, like the writer Michael Kinsley, have pointed this out, but even he admitted that he wasn't sure what conclusion to draw. So here goes: genetic discrimination, however troubling, is both rational and inevitable. And the sooner we get over our hand-wringing, the better.

Start with the analogy to racial discrimination. It's bogus. The point of laws against racial bias is to outlaw irrational discrimination based on irrelevant characteristics. The point of laws against genetic discrimination is to outlaw rational bias based on relevant information. The two principles aren't merely different; they're opposite. We perform individual, rational acts of discrimination all the time. In fact, it would be hard to function without them. Deciding not to put an art historian in charge of a nuclear power plant is not bias but common sense. Similarly, discriminating against a blind person when hiring a baseball umpire is certainly not a function of hostility to blind people in general and wouldn't even be illegal under the Americans with Disabilities Act. Sure, it's discrimination—but it's rational discrimination and is not, and shouldn't be, illegal. So why should genetic discrimination?

The best answer to this is that most genetic information is speculative. It doesn't tell you what a person is; it tells you what she may be. Right now, it

From Andrew Sullivan, "Promotion of the Fittest," *The New York Times Magazine* (July 23, 2000). Copyright © 2000 by Andrew Sullivan. Reprinted by permission of The Wylie Agency.

could tell an employer that a job applicant might have a propensity for heart trouble in the future, or for Parkinson's disease. Within the foreseeable future, it might even reveal that a person's genetic spatial skills are particularly good or that her verbal fluency is genetically high. But it won't tell you what a person has actually made of her natural gifts or whether she might be lucky and avoid certain likely genetic fates. It might tell you that a person has the genes to make a fine pianist, but it won't tell you if he has practiced or even knows how to read music.

Clinton's executive order rested on this distinction. It bans the use of genetic testing to determine if a person has a propensity for being bad at a certain job or for having a specific physical ailment in the future, but it allows such testing to see if a person has an actual existing condition that makes him less able to perform a certain task. So it's O.K. to test if a fighter pilot has a genetic condition that makes him liable now to have a sudden heart attack on the job; but it's not O.K. to test him to see if his genes suggest that he could develop Alzheimer's in preretirement years.

I get the distinction. I just don't see the ethical difference between using genes to hazard future performance and using other means to do so. After all, we already use countless ways of discriminating rationally on the basis of the likelihood of future ability. What else is an SAT score, if not an attempt to predict future performance? Or a garden-variety letter of recommendation? What are these but predictors exactly analogous to genetic testing—not destiny as such, but pretty reliable guides? The real question, then, is, Why should imprecise and often dangerous predictors (like SAT results) be morally acceptable but more precise methods (like genes) be morally repugnant? If anything, genetic testing for future capacities is less objectionable because it's more reliable.

Most of our current worries stem, of course, from insurance. What's to prevent insurers, we fret, from demanding genetic tests to see if someone is more likely to have breast cancer or heart disease than another random person? The result could be the end of insurance pools as we know them. But it's worth noting one thing. Genetic testing is not a reversal of the principle behind insurance; it's just an elaboration of it. All insurance is about predicting the future based on imperfect knowledge of the present. The point of genetic testing is to give us a better idea of the present and future. Young single males, for example, have a harder time getting car insurance than married middle-age women. We accept this principle as a recognition of reality. But why is it less objectionable than testing individuals for a genetic predisposition to high blood pressure? At least that doesn't extrapolate from a general population to an individual.

What's happening is that the veil of ignorance that once covered our inner lives is wearing increasingly thin. The change will thrill and dismay us, whatever our politics. It seems to me, to take one obvious consequence, that socialized medicine is now all but inevitable. It's inevitable not because it's inherently better than an insurance-based system. It almost certainly isn't. It's inevitable because the ignorance on which an insurance-based system necessarily rests is slowly disappearing. We'll either have to force insurers to ignore glaring, easily obtainable facts relevant to their business—and see the numbers of private entrepreneurs prepared to enter the market gradually shrink—or we'll have to make it illegal for individuals with great genetic results to use and market that information to insurers for cheaper coverage. Eventually, as the writer Clive Crook has argued, the private sector will either be so expensive it will be beyond most of our reach or so regulated it will look like a public system anyway. In the long run, only the government will be dumb enough or enlightened enough to mandate a national insurance pool that works.

Simply ban all genetic testing of any kind? That would mean losing a historic chance to cure countless diseases and develop unique health strategies for individuals who will want them. Prevent employers and governments from testing? Sure, but what do you do when private individuals get their own tests done and then bring them to job interviews? How do you practically stop an employer from being influenced by that information in a free society? And if some employers are high-minded enough to keep their eyes shut in a fiercely competitive market, others will realize that ignorance is too costly a financial risk to bear.

The twists won't end there. As the potential for rational discrimination grows, the space for old-fashioned bias may shrink. Men and women will increasingly be judged not by the color of their skin but by the content of their chromosomes. The irrational cruelty of bias will be replaced by the rational cruelty of fate. In retrospect, we may miss the evils we could do something about.

NO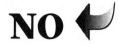

Thomas H. Murray

Genetics and the Moral Mission of Health Insurance

All men are created equal. So reads one of the United States of America's founding political documents. This stirring affirmation of equality was not meant as a claim that all people are equivalent in all respects. Surely the drafters of the Declaration of Independence and the Constitution were as aware then as we are now of the wondrous variety of humankind. People differ in their appearance, their talents, and their character, among other things, and those differences matter enormously.

The commitment to equality embodied in our political tradition is not a claim that people, in fact, are indistinguishable from one another. Rather it is an assertion that before this government, this system of laws and courts, all persons are to be given equal standing, and all persons must be treated with equal regard.

Human genetics, in contrast, is a *science of inequality*—a study of human particularity and difference. One of the most difficult challenges facing us in the coming flood tide of genetic information is how to assimilate these evidences of human differences without undermining our commitment to political, legal, and moral equality.

The information about human differences pouring forth from the science of human genetics provides us with a multitude of opportunities to treat people differently according to some aspect of their genetic makeup. Deciding which uses of this information are just and which are unjust will require us to reexamine the ethical significance of a wide variety of human differences and the larger social purposes of a variety of institutions, among them health, life, and other forms of insurance.

Health insurance in the United States has moved from a system based mostly on community rating where, in a given community, all people pay comparable rates, to a system where the cost to the purchasers of insurance is based on the expected claims—a risk- or experienced-based system. This movement has significant ethical as well as economic overtones. Community rating was a system that reflected a notion of community responsibility for providing health care for its members, where the qualifying principle was community membership. Other differences, such as preexisting risks, did not count as morally

From Thomas H. Murray, "Genetics and the Moral Mission of Health Insurance," *Hastings Center Report*, vol. 22, no. 6 (November–December 1992). Copyright © 1992 by The Hastings Center. Reprinted by permission.

relevant distinctions. Risk- and experience-based systems presume that it is fair to charge different prices, or to refuse to insure people entirely, if they will need expensive health care. Such systems treat predicted need for care as a morally relevant difference among persons that justifies differential access to health insurance, and through it, to health care. But this presumes precisely what is in question: what are good moral reasons for treating people differently with respect to access to health insurance and health care? . . .

Genetics and Distributive Justice

Distributive justice, as the term implies, concerns the distribution of social goods or ills: in its simplest formulation it holds that like cases are to be treated alike and unlike cases are to be treated differently. All depends, obviously, on how we fill in the material conditions of this purely formal statement of comparative justice. When we are asking about a particular occasion of just or unjust treatment, the question commonly takes the form, What makes these cases like or unlike in a morally relevant way? Failure to state a morally relevant reason for treating people differently opens one to the charge that one's action was arbitrary, capricious, and unjust.

Human genetics provides a large and rapidly growing set of differences among persons that may be used to try to justify unequal treatment. For many genetic differences and many distributions of social goods, the moral relevance of the difference seems transparently obvious. Height, for example, is largely determined by genetics. Does it make any sense to say that it was unfair to allow Kareem Abdul Jabaar to play center in the National Basketball Association for many years, but not me, just because he is taller than I am, and our differences in height are genetic, rather than anything we can claim credit for accomplishing? Most people would judge that to be absurd. In this instance a genetic difference—height—constitutes a morally relevant difference that justifies treating people differently. That same difference, however, would not justify treating us differently if, for example, we were accused of a crime, or being judged on our literary accomplishments, or in need of health care. . . .

Having health insurance is a way to pay for . . . treatment—the cost of treating a serious illness can easily exceed an average family's ability to pay for it. Health insurance is, for most people, the means to the end of health care. It is not the good of health care itself. But to the extent that it determines who does and who does not have access to care, and who has the peace of mind that comes with knowing that if care is needed it will be available, access to health insurance is a matter of justice.

Genetic Testing: The Challenge for Health Insurance

Research in human genetics, such as the Genome Project, is likely to increase dramatically our ability to predict whether individuals are at risk for particular diseases. There are tests currently offered for diseases such as Huntington's, where the presence of the gene assures that the individual will develop the disease if he or she lives long enough. There are tests for carrier status such as cystic fibrosis where two copies of the defective gene—one from each parent —must be inherited in order for symptomatic disease to occur. And there will be tests for diseases of complex etiology such as heart disease, cancer, stroke, lung disease, and the like. For certain relatively rare genes there will be a strong connection between having the gene and having the disease. Yet most of the common killing and disabling diseases are more likely to have a complex variety of causes, including perhaps several genes each of which has some predictive relationship with the disease. These risk-oriented genetic predictors potentially are very interesting to employers and insurers.

Genetic information, in fact, is used now by insurers. There may be considerable genetic information in one's medical record. If your policy is being individually underwritten, that entire record can be copied and shipped to the prospective insurer and that information used to justify increasing the price or denying health insurance altogether. But this begs a prior question: should information about genetic differences be used at all in health insurance?

One argument against paying any special attention to genetic predictors of risk is that insurers already use risk predictors that have genetic components. Coronary artery disease is an example. It is well known that people with higher levels of cholesterol, especially the low-density-lipoprotein component, are at higher risk of coronary artery disease and subsequent heart attacks. It also seems clear that an individual's cholesterol level is at least in part determined by genetics. Variations in individual metabolism can have a substantial impact on a person's cholesterol level, such that two people can be equally virtuous (or careless) in diet and exercise and yet have very different cholesterol levels, and, presumably, very different risks for coronary artery disease and heart attack.

In time it is likely that researchers will discover a number of genes that affect cholesterol metabolism and, presumably, cholesterol level, arterial disease, and the risk of a heart attack. We may be able to construct a genetic profile of an individual's risk of heart disease. Does such a predictive index differ in any ethically significant way from today's cholesterol test, which has not evoked similar objections?

Genetic tests differ from a cholesterol test in that the latter, even if significantly influenced by genetics, is still in some measure under the individual's control. The risk of heart attack is affected by a variety of health-related behaviors including diet, exercise, stress, and smoking. To the extent that people can be held responsible for their behavior, their cholesterol level is something for which they have some responsibility. On the other hand, people cannot be said to be responsible for their genes. An old maxim in ethics is "Ought implies can." You should not be held morally accountable for that which you were powerless to influence.

Genetic tests may also have more direct distributional consequences. Alleles occur in different frequencies in different ethnic groups; it would not be surprising to find that an allele associated with an epidemiologically significant disease such as coronary artery disease was more prevalent in some ethnic groups than in others. Alpha-1 antitrypsin deficiency, associated with lung disease, appears to be more common among people of Scandinavian ancestry. If the group in which the allele occurs more often was not historically a target of discrimination, we might not be particularly concerned. If, however, the allele was more common in a group that continues to suffer discrimination, such as sickle-cell trait in people of African descent, we would have good reason for concern. The mere fact that genetic predictors have the potential to affect differentially ethnic groups that experience discrimination does not uniquely distinguish them from other risk predictors. Hypertension, for example, is more prevalent among Americans of African heritage. But the immediate and direct tie between genetics and ethnicity may make genetic testing a more blatant use of a potentially explosive and discriminatory social classification scheme.

A third response to the claim that we need not worry about genetic risk testing because it is essentially similar to things like cholesterol testing is to question the premise that people know about the genetic component of cholesterol. Discussions of cholesterol in the media emphasize the things people can do to lower it. Reminders that cholesterol level is also significantly affected by genetics appear less frequently, and it may well be that most people are unaware that cholesterol level has a substantial genetic component. If people did understand that, perhaps they would be less tolerant of the widespread use of cholesterol testing to determine insurance eligibility, precisely because it was to that extent outside of individuals' control.

There is yet another possibility: that the central notion underlying commercial health insurance underwriting—the greater the likelihood of illness, the more one should pay for coverage—is morally unsound.

Actuarial Fairness

Insurers take a particular view of fairness: actuarial fairness. Actuarial fairness claims that "policyholders with the same expected risk of loss should be treated equally.... An insurance company has the responsibility to treat all its policyholders fairly by establishing premiums at a level consistent with the risk represented by each individual policyholder."[1] This definition of fairness begs the question: Why should we count differences in risk of disease as an ethically relevant justification for treating people differently in their access to health insurance and health care?

Actuarial fairness does have a realm of application in which it seems reasonable. Call it the Lloyds of London model: if two oil tanker companies ask to have their cargoes and vessels insured, one for a trip up the Atlantic to a U.S. port, the other for a voyage through the Arabian Gulf during the height of the war in Kuwait and Iraq, the owner of the first ship would cry foul if she were charged the same extraordinarily high rate as the owner of the second. Most of us, I suspect, would agree that charging the two owners the same rate would be unfair. What makes it so?

For one thing, the two ships are exposed to vastly different risks, and it seems only fair to charge them accordingly. (The process of assessing risks is called underwriting.) Furthermore, the risks were assumed voluntarily. Third, the goal of both owners is profit, and it seems reasonable to ask them to bear the expense of voluntarily assumed risks. We could also ask how commercial insurance divides up the world. In this hypothetical [situation] it divides it into those who prefer prudent business ventures and those willing to take great risks. That does not seem to be an objectionable way to parse the world for the purpose of insuring oil tankers.

In practice, insurers do not behave as if actuarial fairness were an ironclad moral rule. Valid predictors may not be used for a variety of reasons, typically having to do with other notions of fairness—for example, not discriminating on the basis of race, sex, class, or locale, even though these characteristics are related to the likelihood of insurance claims. Deborah Stone, who has studied insurance practices for HIV infection, dismisses the idea of actuarial fairness and argues instead that:

> insurability is the set of policy decisions by insurers about whom to accept. It is not a trait, but a concept of *membership*.... Treated as a scientific fact about individuals, the notion of insurability disguises fundamentally political decisions about membership in a community of mutual responsibility.[2] ...

Underwriting and the Social Purposes of Insurance

The threat genetic testing poses to the future of insurance for health-related risks—including health, life, and disability insurance—compels us to reexamine the social purposes served by insurance. Two points are obvious: first, that different types of insurance can have different purposes; and second, that the purpose of a particular form of insurance must be understood within its social context.

Life insurance, for example, is meant to provide financial security for one's dependents in the event that one dies. In the contemporary United States we must evaluate the role of such insurance in the context of a not particularly generous social welfare system that would otherwise leave the surviving dependents of a deceased breadwinner in very poor financial condition. The typical purchaser is an individual with one or more dependents who are unlikely to become financially independent in the immediate future. The benefits from life insurance are intended to tide survivors over until they can become financially self-sufficient, or live out their lives decently; they are not meant to provide windfalls to friends of the deceased. To the extent that life insurance is perceived as serving a need rather than being merely a commodity, we are likely to regard it as something that ought to be available to all. Our public policies toward life insurance suggest we view it otherwise, however. We prohibit certain actuarially valid distinctions such as ethnicity in setting life insurance rates. But we do not require that all persons, whatever their age, employment, or health, be permitted to buy life insurance at identical prices or at all. In consequence, the financial dependents of a person unable to obtain life insurance may suffer devastating changes in their life prospects if the principal earner dies.

Does the Lloyds of London model fit health care? Despite the current enthusiasm for tying voluntary behavior to health, most illness and disability is neither chosen nor in any sense "deserved," distinguishing it from the risks of shipping oil in a war zone. Neither is the goal of health care for those who seek it profit. Daniels argues that "justice requires that we protect *fair equality of opportunity* for individuals in a society." Reasonable access to health care in the contemporary United States is a necessary condition for fair equality of opportunity to pursue other goods that life affords. The social purpose of health insurance, understood in this way, is to provide access to the health care that people need to have a fair opportunity in life.

Lastly, how does underwriting in health insurance divide the world? It sets off the well from the ill and those likely to become ill. For insurers, the concept of actuarial fairness provides a rationale for charging much higher rates or declining to insure persons with a substantial possibility of illness or disability, reasoning that such persons should bear the costs associated with their particular risks. Persons at risk could find it difficult to obtain insurance at affordable rates, or at all. . . .

Implications for Policy

The era of predictive genetic testing coincides with a period of grave public concern about health care. . . .

There is little doubt that the current ragged system of private and public programs, with its many holes and frayed edges, must be changed. The conviction that health care ought to be available to those who need it seems to be widely shared. That conviction, together with a growing sense that the current patchwork is failing, may be strong enough to overcome the citizenry's hesitations about government inefficiency. Indeed, it seems likely that private health insurance would not have survived this long if not for government intervention. Tax subsidies for employer-sponsored health insurance programs amounted to $39.5 billion in 1991.[3] In addition, we provide direct government coverage for the health needs of people that commercial insurers want to avoid: Medicare, for those much more likely to need health care; and Medicaid, for some of those unable to pay for their own insurance.

Public programs such as Medicare and Medicaid tell us something important about our moral convictions on health care. They suggest that we are not content to allow the old and the poor simply to languish without access to care. Had we not passed such legislation, we well might have overturned or radically restructured the existing system of commercial health insurance decades ago.

There are good reasons to doubt that actuarial fairness is an adequate description of genuine fairness in health insurance. It may be a sufficient principle for commercial insurance against losses of ships at sea, but even a brief inquiry into the social purpose of health insurance suggests that apportioning by risks, as actuarial fairness dictates, fails to accomplish the primary social goals of health insurance. Genetic tests, like other predictors of the need for health care, are not good reasons for treating people differently with respect to access to health insurance.

References

Karen A. Clifford and R. P. Iuculano, "AIDS and Insurance: The Rationale for AIDS-Related Testing," *Harvard Law Review* 100 (1987): 1806–24.

Deborah A. Stone, "AIDS and the Moral Economy of Insurance," *American Prospect* 1 (1990): 62–73.

John K. Iglehart, "The American Health Care System: Private Insurance," *NEJM* 326 (1992): 1715–20.

POSTSCRIPT

Should Information From Genetic Testing Be Available to Employers and Insurers?

The federal Health Insurance Portability and Accountability Act, signed by President Bill Clinton in August 1996, declares that genetic information itself is not a preexisting condition. The law provides that someone who has had a genetic test predicting a high risk of developing a disease later in life but who is not yet ill cannot be denied insurance on the grounds of the test alone. However, insurance rates are not covered by the law. On the state level, in 1996 a comprehensive Genetic Privacy Act intended to protect the rights of people who choose to obtain predictive genetic testing was passed in New Jersey. In 1993 the Human Genome Project's Task Force on Genetic Information and Insurance recommended that "information about past, present or future health status, including genetic information, should not be used to deny health care coverage or services to anyone."

In "Genetic Testing and the Social Responsibility of Private Health Insurance Companies," *Journal of Law, Medicine and Ethics* (Spring 1993), Nancy S. Jecker argues that "socially responsible insurance companies will avoid genetic discrimination." The existence of discrimination as a consequence of genetic testing is documented in an article by Paul R. Billings et al. in the *American Journal of Human Genetics* (vol. 50, 1992). The American Medical Association's position on the use of genetic testing by employers, outlined in the *Journal of the American Medical Association* (October 2, 1991), is that it generally opposes genetic testing by employers, but it recognizes a limited exception in excluding workers who have a genetic susceptibility to occupational illness.

Karen Rothenberg and colleagues from the Committee on Genetic Information and the Workplace of the National Action Plan on Breast Cancer, which is coordinated by the U.S. Public Health Service Office on Women's Health, and the National Institutes of Health/Department of Energy Working Group on Ethical, Legal, and Social Implications of Human Genome Research, offer guidelines for restricting the use of genetic information in "Genetic Information and the Workplace: Legislative Approaches and Policy Challenges," *Science,* (March 21, 1997). For more general readings on genetic screening and insurance, see Pat Milmoe McCarrick, *Genetic Testing and Genetic Screening* (Scope Note No. 22, Kennedy Institute of Ethics, 1993, updated 1999) at http://www.georgetown.edu/research/nrcbl/scopenotes/sn22.htm.

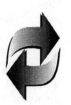

ISSUE 14

Should Parents Always Be Told of Genetic-Testing Availability?

YES: Mary Z. Pelias, from "Duty to Disclose in Medical Genetics: A Legal Perspective," *American Journal of Medical Genetics* (vol. 39, 1991)

NO: Diane E. Hoffmann and Eric A. Wulfsberg, from "Testing Children for Genetic Predispositions: Is It in Their Best Interest?" *Journal of Law, Medicine and Ethics* (vol. 23, no. 4, 1995)

ISSUE SUMMARY

YES: Mary Z. Pelias, attorney and professor of genetics, argues that parental autonomy and family privacy should govern decisions about whether or not to test children for genetic predispositions to disease and that physicians and genetic counselors have an obligation to disclose full information.

NO: Law professor Diane E. Hoffmann and pediatrician Eric A. Wulfsberg assert that caution and restraint should govern decisions on testing for genetic predispositions in children and that safeguards should be adopted to diminish the potentially negative effects of testing and to protect children's best interests.

Among the most dramatic results of the Human Genome Project, which is designed to determine the complete chemical sequence of human DNA, is the identification of an ever-increasing number of genetically linked conditions. To date, more than 900 genes associated with disease have been found. One example is Huntington's disease, a disorder that leads to mental and neurological deterioration and eventually death. About 100,000 people in the United States are at risk for this disease, which typically begins to be noticed in the patient's late 30s or early 40s. Another genetically linked condition is adult polycystic kidney disease, which accounts for about 10 percent of all end-stage renal disease in the United States. Still another condition is alpha1-antitrypsin deficiency, an enzyme deficiency that leads to a high risk of early-onset emphysema in at-risk individuals of Scandinavian ancestry. Genes linked to particular forms of breast cancer and colon cancer have also been identified, and genes that predict a high risk of other forms of cancer, heart disease, and Alzheimer's disease are likely to be found before long.

Tests for detecting predisposition to a number of genetic disorders are already available, and others are likely to enter the marketplace in coming years. Screening of newborns for some genetically linked or maternally transmitted diseases, especially those that are treatable and likely to manifest symptoms in childhood, is well established, although in some cases it remains controversial. In many states, newborns are routinely screened for sickle-cell disease, a blood condition that targets African Americans in particular, and for phenylketonuria (PKU), a rare but treatable enzyme deficiency that affects a child's ability to absorb certain types of nutrition. Some forms of screening are used primarily to aid reproductive decision making—the goal is to determine if one or both partners carry a disease-linked gene that may put their offspring at risk. Tay-Sachs disease, which primarily affects Jewish families from Eastern Europe and kills affected infants within a few years, is one example. As a result of prenatal screening, fewer babies have been born with Tay-Sachs disease since 1989. A DNA test was also initiated for cystic fibrosis; it has been used primarily by couples with a family history that puts them at risk. Cystic fibrosis is the most common life-threatening genetic disorder to affect people of European descent, but other population groups may be affected as well. About 8 million Americans are believed to carry the cystic fibrosis gene.

For adults, the decision to be tested for genetic conditions is difficult and troubling, carrying as it does the risks of learning negative information, the potential for insurance and employment discrimination, and the sense that life choices have become restricted. Decisions about whether or not to test one's children are even weightier. While testing for a genetic condition for which treatment exists (as is now the case with sickle-cell disease) involves one set of considerations, testing for a condition that cannot be treated or may not show up until the individual is well into adulthood, if at all, involves markedly different and more complex decision making.

The authors of the following selections take opposing views as to whether or not children should be tested for genes that may predict illness and as to who should decide. Mary Z. Pelias invokes the long history of patient and parental autonomy, full disclosure, and informed consent in contending that physicians' withholding of genetic testing for children is a form of medical paternalism. Diane E. Hoffmann and Eric A. Wulfsberg call on another long-standing tradition—protecting the best interests of children—in urging restraint and caution in utilizing testing that may have serious negative effects with no balancing benefits.

229

Mary Z. Pelias

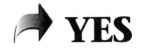 **YES**

Duty to Disclose in Medical Genetics: A Legal Perspective

Implications in Medical Genetics: Testing and Counseling for Deleterious Genes

The power of geneticists to detect the presence of deleterious genes has increased rapidly with progressive refinements in the use of DNA markers. As technical knowledge expands, so does the power of the geneticist to influence the lives of clients who seek counseling about their own genetic status or the status of their children. In this developing context, the geneticist may experience most vividly the contrast between the beneficent care-giver and the client whose autonomy must be respected. Here, depending on the law of the state where a lawsuit arises, the geneticist may appreciate the full impact of the judicial mandate to impart all information that is material to a patient's decision-making process (Canterbury v. Spence, 1972).

Nowhere has the power of the medical geneticist been expressed more clearly than in recent suggestions about predictive testing for the gene that causes Huntington disease. Several authors have recommended that predictive testing should be unavailable both for minor children and for couples who seek prenatal testing but equivocate about terminating a high risk pregnancy (Bloch and Hayden, 1990; Committee of IHA and WFN, 1990). Parents of minor children would be classified as third parties, whose interests in their own minor children are equated with interests of "adoption agencies, educational institutions, insurance companies, and other third parties." Limiting the interests of parents by classifying them as third parties is proposed as a means of protecting the privacy and autonomy of the minor child. Genetic counseling would be directed toward discouraging parents and at-risk couples from seeking information. Since no immediate advantage can be predicted for minor children whose genetic status is investigated, the refusal by professionals to test children or at-risk couples is viewed as a policy that supports the best interests of family life and the emotional and psychological security of children who may harbor the gene. These arguments against disclosure rest on the facts that Huntington disease is a late-onset disorder and that no treatment is presently available.

From Mary Z. Pelias, "Duty to Disclose in Medical Genetics: A Legal Perspective," *American Journal of Medical Genetics,* vol. 39 (1991). Copyright © 1991 by Wiley-Liss, Inc., a subsidiary of John Wiley & Sons, Inc. Reprinted by permission.

These suggestions must have resulted from considerable deliberation, and they are unquestionably sincere. However, they raise serious questions about paternalism in genetic counseling and about the duty of a counselor to his client. They also challenge the principles of parental autonomy and of the privacy of the family unit in our culture. The fundamental issue is neither the nature of the specific genetic disease nor the availability of any treatment but, rather, a renewed tension between the beneficence model of patient care and the rights of parents to their own autonomy and to the protection of their family units.

Although references to constitutional history may have only peripheral interest in suits of professional negligence, the holdings of the Supreme Court are nonetheless regarded as reflections of the values of our society. On several occasions the Supreme Court has affirmed the sanctity of the family unit, so that courts and legislatures are now loathe to interfere with this most basic social group. The scope of "liberty" guaranteed to every American by the fourteenth amendment was addressed in a frequently quoted case involving the role of parents in making educational decisions for their children:

> Without doubt, [liberty] denotes not merely freedom from bodily restraint but also the right of the individual to contract, to engage in any of the common occupations of life, to acquire useful knowledge, to marry, establish a home and bring up children, to worship God according to the dictates of his own conscience, and generally to enjoy those privileges long recognized at common law as essential to the orderly pursuit of happiness by free men (Meyer v. Nebraska, 1923).

This holding was reinforced when the Court later affirmed "the liberty of parents and guardians to direct the upbringing and education of children under their control" (Pierce v. Society of Sisters, 1925). More recently, in the context of making medical decisions for minor children, the Court noted that "[s]tate law vests decisional responsibility in the parents, in the first instance" (Bowen v. American Hosp. Ass'n, 1986). This judicial thrust was supported by the President's Commission for the Study of Ethical problems in Medicine and Biomedical and Behavioral Research when it noted that

> [T]here is a presumption, strong but rebuttable, that parents are the appropriate decisionmakers for their infants. Traditional law concerning the family, buttressed by the emerging right of privacy, protects a substantial range of discretion for parents (President's Commission, 1983).

Considerations by both the judicial and administrative branches of federal government have thus affirmed the role of parents as the primary decision makers in the lives of their children. Any attempt to usurp the parental role contradicts this clearly expressed public policy, and justification of such an effort would indeed have to be compelling in order to survive a constitutional challenge. The geneticist who defines parents as "third parties" in relation to their own children and assumes the right to make parental decisions acts without regard to our history of protecting the parental prerogative.

A more realistic hazard for the medical geneticist lies in the possibility of being sued in tort for failure to disclose all information material to the plaintiff's decision-making process. When a practicing geneticist assumes the role of guardian of the privacy and autonomy of children who may have deleterious genes, he assumes the role of the parents of these children. If the geneticist then fails to disclose complete information to the parents of these children, he risks allegations of injury to both the parents and the child. Parents deprived of complete information about the genetic status of their children will assert that their parental autonomy was compromised when they were deprived of the chance to explore every available opportunity for their child with a deleterious gene. Children will also claim injury resulting from these diminished opportunities. Parents denied prenatal testing when they refuse to commit to aborting an affected, or high risk, fetus, will have actions in wrongful birth, and children born to these parents may have actions in wrongful life.[1] The plaintiffs may demonstrate that these lost opportunities should be compensable and may well recover substantial damages.

Beyond the practical aspects of litigation may lie a far greater hazard to the profession of medical genetics. Most medical geneticists have adopted a policy of non-directive counseling aimed at communicating information and helping clients understand and cope with their situations (Fraser, 1974; Ad Hoc Committee on Genetic Counseling, 1975). If medical geneticists now adopt a policy of limiting the information available for disclosure, or if counseling becomes so directive as to solicit an agreement to terminate an affected pregnancy in return for prenatal testing, it can only be a matter of time before these situations are exposed in court and exploited in the media. Such exposure and exploitation could severely damage the credibility of the profession. This risk can be avoided, however, by respecting the autonomy of clients and adopting a policy and a practice of full, unconditional disclosure.

Another question of disclosure that arises in the context of testing for deleterious genes is whether the geneticist has any obligation, or right, to disclose genetic information to third parties, including collateral relatives who participate in a study, or schools, employers, or insurance companies. With respect to disclosure to participating collateral relatives, 3 facts must be considered. First, both the client and the relative are protected by their rights to privacy and to personal autonomy. Second, any exchange between a physician and his patient is confidential. The only legal precedent for breaking this confident is knowledge by the physician that the patient poses a foreseeable danger to an identifiable third party, in particular, a psychiatrist's knowledge of a patient's threats of bodily harm to his former girlfriend (Tarasoff v. Regents of the Univ. of Cal., 1976; Davis v. Lhim, 1983). Third, while the geneticist may not discover information that is immediately life-threatening, as in *Tarasoff* or *Davis*, the information may well have a significant influence on a relative's family planning decisions and on the children who are born to that relative. With these facts in mind, then, the geneticist should have the consent of both his client and the participating collateral relative before revealing any information to the relative. Any fortuitous information about non-participating relatives should ideally be kept in confidence until an inquiry is initiated by that relative himself. Certainly the geneticist is in a position to encourage communication among family members, but he is obliged to respect the privacy, autonomy, and confidentiality of those with whom he has direct contact....

Summary and Conclusions

During the past century the physician-patient relationship has evolved from the beneficent approach to providing health care to an approach that gives great deference to the patient's moral and legal right to personal autonomy. Decisions formerly made by health care providers for the benefit of their patients are now made by patients themselves. This shift in decision-making prerogative has been accompanied by the evolution of the legal doctrine of informed consent. Care-givers are now required to impart information that meets either the standard of care practiced among professionals or the standard of care determined to include all information material to a patient's decision. Professional conduct that fails to meet the applicable standard of care constitutes a breach of duty owed to the patient. If the patient is injured as a result of this breach, he may sue in tort for medical negligence to recover his damages.

Full disclosure and communication of genetic information often involves information that is unpleasant, even devastating, to counseling clients. The hard reality of genetic counseling is that clients must often learn of poor prognoses, limited if any treatment options, and diminished life expectancy of loved ones. This reality applies equally to chromosomal problems and to single gene disorders, whether dominant or recessive, across the full range of hereditary problems that affect human beings. Geneticists who intentionally restrict information that is sought by clients place themselves at risk of being sued for inadequate disclosure under the doctrine of informed consent. Geneticists who make decisions on behalf of minor children also disregard the constitutional status of parents as the primary decision-makers for their own children. Beyond the detriment to the immediate parties in genetic counseling, however, lies a grave risk to the profession of medical genetics of allegations of directive counseling aimed at controlling the lives and the reproductive decisions of genetic counseling clients. These dangers must be avoided. They will be best avoided by recognizing a policy of full disclosure to clients who seek information about any hereditary problem.

Respect for patient autonomy and the need for full disclosure in the treatment of genetic disease has also acquired new facets as medical and surgical therapies have become more refined. While parents are usually regarded as the sole decision-makers for their children in questions about treatment, there has recently been a growing recognition in the legislatures and courts of the ability of mature minors to understand and to participate in these decisions. This ability is recognized both in accepting and in refusing a proposed course of treatment. Full disclosure is also mandated when experimental treatment regimes are proposed, with the additional caveat that this is a controversial area, with no professional consensus about ethical standards. Such tenuous treatment situations demand utmost sensitivity to the needs and expectations of all persons involved. Failure of the geneticist to disclose all available information to clients, or patients, who must make critical decisions will be an invitation for allegations of malpractice.

The doctrine of informed consent may eventually be extended to include a duty of the medical geneticist to re-contact counseling clients when new information is amassed that could be material in decisions made by these persons. Based on relevant case law, the geneticist, as the knowledgeable professional, may be required to disclose new information, but he can mitigate the chances of litigation by including his clients in the counseling process, by stressing the importance of communicating changes of address and status, and by making good faith efforts to re-contact patients who seem to have disappeared.

The history of medical genetics acknowledges the difficult aspects of genetic counseling, but it also supports the need for candid and complete disclosure of information to counseling clients. For many years one thrust of counseling has been to help families "make the best possible adjustment to the disorder in an affected family member" (Committee on Genetic Counseling, 1975). How one family deals with genetic information may differ greatly from the way another family deals with the same information, and these decisions are appropriately made within the privacy of each family. The geneticist should continue to serve as the trustee of genetic information. Counseling clients and patients, as the beneficiaries of this trust, are morally and legally entitled to full disclosure and to the right to give truly informed consent.

Note

1. Wrongful life actions are brought by children who are born with defects that could have been predicted or detected prenatally. These children claim that it would be better not to be born at all than to be born to a life of suffering and pain. The success of wrongful life actions is considerably more dubious than the success of wrongful birth actions because the courts have demonstrated a reluctance to make judgments about the value of a diminished life in relation to not being born at all (Pelias, 1986).

References

Bloch M., Hayden MR (1990): Opinion: Predictive testing for Huntington disease in childhood: Challenges and implications. Am J Hum Genet 46:1–4.

Bowen v. American Hospital Association, 476 U.S. 610 (1986).

Canterbury v. Spence, 464 F.2d 772 (D.C. Cir. 1972).

Committee of the International Huntington Association and the World Federation of Neurology (1990): Ethical issues policy statement on Huntington's disease molecular genetics predictive test. J. Med Genet 27:34–38.

Committee on Genetic counseling (1975): Genetic counseling. Am J Hum Genet 27:240–242.

Davis v. Lhim, 124 Mich. App. 291, 335 N.W.2d 481 (1983).

Fraser FC (1974): Genetic counseling. Am J Hum Genet 26:636–659.

Meyer v. Nebraska, 262 U.S. 390 (1923).

Pelias MZ (1986): Torts of wrongful birth and wrongful life: A review. Am J Med Genet 25:71–80.

Pierce v. Society of Sisters, 268 U.S. 510 (1925).

President's Commission (1983): Report of the President's Commission for the Study of Ethical Problems in Medicine and Biomedical and Behavioral Research. Washington, D.C.: Government Printing Office.

Tarasoff v. Regents of Univ. of Cal., 17 Cal. 3d 425, 131 Cal. Rptr. 14, 551 P.2d 334 (1976).

Diane E. Hoffmann and
Eric A. Wulfsberg

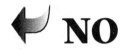 **NO**

Testing Children for Genetic Predispositions: Is It in Their Best Interest?

Researchers summoned a Baltimore County woman to an office at the Johns Hopkins School of Public Health last spring to tell her the bad news. They had found a genetic threat lurking in her 7-year-old son's DNA—a mutant gene that almost always triggers a rare form of colon cancer. It was the same illness that led surgeons to remove her colon in 1979. While the boy, Michael, now 8, is still perfectly healthy, without surgery he is almost certain to develop cancer by age 40.

This genetic fortune-telling was no parlor trick. It was the product of astonishing advances in recent decades in understanding how genes build and regulate our bodies. And as scientists pinpoint new genes and learn to forecast the onset of more inherited disorders, millions of people are likely to demand their medical prognosis.[1]

Testing healthy newborns and children for genetic DNA abnormalities that will not manifest disease symptoms for many years, if ever, is now rarely done. However, the entry of such tests into the marketplace is raising the specter of their widespread use. Tests that predict the likelihood of cancer are attracting the greatest attention, and they may be the first such tests to be administered on a large-scale basis.[2] Currently, tests are available for predisposition to breast cancer, colon cancer, melanoma, and thyroid cancer.[3]

Marketing these tests to the general population is highly controversial, with proponents arguing that people have a right to know if they or their children are at increased risk and that it would be unethical to deny them that information. Much of the advocacy for widespread use of the tests comes from the biotechnology companies offering them.[4] For example, a recent news article about marketing these genetic tests described the question of testing children as "delicate." Yet it also reported, in a letter to dermatologists on testing for melanoma predisposition, that the manufacturer of the tests believed "[e]arly screening with this easy and painless test is particularly useful when testing children."[5]

From Diane E. Hoffmann and Eric A. Wulfsberg, "Testing Children for Genetic Predispositions: Is It in Their Best Interest?" *Journal of Law, Medicine and Ethics*, vol. 23, no. 4 (1995), pp. 331–344. Copyright © 1995 by The American Society of Law, Medicine and Ethics. Reprinted by permission.

Some advocates of testing children go so far as to state that a geneticist has a medical and legal duty to advise parents about presymptomatic testing procedures for some (even late-onset) diseases and either to administer the procedure or to refer the child to a colleague for administration (presuming the child meets certain pre-administration criteria).[6] Others describe the effort to keep the tests from patients as medical paternalism.[7] Opponents have characterized the initiative to market the genetic tests as "alarming," arguing that this area of genetic testing is still in the research phase and that the tests should not be marketed now.[8] Others argue that, due to the uncertain psychological consequences for children of predictive testing, such testing should not generally be done at this time or should be restricted.[9]

We support those who express caution and urge restraint[10] in conducting predictive genetic tests on children, and we suggest policy recommendations to safeguard children's interests from possible negative effects of such testing. Many of our suggestions are consistent with the recently published joint statement of the American Society of Human Genetics (ASHG) and the American College of Medical Genetics (ACMG) on genetic testing of children and adolescents.[11] . . .

Throughout, we use the term *genetic disease* to refer to that rare group of disorders in which an abnormality (or abnormalities) in the genetic code (DNA) of an individual is associated with a near certainty of developing disease. In contrast, we use *genetic predisposition* to refer to an abnormality in the genetic code of an individual that results in an increased risk of developing a disease.

Current Testing of Newborns and Children

Little genetic testing of children is currently performed, other than newborn screening for a small number of treatable genetic diseases that are expected to cause symptoms if not treated during infancy. When testing is performed on older children, it is generally limited to those few individuals who either are suspected of having a genetic disease or are in families at high risk for having a genetic disease. Several attempts have been made to categorize reasons to do genetic testing on infants and children.[12] Using the work of Wertz et al. and Fost as a starting point, we employ a comprehensive list of seven categories: (1) testing of immediate benefit to the infant or minor, including newborn screening, disease testing for a symptomatic condition in the child, or presymptomatic testing for which treatment during childhood is available and beneficial; (2) reproductive-associated testing and counseling for older adolescents that is mainly genetic carrier rather than genetic disease testing; (3) testing for the benefit of other family members' reproductive decision making, where it may be necessary to test both affected and unaffected family members to understand the inheritance of a genetic disease; (4) research-related testing that is generally conducted under informed consent protocols approved by institutional review boards; (5) testing by insurance companies for the purpose of excluding individuals from coverage; (6) presymptomatic testing to predict

a child's future risk of developing a genetic disease or of having a genetic predisposition for which no current treatment or effective prevention exists; and
(7) testing for carrier status at an age when the child cannot procreate.

Predictive Testing

Our primary focus is category (6)—testing for presymptomatic genetic diseases
or predispositions. While a relatively recent survey indicates that many British
geneticists and pediatricians would presymptomatically test children for a genetic condition at the request of the parents and with little immediate benefit to
the child,[13] many ethicists and professional genetics societies agree that testing
children for genetic diseases, predispositions, or carrier status is only appropriate when a clear and timely benefit to the minor exists.[14] And the debate,
in large part, has focused on determining what constitutes a clear and timely
benefit and who would benefit from the information. While many professionals argue that there is insufficient benefit to the child to warrant widespread
screening or even high-risk family testing for most genetic diseases during
childhood,[15] some argue that the information may be beneficial to the child's
family. Whether this benefit would outweigh the negative aspects of being
identified as having a disease, such as being treated differently by one's parents (no college fund or other long-term plans), has significant ramifications
for the appropriateness of predictive testing....

Psychological Impact

Concerns about testing children solely for predictive purposes have focused
largely on the potential psychological implications to the child, especially in
cases of predisposition to an incurable disease.[16] Wertz et al. have summarized
some of the psychological and emotional consequences of such testing. They
argue that in requesting testing, parents typically think only of the benefits of
a negative test result and not of the potentially damaging effects of a positive
result:

> "Planning for the future," perhaps the most frequently given reason for test-
> ing, may become "restricting the future" (and also the present) by shifting
> family resources away from a child with a positive diagnosis.... In families
> with a chronically ill child, there is less socialization to future roles for all
> the children, including those who are "healthy." Parents are less likely to say
> "When you grow up ..." or "When you have children of your own..." to
> any of their children, because they cannot say these words to the ill child....
> "Alleviation of anxiety," another reason commonly given by parents for pre-
> dictive genetic testing, does not necessarily benefit the children. A positive
> diagnosis may create serious risks of stigmatization, loss of self-esteem, and
> discrimination [by] family or by institutional third parties such as employ-
> ers or insurers. Testing may disrupt parent-child or sibling-sibling bonds,
> may lead to scapegoating a child with a positive result or to continued
> anxiety over a child despite a negative result....[17]

Identifying a child with a genetic predisposition may lead to the "vulnerable child syndrome" in which parents become overprotective and unnecessarily restrict a child's activities.[18] Also, those who test negative have been shown to experience "survivor guilt."[19] Given these concerns, the International Huntington's Disease Association and the World Federation of Neurology have issued policy statements recommending that minors not be tested for Huntington's disease,[20] and the National Kidney Foundation has recommended that minors not be tested for the gene for adult polycystic kidney disease except in specific circumstances where preventive measures are applicable for stroke.[21] . . .

Should Physicians Disclose the Availability of Presymptomatic Genetic Tests for Children?

The controversy surrounding presymptomatically testing children for genetic disease may soon cause anxiety for some physicians as to whether they must or should disclose the availability of genetic tests to parents of healthy children. Physicians may be concerned about potential liability for failure to inform parents about such tests. Some have contributed to this concern by arguing that physicians may have a legal duty to disclose the availability of these tests.[22] They rely erroneously on case law on prenatal testing and wrongful birth. In these cases, parents have successfully claimed that had they known about the test, they would have consented to it; and, if it had indicated that their fetus had a serious genetic condition, they would have terminated the pregnancy. Instead, the physician's failure to inform them of the test resulted in their having a child with a severe genetic abnormality that could have been detected.[23]

The problem with this analogy is that, in the prenatal context, parents could use the information to make a decision to terminate the pregnancy. In the context of testing children for a genetic predisposition for which the parent can do nothing to alter the likely manifestation of the disease, the physician would be not be legally liable. Liability would only attach when a beneficial intervention exists and failure to test or to test in a timely manner would result in harm to the child.

Thus, for a genetic disease for which we have no effective preventive intervention or treatment, a physician would have no legal duty and should not fear liability for failure to inform parents of a genetic test. We argue that this is the case both when there is no family history or probable cause for believing the child has a genetic predisposition and when there is a family history of the disease. While courts have made a distinction between informing parents about a test for a genetic disease when there is and is not a family history of the disease,[24] these cases are based on the prenatal testing paradigm, in which parents have the option of terminating the pregnancy.

We argue further that, as a policy matter, a physician should not be obligated to disclose the availability of the tests under these circumstances. Where no family history of a genetic condition exists, requiring disclosure of all available tests would take considerable time on the part of a physician or other health professional for no likely benefit to the child or parents. Disclosure in this circumstance arguably wastes resources, and it has the potential for psychological harm....

Should Physicians Perform Predictive Genetic Testing on Children?

With the increased availability of tests for genetic predispositions, physicians will undoubtedly encounter parents who have read about the tests and request one or more of them for their child. Do physicians have a legal duty to perform such tests? More importantly, *should* physicians perform such tests?

As to the first question, physicians are under no legal obligation to provide the test. They are free not to provide a treatment or diagnostic test to a patient under most circumstances. In some cases, if the treatment or diagnostic test is considered part of standard medical care, a physician would need to inform a patient of it but would not be required to provide it. In some jurisdictions, under certain circumstances, they may have a legal obligation to refer the patient to another provider who would provide the test or treatment.[25] In a recent article, Clayton ably dispels the myth that parents have a constitutional right to demand medical treatment or testing for their child, as well as the belief held by some physicians that they will be liable under tort law for failure to provide the tests.[26] Her persuasive analysis should provide comfort to physicians who refuse to test children for genetic predispositions.

As to whether a physician *should* provide such tests for genetic dispositions, we argue generally that such tests should not be provided but that a distinction may be made between cases in which there is and is not a family history of a genetic disease. If there is no family history or other risk factors, to test a healthy child for predisposition to genetic diseases is simply a fishing expedition with no foundation. If there is a family history, we concur with the ASHG-ACMG position that the decision to test should be made by a physician in discussion with the child and the child's parents.

In very young children, testing should be delayed in most cases until the child can understand the implications of the test. For example, where a mother and her three-year-old daughter visit a pediatrician for the first time and a medical history of the child reveals that the mother's mother and sister both had breast cancer, the physician should inform the mother about the availability of the test for herself, and might suggest that, if interested in it, she talk to her internist who can refer her to a geneticist. With respect to her three year old, the physician should simply state that, at some time in the future (when the child is sufficiently mature to understand the information), the child's mother might want to talk to her daughter about the family history and the test and to let the daughter decide if she would like to have the test done and, if so, when.

In some cases, however, parents may persistently demand a test for their child. Some have argued that to deny the parents the test is medical paternalism and flies in the face of our general deference to parents regarding medical decision making for their children.[27] The law clearly gives parents this authority and assumes that parents will act in their child's best interests when making such decisions. Very seldom, in fact, are parents denied the right to make medical decisions for their children, and, when denied, the cases usually involve questions of parental abuse or neglect. But cases deferring to parental decision making are not analogous to the case of genetic testing. Virtually all cases of deference to parental decision making involve circumstances in which a medical professional is recommending a course of treatment for a child, for example, surgery or chemotherapy, and the parents refuse it. Although parental decision making can be taken away when failure to provide the treatment would threaten the child's life, in virtually all other cases the parents have the right to decide not to consent to a proposed treatment.

This stands in stark contrast to cases in which the parent wants a treatment or procedure for the child that is not recommended by the physician. An example might be a common parental request to have the child's blood type determined. Pediatricians generally will not draw a child's blood simply to satisfy the parents' curiosity—he/she must have a medical reason to perform the test. Genetic tests may be somewhat more complex, and physicians may need guidance in determining where or under what circumstances a test should or might be provided.... We recommend that ... guidelines not be rigid, however, so that physicians have some latitude in deciding whether testing is warranted in a particular case. This flexibility should also allow a physician to converse with a child's parents or a child (if sufficiently mature) regarding the desire for the testing.

Although parents generally know their child best and care most about the child's welfare, we believe that physicians and health care providers have an obligation to provide them with sufficient information to make a true informed decision about the benefits and risks associated with testing for a genetic predisposition. If parents, despite a statement from their child's physician that the physician does not generally perform predictive genetic testing, want the test performed, we recommend that the physician refer them to an appropriately trained genetic counselor or another physician who can objectively explain the risks and benefits of such testing. If they still desire the testing, the health care provider must obtain their informed consent....

Safeguards Protecting Children—A Recommendation

Given concerns about testing children for genetic predispositions, we urge adoption of safeguards to ensure that the tests are administered consistent with the child's best interests. While an argument can be made that safeguards should be in place for all tested, children are particularly vulnerable to the potential negative effects of predisposition testing. The most compelling argument for this is the impact a positive test result may have on how a child will be treated by his parents, family, and, potentially, society. Few empirical studies have been done on this issue..., but caution in this type of testing is now warranted, and professional societies must play a role in encouraging physicians to exercise restraint in this area....

Where the guidelines indicate that testing might be appropriate and the parents want that genetic testing performed, we recommend that the child's physician, if not qualified himself, refer the child and his/her parents to a genetic counselor or knowledgeable physician to discuss the test risks (including the psychological risks and the potential impact on family dynamics). We urge that counselors discuss with parents the risk of overvaluing information that can be obtained from genetic tests and not discount the subtle ways in which this information might psychologically harm a child by virtue of treatment by family, friends, and school systems. Finally, counselors should help parents to think through how they will use the information and at what point and under what conditions they will tell their child about a positive test result. The family, after meeting with the counselor, may still desire the test, but the additional counseling and discussion should clarify the issues and make parents more knowledgeable about the risks of the tests.

In addition, all parents seeking genetic testing of a child should give written consent to the procedure. State departments of public health (or comparable agencies) should consider designing model consent forms that list the potential risks and benefits of the proposed test, including the psychological risks and the impact on family dynamics. Forms prepared by some state health departments for HIV testing may serve as models. We also recommend, in all cases where a child tests positive for a genetic predisposition, that the child (if sufficiently mature) and his parents be provided the opportunity to meet with a genetic counselor or knowledgeable physician to explain the results. If necessary, psychological counseling should also be made available to the family.

As regards follow-up, physicians who offer or perform a predictive genetic test on a child have an obligation to tell the family that they should check back periodically with the physician to determine whether any new developments might benefit the child. Physicians should also know about possible resources for the family, including toll-free numbers, family support groups, or disease registries, that could assist them in keeping up-to-date regarding their child's condition. Finally, for certain life-threatening conditions or conditions that have the potential to affect the quality of a child's life significantly, registries should be established by national public health agencies or private disease associations. These registries would be voluntary, would track cases of genetic predispositions, and would inform registrants of new developments that could benefit them.

Conclusion

The availability of more and more genetic tests will create unique dilemmas for parents, their children, and their health care providers. We advise caution in the administration of these tests to children when such testing is solely for predictive purposes. Professional associations must take a strong stand on this issue and should provide physicians with guidance as to when they should disclose the availability of tests to families as well as to when it would be appropriate to perform such tests. If a predictive test is appropriate for a child, based on established guidelines, safeguards must be in place to ensure accurate and informed decision making by parents and child (if sufficiently mature). Finally, if predictive testing is done on a young child, resources should be made available, through government funding or private agencies, to assist parents in keeping informed about their child's condition and any beneficial interventions. In addition to the establishment of registries for some conditions, public health education and information dissemination strategies should be implemented to ensure that when new information is available, it reaches a large segment of the population. This way, parents of children like Michael, with the predisposing gene for colon cancer, will bring their children in to see a physician when a treatment or cure for colon cancer is available.

Acknowledgments

Research for this paper was supported by a grant (RO1HG00419) from the National Institutes of Health Center for Human Genome Research. The authors are grateful for the comments of Robert Wachbroit and Karen Rothenberg on an earlier draft.

Notes

1. D. Birch, "Genetic Fortune-Telling," *Baltimore Sun*, May 9, 1995, at A1.

2. Tests are also predicted to be available for predispositions to "complex conditions and behaviors," such as "mental illness, Alzheimer's disease, hyperactivity, heart disease, ... and susceptibility to alcoholism, addiction, and even violence." Some have described those persons who test positive for these conditions as the "pre-symptomatically ill" or the "person 'at-risk'." R. C. Dreyfuss and D. Nelkin, "The Jurisprudence of Genetics," *Vanderbilt Law Review*, 45 (1992): at 318.

3. According to newspaper reports, the tests cost approximately $800 for the first family member and $250 for each additional member. They are being offered under research protocols to cancer families by at least one biotechnology company. See G. Kolata, "Tests to Assess Risks for Cancer Raising Questions," *New York Times*, Mar. 27, 1995, at A1.

4. See M. R. Natowicz and J. S. Alper, "Genetic Screening: Triumphs, Problems, and Controversies," *Journal of Public Health Policy*, 12 (1991): at 485.

5. Kolata, *supra* note 3, at A9.

6. See, for example, N. F. Sharpe, letter, "Pre-Symptomatic Testing for Huntington Disease: Is There a Duty to Test Those Under the Age of Eighteen Years?," *American Journal of Medical Genetics*, 46 (1993): 250–53.

7. M. Z. Pelias, "Duty to Disclose in Medical Genetics: A Legal Perspective," *American Journal of Medical Genetics*, 39 (1991): at 350.

8. Kolata, *supra* note 3.

9. See, for example, N. Fost, "Genetic Diagnosis and Treatment: Ethical Considerations," *American Journal of Diseases of Children*, 147 (1993): 1190–95; D. C. Wertz et al., "Genetic Testing for Children and Adolescents: Who Decides?," *JAMA*, 272 (1994): 875–82; and P. S. Harper and A. Clarke, "Viewpoint: Should We Test Children for 'Adult' Genetic Disease?," *Lancet*, 335 (1990): 1205–06.

10. *Id.*

11. American Society of Human Genetics and American College of Medical Genetics, "Points to Consider: Ethical, Legal, and Psychosocial Implications of Genetic Testing in Children and Adolescents," *American Journal of Human Genetics*, 57 (1995): 1233–41.

12. Wertz et al., *supra* note 9; and Fost, *supra* note 9.

13. *Id.*

14. The Committee on Assessing Genetic Risks, which was appointed by the Institute of Medicine, recommends that "[c]hildren should generally be tested only for genetic disorders for which there exists an effective curative or preventive treatment that must be instituted early in life to achieve maximum benefit." See Institute of Medicine, L. B. Andrews et al., eds., *Assessing Genetic Risks: Implications for Health and Social Policy* (Washington, D.C.: National Academy Press, 1994): at 10. Detailed statements on the testing of children have been prepared by the Working Party of the Clinical Genetics Society in the United Kingdom and, more recently, by ASHG and ACMG, see *supra* note 11. The Working Party makes several recommendations, including the following:

> (1) The predictive genetic testing of children is clearly appropriate where onset of the condition regularly occurs in childhood or there are useful medical interventions that can be offered (for example, diet, medication, surveillance for complications). (2) In contrast, the working party believes that predictive testing for an adult onset disorder should generally not be undertaken if the child is healthy and there are no medical interventions established as useful that can be offered in the event of a positive test result.

A. Clarke, Working Party of the Clinical Genetics Society, "The Genetic Testing of Children," *Journal of Medical Genetics*, 31 (1994): at 785.

15. Clarke, *supra* note 14; but see Harper and Clarke, *supra* note 9.

16. Wertz et al., *supra* note 9; and Clarke, *supra* note 14.

17. Wertz et al., *supra* note 9, at 878, citing J. H. Fanos, *Developmental Consequences for Adulthood of Early Sibling Loss* (Ann Arbor: University of Michigan Microfilms, 1987), and J. Dunn, *Sisters and Brothers* (Cambridge: Harvard University Press, 1985).

18. Fost, *supra* note 9, at 1193, citing A. Tluczek et al., "Parents' Knowledge of Neonatal Screening and Response to False-Positive Cystic Fibrosis Screening," *Journal of Developmental and Behavioral Pediatrics*, 13 (1992): 181–86.

19. D. Ball et al., "Predictive Testing of Adults and Children," in A. Clarke, ed., *Genetic Counselling: Practice and Principles* (London: Routledge, 1994): at 70.

20. *Id.* at 74.

21. Wertz et al., *supra* note 9, at 876, citing A. Gabow et al., "Gene Testing in Autosomal Dominant Adult Polycystic Kidney Disease: Results of a National Kidney Foundation Workshop," *American Journal of Kidney Diseases*, 13 (1989): 85–87. Also, according to Biesecker et al., the long-term outcome of polycystic kidney disease is not altered by early identification. The impetus for testing individuals for the disease comes primarily from "efforts to identify unaffected living related renal transplant donors at an age where renal ultrasound will not accurately identify all pre-symptomatic carriers; this can result in the identification of carriers for a disease in which early clinical intervention does not alter the course." The National Kidney Foundation only endorses testing presymptomatically for the disease as part of evaluation for renal transplant donation. B. B. Biesecker et al., "Genetic Counseling for Families with Inherited Susceptibility to Breast and Ovarian Cancer," *JAMA*, 269 (1993): at 1971.

22. See, for example, Pelias, *supra* note 7; and Sharpe, *supra* note 6.

23. See, for example, *Berman v. Allan*, 404 A.2d 8, 15 (N.J. 1979) (court held that parents of a congenitally defective child had a valid claim for compensation for their mental and emotional suffering over the birth of the child when the claim was

based on the failure of the expectant mother's doctors to inform the parents of the availability of the diagnostic procedure known as amniocentesis); see also *Phillips v. United States*, 566 F. Supp. 1 (D.S.C. 1981); and *Becker v. Schwartz*, 386 N.E.2d 807 (N.Y. 1978). These cases are often referred to as wrongful birth cases.

24. See, for example, *Munro v. Regents of the University of Cal.*, 263 Cal. Rptr. 878, 882 (Cal. Ct. App. 1989) (doctor did not commit medical malpractice in failing to check whether pregnant woman and her husband were carriers of Tay-Sachs disease, even though the couple's child was later born with Tay-Sachs, when defendants submitted expert evidence that the couple did not meet the profile characteristics necessary to warrant performing a Tay-Sachs carrier screening test); see also *Roth v. Group Health Ass'n, Inc.*, Dkt. No. 88-1005 (D.D.C., settled June 12, 1989) (woman who knew she had a genetic defect in her family sued her doctor and HMO for failing to perform amniocentesis because she was under the age of thirty-five; when her child was born with the defect, she filed a malpractice suit and received a $925,000 settlement).

25. See, for example, Md. Code Ann., Health-Gen. §5-613(a) (1994) (if a patient or his agent or surrogate requests that everything be done for a seriously ill patient, including CPR, and the treating physician believes that CPR would be medically ineffective, the physician must inform the patient of the option to transfer the patient to another provider and must assist in that process).

26. E. W. Clayton, "Removing the Shadow of the Law from the Debate about Genetic Testing of Children," *American Journal of Medical Genetics*, 57 (1995): at 630–32.

27. Pelias, *supra* note 7.

POSTSCRIPT

Should Parents Always Be Told of Genetic-Testing Availability?

Most of the major organizations that have analyzed the issues raised by genetic testing of children for adult-onset diseases have urged caution. In June 1995 the American Medical Association's Council on Ethical and Judicial Affairs said, "If parents have complete freedom to consent to genetic testing for their children, the testing may disclose information that precipitates discrimination against the children. Even if no discrimination results, the parents have preempted their children's right to decide, upon maturity, that they would prefer not to know their genetic status. Accordingly, unless there are important benefits for a child from diagnostic testing, the risks of testing suggest that parents should not be able to require genetic testing of their child." In a 1995 resolution the National Society of Genetic Counselors emphasized the need to explore the psychological and social risks and benefits for both the children and the parents that are inherent in early genetic identification. The society concluded, "Until more data is gathered on the impact of this type of testing, extreme caution should be taken regarding the use of such tests."

Nonetheless, the scientific field of genetics is advancing rapidly, as Philip Kitcher indicates in *The Lives to Come: The Genetic Revolution and Human Possibilities* (Simon & Schuster, 1996). For a historical perspective, see *Controlling Human Heredity: 1865 to the Present* by Diane B. Paul (Humanities Press, 1995). Peter S. Harper and Angus Clarke, in "Should We Test Children for 'Adult' Genetic Diseases," *The Lancet* (May 19, 1990), urge a fuller debate of the ethical and professional issues involved with widespread testing of a significant number of disorders and careful consideration of individual circumstances. The issues raised by testing are also explored at both the professional and societal level in Eric T. Juengst, "The Ethics of Prediction: Genetic Risk and the Physician-Patient Relationship," *Genome Science and Technology* (vol. 1, no. 1, 1995). In "Genetic Testing for Children and Adolescents: Who Decides?" *Journal of the American Medical Association* (September 21, 1994), Dorothy C. Wertz, Joanna H. Fanos, and Philip R. Reilly propose guidelines for predictive genetic testing and counseling. Lisa Geller provides an update of genetic testing issues in "Individual, Family, and Society Dimensions of Genetic Discrimination," *Science and Engineering Ethics* (vol. 2, 1996). In their book *Morality and the New Genetics* (Jones & Barlett, 1996), Bernard Gert et al. show how a philosophical analysis can be used to contend with the moral issues that arise from the new genetics.

Articles on testing for specific genetic diseases include "Consensus Statement on Predictive Testing for Alzheimer Disease," *Alzheimer Disease and As-*

sociated Disorders (vol. 9, no. 4, 1995); Barbara B. Biesecker et al., "Genetic Counseling for Families With Inherited Susceptibility to Breast and Ovarian Cancer," *Journal of the American Medical Association* (April 21, 1993); Eric Kodish et al., "Genetic Testing for Cancer Risk: How to Reconcile the Conflicts," *Journal of the American Medical Association,* (January 21, 1998); Benjamin S. Wilfond and Kathleen Nolan, "National Policy Development for the Clinical Application of Genetic Diagnostic Technologies: Lessons From Cystic Fibrosis," *Journal of the American Medical Association* (December 22/29, 1993); Riyana Babul et al., "Attitudes Toward Direct Predictive Testing for the Huntington Disease Gene: Relevance for Other Adult-Onset Diseases," *Journal of the American Medical Association* (November 17, 1993); and Sandi Wiggins et al., "The Psychological Consequences of Predictive Testing for Huntington's Disease," *The New England Journal of Medicine* (November 12, 1992). A personal account of the decision to be tested for Huntington's disease, Catherine V. Hayes's "Genetic Testing for Huntington's Disease—A Family Issue," also appears in the November 12, 1992, issue of *The New England Journal of Medicine.* An article that demonstrates how screening for sickle-cell disease can decrease patient mortality is Elliott Vichinsky et al., "Newborn Screening for Sickle Cell Disease: Effect on Mortality," *Pediatrics* (June 1988). The issue of prenatal testing is explored in *Women and Prenatal Testing: Facing the Challenges of Genetic Technology* edited by Karen H. Rothenberg and Elizabeth J. Thomson (Ohio State University Press, 1994). Gary N. McAbee, Jack Sherman, and Barbara Davidoff-Feldman discuss recent court decisions that support the belief that it is a physician's duty to warn third parties who may be at risk for a genetic disease in "Physician's Duty to Warn Third Parties About the Risk of Genetic Diseases," *Pediatrics* (July 1998). In one case, *Pate v. Threlkel* in Florida, the physician was deemed responsible only for warning the patient; in another, *Safer v. Pack* in New Jersey, the physician had to directly warn the third party at risk. Leonard J. Deftos also sees the same trend in "The Evolving Duty to Disclose the Presence of Genetic Disease to Relatives," *Academic Medicine* (September 1998). He states that physicians who care for patients and their families, not lawyers and ethicists with no clinical training, should develop guidelines for disclosure. Also see Ellen Clayton Wright, "Genetic Testing in Children," *Journal of Medicine and Philosophy* (vol. 22, no. 3, 1997).

On the Internet ...

New Scientist

This site offers pro and con views on the issue of animal experimentation. It also contains letters from readers of *New Scientist* articles on animal experimentation.

```
http://www.newscientist.com/nsplus/insight/animal/
animal.html
```

ABC News.com: Sham Surgery

This site contains two articles regarding sham surgery. You may also find links to *The New England Journal of Medicine* and the NIH Office of Protection From Research Risks.

```
http://www.abcnews.go.com/sections/living/DailyNews/
shamsurgery092499_feature.html
```

PART 6

Human and Animal Experimentation

*T*he goal of scientific research is knowledge that will benefit society. But achieving that goal may subject humans and animals to some risks. Questions arise about not only how research should be conducted but whether or not it should be conducted at all. What, for example, are the justifications for using placebos in research? This section contends with issues that will shape the future of experimental science.

- Should Animal Experimentation Be Permitted?

- Is Sham Surgery Ethically Acceptable in Clinical Research?

ISSUE 15

Should Animal Experimentation Be Permitted?

YES: Jerod M. Loeb et al., from "Human vs. Animal Rights: In Defense of Animal Research," *Journal of the American Medical Association* (November 17, 1989)

NO: Tom Regan, from "Ill-Gotten Gains," in Donald Van DeVeer and Tom Regan, eds., *Health Care Ethics: An Introduction* (Temple University Press, 1987)

ISSUE SUMMARY

YES: Jerod M. Loeb and his colleagues, representing the American Medical Association's Group on Science and Technology, assert that concern for animals, admirable in itself, cannot impede the development of methods to improve the welfare of humans.

NO: Philosopher Tom Regan argues that conducting research on animals exacts the grave moral price of failing to show proper respect for animals' inherent value, whatever the benefits of the research.

In 1865 the great French physiologist Claude Bernard wrote, "Physicians already make too many dangerous experiments on man before carefully studying them in animals." In his insistence on adequate animal research before trying a new therapy on human beings, Bernard established a principle of research ethics that is still considered valid. But in the past few decades this principle has been challenged by another view—one that sees animals not as tools for human use and consumption but as moral agents in their own right. Animal experimentation, according to this theory, cannot be taken for granted but must be justified by ethical criteria at least as stringent as those that apply to research involving humans.

Philosophers traditionally have not ascribed any moral status to animals. Like St. Thomas Aquinas before him, René Descartes, a seventeenth-century French physiologist and philosopher, saw no ethical problem in experimentation on animals. Descartes approved of cutting open a fully conscious animal because it was, he said, a machine more complex than a clock but no more capable of feeling pain. Immanuel Kant argued that animals need not be treated as ends in themselves because they lacked rationality.

Beginning in England in the nineteenth century, antivivisectionists (people who advocate the abolition of animal experimentation) campaigned, with varying success, for laws to control scientific research. But the internal dissensions in the movement and its frequent lapses into sentimentality made it only partially effective. At best the antivivisectionists achieved some legislation that mandated more humane treatment of animals used for research, but they never succeeded in abolishing animal research or even in establishing the need for justification of particular research projects.

The more recent movement to ban animal research, however, is both better organized politically and more rigorously philosophical. The movement, often called animal liberation or animal rights, is similar in principle to the civil rights movement of the 1960s. Just as blacks, women, and other minorities sought recognition of their equal status, animal advocates have built a case for the equal status of animals.

Peter Singer, one of the leaders of this movement, has presented an eloquent case that we practice not only racism and sexism in our society but also "speciesism." That is, we assume that human beings are superior to other animals; we are prejudiced in favor of our own kind. Experimenting on animals and eating their flesh are the two major forms of speciesism in our society. Singer points out that some categories of human beings—infants and mentally retarded people—rate lower on a scale of intelligence, awareness, and self-consciousness than some animals. Yet we would not treat these individuals in the way we do animals. He argues that "all animals are equal" and that the suffering of an animal is morally equal to the suffering of a human being.

Proponents of animal research counter that such views are fundamentally misguided, that human beings, with the capacity for rational thought and action, are indeed a superior species. They contend that, while animals deserve humane treatment, the good consequences of animal research (i.e., knowledge that will benefit human beings) outweigh the suffering of individual animals. No other research techniques can substitute for the reactions of live animals, they declare.

In the selections that follow, Jerod M. Loeb and his colleagues reaffirm the American Medical Association's defense of animal research because it is essential for medical progress and it would be unethical to deprive humans and animals of advances in medicine that result from this research. Tom Regan disputes the view that benefit to humans justifies research on animals. Pointing to their inherent value, he says that "whatever our gains, they are ill-gotten," and he calls for an end to such research.

Jerod M. Loeb et al.

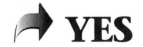 **YES**

Human vs. Animal Rights:
In Defense of Animal Research

Research with animals is a highly controversial topic in our society. Animal rights groups that intend to stop all experimentation with animals are in the vanguard of this controversy. Their methods range from educational efforts directed in large measure to the young and uninformed, to promotion of restrictive legislation, filing lawsuits, and violence that includes raids on laboratories and death threats to investigators. Their rhetoric is emotionally charged and their information is frequently distorted and pejorative. Their tactics vary but have a single objective—to stop scientific research with animals.

The resources of the animal rights groups are extensive, in part because less militant organizations of animal activists, including some humane societies, have been infiltrated or taken over by animal rights groups to gain access to their fiscal and physical holdings. Through bizarre tactics, extravagant claims, and gruesome myths, animal rights groups have captured the attention of the media and a sizable segment of the public. Nevertheless, people invariably support the use of animals in research when they understand both sides of the issue and the contributions of animal research to relief of human suffering. However, all too often they do not understand both sides because information about the need for animal research is not presented. When this need is explained, the presentation often reveals an arrogance of the scientific community and an unwillingness to be accountable to public opinion.

The use of animals in research is fundamentally an ethical question: is it more ethical to ban all research with animals or to use a limited number of animals in research under humane conditions when no alternatives exist to achieve medical advances that reduce substantial human suffering and misery? . . .

Animals in Scientific Research

Animals have been used in research for more than 2000 years. In the third century BC, the natural philosopher Erisistratus of Alexandria used animals to study bodily function. In all likelihood, Aristotle performed vivisection on animals. The Roman physician Galen used apes and pigs to prove his theory that veins carry blood rather than air. In succeeding centuries, animals were employed to

From Jerod M. Loeb, William R. Hendee, Steven J. Smith, and M. Roy Schwarz, "Human vs. Animal Rights: In Defense of Animal Research," *Journal of the American Medical Association,* vol. 262, no. 19 (November 17, 1989), pp. 2716–2720. Copyright © 1989 by The American Medical Association. Reprinted by permission.

confirm theories about physiology developed through observation. Advances in knowledge from these experiments include demonstration of the circulation of blood by Harvey in 1622, documentation of the effects of anesthesia on the body in 1846, and elucidation of the relationship between bacteria and disease in 1878.[1] In his book *An Introduction to the Study of Experimental Medicine* published in 1865, Bernard[2] described the importance of animal research to advances in knowledge about the human body and justified the continued use of animals for this purpose.

In this century, many medical advances have been achieved through research with animals.[3] Infectious diseases such as pertussis, rubella, measles, and poliomyelitis have been brought under control with vaccines developed in animals. The development of immunization techniques against today's infectious diseases, including human immunodeficiency virus disease, depends entirely on experiments in animals. Antibiotics that control infection are always tested in animals before use in humans. Physiological disorders such as diabetes and epilepsy are treatable today through knowledge and products gained by animal research. Surgical procedures such as coronary artery bypass grafts, cerebrospinal fluid shunts, and retinal reattachments have evolved from experiments with animals. Transplantation procedures for persons with failed liver, heart, lung, and kidney function are products of animal research.

Animals have been essential to the evolution of modern medicine and the conquest of many illnesses. However, many medical challenges remain to be solved. Cancer, heart disease, cerebrovascular disease, dementia, depression, arthritis, and a variety of inherited disorders are yet to be understood and controlled. Until they are, human pain and suffering will endure, and society will continue to expend its emotional and fiscal resources in efforts to alleviate or at least reduce them.

Animal research has not only benefited humans. Procedures and products developed through this process have also helped animals.[4,5] Vaccines against rabies, distemper, and parvovirus in dogs are a spin-off of animal research, as are immunization techniques against cholera in hogs, encephalitis in horses, and brucellosis in cattle. Drugs to combat heartworm, intestinal parasites, and mastitis were developed in animals used for experimental purposes. Surgical procedures developed in animals help animals as well as humans.

Research with animals has yielded immeasurable benefits to both humans and animals. However, this research raises fundamental philosophical issues concerning the rights of humans to use animals to benefit humans and other animals. If these rights are granted (and many people are loath to do so), additional questions arise concerning the way that research should be performed, the accountability of researchers to public sentiment, the nature of an ethical code for animal research, and who should compose and approve the code. Today, some animal activists are asking whether humans have the right to exercise dominion over animals for any purpose, including research. Others suggest that because humans have dominion over other forms of life, they are obligated to protect and preserve animals and ensure that they are not exploited. Still others agree that animals can be used to help people, but only under circumstances that are so structured as to be unattainable by most researchers. These attitudes may all differ, but their consequences are similar. They all threaten to diminish or stop animal research.

Challenge to Animal Research

Challenges to the use of animals to benefit humans are not new—their origins can be traced back several centuries. With respect to animal research, opposition has been vocal in Europe for more than 400 years and in the United States for at least 100 years.[6]

Most of the current arguments against research with animals have historic precedents that must be grasped to understand the current debate. These precedents originated in the controversy between Cartesian and utilitarian philosophers that extended from the 16th to the 18th centuries.

The Cartesian-utilitarian debate was opened by the French philosopher Descartes, who defended the use of animals in experiments by insisting the animals respond to stimuli in only one way—"according to the arrangement of their organs."[7] He stated that animals lack the ability to reason and think and are, therefore, similar to a machine. Humans, on the other hand, can think, talk, and respond to stimuli in various ways. These differences, Descartes argued, make animals inferior to humans and justify their use as a machine, including as experimental subjects. He proposed that animals learn only by experience, whereas humans learn by "teaching-learning." Humans do not always have to experience something to know that it is true.

Descartes' arguments were countered by the utilitarian philosopher Bentham of England. "The question," said Bentham, "is not can they reason? nor can they talk? but can they suffer?"[8] In utilitarian terms, humans and animals are linked by their common ability to suffer and their common right not to suffer and die at the hands of others. This utilitarian thesis has rippled through various groups opposed to research with animals for more than a century.

In the 1970s, the antivivisectionist movement was influenced by three books that clarified the issues and introduced the rationale for increased militancy against animal research. In 1971, the anthology *Animals, Men and Morals*, by Godlovitch et al,[9] raised the concept of animal rights and analyzed the relationships between humans and animals. Four years later, *Victims of Science*, by Ryder,[10] introduced the concept of "speciesism" as equivalent to fascism. Also in 1975, Singer[11] published *Animal Liberation: A New Ethic for Our Treatment of Animals*. This book is generally considered the progenitor of the modern animal rights movement. Invoking Ryder's concept of speciesism, Singer deplored the historic attitude of humans toward nonhumans as a "form of prejudice no less objectionable than racism or sexism." He urged that the liberation of animals should become the next great cause after civil rights and the women's movement.

Singer's book not only was a philosophical treatise; it also was a call to action. It provided an intellectual foundation and a moral focus for the animal rights movement. These features attracted many who were indifferent to the emotional appeal based on a love of animals that had characterized antivivisectionist efforts for the past century. Singer's book swelled the ranks of the antivivisectionist movement and transformed it into a movement for animal rights. It also has been used to justify illegal activities intended to impede animal research and instill fear and intimidation in those engaged in it. . . .

Defense of Animal Research

The issue of animal research is fundamentally an issue of the dominion of humans over animals. This issue is rooted in the Judeo-Christian religion of western culture, including the ancient tradition of animal sacrifice described in the Old Testament and the practice of using animals as surrogates for suffering humans described in the New Testament. The sacredness of human life is a central theme of biblical morality, and the dominion of humans over other forms of life is a natural consequence of this theme.[12] The issue of dominion is not, however, unique to animal research. It is applicable to every situation where animals are subservient to humans. It applies to the use of animals for food and clothing; the application of animals as beasts of burden and transportation; the holding of animals in captivity such as in zoos and as household pets; the use of animals as entertainment, such as in sea parks and circuses; the exploitation of animals in sports that employ animals, including hunting, racing, and animal shows; and the eradication of pests such as rats and mice from homes and farms. Even provision of food and shelter to animals reflects an attitude of dominion of humans over animals. A person who truly does not believe in human dominance over animals would be forced to oppose all of these practices, including keeping animals as household pets or in any form of physical or psychological captivity. Such a posture would defy tradition evolved over the entire course of human existence.

Some animal advocates do not take issue with the right of humans to exercise dominion over animals. They agree that animals are inferior to humans because they do not possess attributes such as a moral sense and concepts of past and future. However, they also claim that it is precisely because of these differences that humans are obligated to protect animals and not exploit them for the selfish betterment of humans.[13] In their view, animals are like infants and the mentally incompetent, who must be nurtured and protected from exploitation. This view shifts the issues of dominion from one of rights claimed by animals to one of responsibilities exercised by humans.

Neither of these philosophical positions addresses the issue of animal research from the perspective of the immorality of not using animals in research. From this perspective, depriving humans (and animals) of advances in medicine that result from research with animals is inhumane and fundamentally unethical. Spokespersons for this perspective suggest that patients with dementia, stroke, disabling injuries, heart disease, and cancer deserve relief from suffering and that depriving them of hope and relief by eliminating animal research is an immoral and unconscionable act. Defenders of animal research claim that animals sometimes must be sacrificed in the development of methods to relieve pain and suffering of humans (and animals) and to affect treatments and cures of a variety of human maladies.

The immeasurable benefits of animal research to humans are undeniable. One example is the development of a vaccine for poliomyelitis, with the result that the number of cases of poliomyelitis in the United States alone declined from 58,000 in 1952 to 4 in 1984. Benefits of this vaccine worldwide are even more impressive.

Every year, hundreds of thousands of humans are spared the braces, wheelchairs, and iron lungs required for the victims of poliomyelitis who survive this infectious disease. The research that led to a poliomyelitis vaccine required the sacrifice of hundreds of primates. Without this sacrifice, development of the vaccine would have been impossible, and in all likelihood the poliomyelitis epidemic would have continued unabated. Depriving humanity of this medical advance is unthinkable to almost all persons. Other diseases that are curable or treatable today as a result of animal research include diphtheria, scarlet fever, tuberculosis, diabetes, and appendicitis.[3] Human suffering would be much more stark today if these diseases, and many others as well, had not been amendable to treatment and cure through advances obtained by animal research.

Issues in Animal Research

Animal rights groups have several stock arguments against animal research. Some of these issues are described and refuted herein.

The Clinical Value of Basic Research

Persons opposed to research with animals often claim that basic biomedical research has no clinical value and therefore does not justify the use of animals. However, basic research is the foundation for most medical advances and consequently for progress in clinical medicine. Without basic research, including that with animals, chemotherapeutic advances against cancer (including childhood leukemia and breast malignancy), beta-blockers for cardiac patients, and electrolyte infusions for patients with dysfunctional metabolism would never have been achieved.

Duplication of Experiments

Opponents of animal research frequently claim that experiments are needlessly duplicated. However, the duplication of results is an essential part of the confirmation process in science. The generalization of results from one laboratory to another prevents anomalous results in one laboratory from being interpreted as scientific truth. The cost of research animals, the need to publish the results of experiments, and the desire to conduct meaningful research all function to reduce the likelihood of unnecessary experiments. Furthermore, the intense competition of research funds and the peer review process lessen the probability of obtaining funds for unnecessary research. Most scientists are unlikely to waste valuable time and resources conducting unnecessary experiments when opportunities for performing important research are so plentiful....

The Use of Primates in Research

Animal activists often make a special plea on behalf of nonhuman primates, and many of the sit-ins, demonstrations, and break-ins have been directed at primate research centers. Efforts to justify these activities invoke the premise that primates are much like humans because they exhibit suffering and other emotions.

Keeping primates in cages and isolating them from others of their kind is considered by activists as cruel and destructive of their "psychological well-being." However, the opinion that animals that resemble humans most closely and deserve the most protection and care reflects an attitude of speciesism (i.e., a hierarchical scheme of relative importance) that most activists purportedly abhor. This logical fallacy in the drive for special protection of primates apparently escapes most of its adherents.

Some scientific experiments require primates exactly because they simulate human physiology so closely. Primates are susceptible to many of the same diseases as humans and have similar immune systems. They also possess intellectual, cognitive, and social skills above those of other animals. These characteristics make primates invaluable in research related to language, perception, and visual and spatial skills.[14] Although primates constitute only 0.5% of all animals used in research, their contributions have been essential to the continued acquisition of knowledge in the biological and behavioral sciences.[15]

Do Animals Suffer Needless Pain and Abuse?

Animal activists frequently assert that research with animals causes severe pain and that many research animals are abused either deliberately or through indifference. Actually, experiments today involve pain only when relief from pain would interfere with the purpose of the experiments. In any experiment in which an animal might experience pain, federal law requires that a veterinarian must be consulted in planning the experiment, and anesthesia, tranquilizers, and analgesics must be used except when they would compromise the results of the experiment.[16]

In 1984, the Department of Agriculture reported that 61% of research animals were not subjected to painful procedures, and another 31% received anesthesia or pain-relieving drugs. The remaining 8% did experience pain, often because improved understanding and treatment of pain, including chronic pain, were the purpose of the experiment.[14] Chronic pain is a challenging health problem that costs the United States about $50 billion a year in direct medical expenses, lost productivity, and income.[15]

Alternatives to the Use of Animals

One of the most frequent objections to animal research is the claim that alternative research models obviate the need for research with animals. The concept of alternatives was first raised in 1959 by Russell and Burch[17] in their book, *The Principles of Humane Experimental Technique.* These authors exhorted scientists to reduce the pain of experimental animals, decrease the number of animals used in research, and replace animals with nonanimal models whenever possible.

However, more often than not, alternatives to research animals are not available. In certain research investigations, cell, tissue, and organ cultures and computer models can be used as adjuncts to experiments with animals, and occasionally as substitutes for animals, at least in preliminary phases of the investigations. However, in many experimental situations, culture techniques and computer models are wholly inadequate because they do not encompass the physiological complexity of the whole animal. Examples where animals are essential to research include development of a vaccine against human immunodeficiency virus, refinement of organ transplantation techniques, investigation of mechanical devices as replacements for and adjuncts to physiological organs, identification of target-specific pharmaceuticals for cancer diagnosis and treatment, restoration of infarcted myocardium in patients with cardiac disease, evolution of new diagnostic imaging technologies, improvement of methods to relieve mental stress and anxiety, and evaluation of approaches to define and treat chronic pain. These challenges can only be addressed by research with animals as an essential step in the evolution of knowledge that leads to solutions. Humans are the only alternatives to animals for this step. When faced with this alternative, most people prefer the use of animals as the research model.

Comment

Love of animals and concern for their welfare are admirable characteristics that distinguish humans from other species of animals. Most humans, scientists as well as laypersons, share these attributes. However, when the concern for animals impedes the development of methods to improve the welfare of humans through amelioration and elimination of pain and suffering, a fundamental choice must be made. This choice is present today in the conflict between animal rights activism and scientific research. The American Medical Association made this choice more than a century ago and continues to stand squarely in defense of the use of animals for scientific research. In this position, the Association is supported by opinion polls that reveal strong endorsement of the American public for the use of animals in research and testing.[18] . . .

The American Medical Association believes that research involving animals is absolutely essential to maintaining and improving the health of people in America and worldwide.[6] Animal research is required to develop solutions to human tragedies such as human immunodeficiency virus disease, cancer, heart disease, dementia, stroke, and congenital and developmental abnormalities. The American Medical Association recognizes the moral obligation of investigators to use alternatives to animals whenever possible, and to conduct their research with animals as humanely as possible. However, it is convinced that depriving humans of medical advances by preventing research with animals is philosophically and morally a fundamentally indefensible position. Consequently, the American Medical Association is committed to the preservation of animal research and to the conduct of this research under the most humane conditions possible.[19,20]

References

1. Rowan AN, Rollin BE. Animal research—for and against: a philosophical, social, and historical perspective. *Perspect Biol Med.* 1983; 27:1–17.
2. Bernard C, Green HC, trans. *An Introduction to the Study of Experimental Medicine.* New York, NY: Dover Publications Inc; 1957.
3. Council on Scientific Affairs. Animals in research. *JAMA,* 1989; 261:3602–3606.
4. Leader RW, Stark D. The importance of animals in biomedical research. *Perspect Biol Med.* 1987; 30:470–485.
5. Kransney JA. Some thoughts on the value of life. *Buffalo Physician,* 1984; 18:6–13.
6. Smith SJ, Evans RM, Sullivan-Fowler M, Hendee WR. Use of animals in biomedical research: historical role of the American Medical Association and the American physician. *Arch Intern Med.* 1988; 148:1849–1853.
7. Descartes R. *'Principles of Philosophy,' Descartes: Philosophical Writings.* Anscombe E, Geach PT, eds. London, England: Nelson & Sons; 1969.
8. Bentham J. *Introduction to the Principles of Morals and Legislation.* London, England: Athlone Press; 1970.
9. Godlovitch S, Godlovitch, Harris J. *Animals, Men and Morals.* New York, NY: Taplinger Publishing Co Inc; 1971.
10. Ryder R. *Victims of Science.* London, England: Davis-Poynter; 1975.
11. Singer P. *Animal Liberation: A New Ethic for Our Treatment of Animals.* New York, NY: Random House Inc; 1975.
12. Morowitz HJ, Jesus, Moses, Aristotle and laboratory animals. *Hosp Pract.* 1988; 23:23–25.
13. Cohen C. The case for the use of animals in biomedical research. *N Engl J Med.* 1986; 315: 865–870.
14. *Alternatives to Animal Use in Research, Testing, and Education.* Washington, DC: Office of Technology Assessment; 1986. Publication OTA-BA-273.
15. Committee on the Use of Laboratory Animals in Biomedical and Behavioral Research. *Use of Laboratory Animals in Biomedical and Behavioral Research.* Washington, DC: National Academy Press; 1988.
16. *Biomedical Investigator's Handbook.* Washington, DC: Foundation for Biomedical Research; 1987.
17. Russell WMS, Burch RL. *The Principles of Humane Experimental Technique.* Springfield, Ill: Charles C Thomas Publisher; 1959.
18. Harvey LK, Shubat SC. *AMA Survey of Physician and Public Opinion on Health Care Issues.* Chicago, Ill: American Medical Association; 1989.
19. Smith SJ, Hendee WR. Animals in research. *JAMA* 1988; 259:2007–2008.
20. Smith SJ, Loeb JM, Evans RM, Hendee WR. Animals in research and testing; who pays the price for medical progress? *Arch Ophthalmol.* 1988; 106:1184–1187.

Tom Regan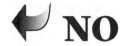

Ill-Gotten Gains

The Story

Late in 1981 a reporter for a large metropolitan newspaper (we'll call her Karen to protect her interest in remaining anonymous) gained access to some previously classified government files. Using the Freedom of Information Act, Karen was investigating the federal government's funding of research into the short- and long-term effects of exposure to radioactive waste. It was with understandable surprise that, included in these files, she discovered the records of a series of experiments involving the induction and treatment of coronary thrombosis (heart attack). Conducted over a period of fifteen years by a renowned heart specialist (we'll call him Dr. Ventricle) and financed with federal funds, the experiments in all likelihood would have remained unknown to anyone outside Dr. Ventricle's sphere of power and influence had not Karen chanced upon them.

Karen's surprise soon gave way to shock and disbelief. In case after case she read of how Ventricle and his associates took otherwise healthy individuals, with no previous record of heart disease, and intentionally caused their heart to fail. The methods used to occasion the "attack" were a veritable shopping list of experimental techniques, from massive doses of stimulants (adrenaline was a favorite) to electrical damage of the coronary artery, which, in its weakened state, yielded the desired thrombosis. Members of Ventricle's team then set to work testing the efficacy of various drugs developed in the hope that they would help the heart withstand a second "attack." Dosages varied, and there were the usual control groups. In some cases, certain drugs administered to "patients" proved more efficacious than cases in which others received no medication or smaller amounts of the same drugs. The research came to an abrupt end in the fall of 1981, but not because the project was judged unpromising or because someone raised a hue and cry about the ethics involved. Like so much else in the world at that time, Ventricle's project was a casualty of austere economic times. There simply wasn't enough federal money available to renew the grant application.

One would have to forsake all the instincts of a reporter to let the story end there. Karen persevered and, under false pretenses, secured an interview

Excerpted and adapted from Tom Regan, "Ill-Gotten Gains," in Donald Van DeVeer and Tom Regan, eds., *Health Care Ethics: An Introduction* (Temple University Press, 1987). Copyright © 1987 by Temple University. Reprinted by permission.

with Ventricle. When she revealed that she had gained access to the file, knew in detail the largely fruitless research conducted over fifteen years, and was incensed about his work, Ventricle was dumbfounded. But not because Karen had unearthed the file. And not even because it was filed where it was (a "clerical error," he assured her). What surprised Ventricle was that anyone would think there was a serious ethical question to be raised about what he had done. Karen's notes of their conversation include the following:

Ventricle: But I don't understand what you're getting at. Surely you know that heart disease is the leading cause of death. How can there be any ethical question about developing drugs which *literally* promise to be life-saving?

Karen: Some people might agree that the goal—to save life—is a good, a noble end, and still question the means used to achieve it. Your "patients," after all, had no previous history of heart disease. *They* were healthy before you got your hands on them.

Ventricle: But medical progress simply isn't possible if we wait for people to get sick and then see what works. There are too many variables, too much beyond our control and comprehension, if we try to do our medical research in a clinical setting. The history of medicine shows how hopeless that approach is.

Karen: And I read, too, that upon completion of the experiment, assuming that the "patient" didn't die in the process—it says that those who survived were "sacrificed." You mean killed?

Ventricle: Yes, that's right. But always painlessly, always painlessly. And the body went immediately to the lab, where further tests were done. Nothing was wasted.

Karen: And it didn't bother you—I mean, you didn't ever ask yourself whether what you were doing was wrong? I mean...

Ventricle: (interrupting): My dear young lady, you make it seem as if I'm some kind of moral monster. I work for the benefit of humanity, and I have achieved some small success, I hope you will agree. Those who raise cries of wrongdoing about what I've done are well intentioned but misguided. After all, I use animals in my research—chimpanzees, to be more precise— not human beings.

The Point

The story about Karen and Dr. Ventricle is just that—a story, a small piece of fiction. There is no real Dr. Ventricle, no real Karen, and so on. But there *is* widespread use of animals in scientific research, including research like our imaginary Dr. Ventricle's. So the story, while its details are imaginary—while it is, let it be clear, a literary device, not a factual account—is a story with a point. Most people reading it would be morally outraged if there actually were a Dr. Ventricle who did coronary research of the sort described on otherwise healthy human beings. Considerably fewer would raise a morally quizzical eyebrow when informed of such research done on animals, chimpanzees, or whatever. The story has a point, or so I hope, because, catching us off-guard, it brings this difference home to us, gives it life in our experience, and, in doing so, reveals something about ourselves, something about our own constellation of values. If we think what Ventricle did would be wrong if done to human beings but all right if done to chimpanzees, then we must believe that there are different moral standards that apply to how we may treat the two—human beings and chimpanzees. But to acknowledge this difference, if acknowledge it we do, is only the beginning, not the end, of our moral thinking. We can meet the challenge to think well from the moral point of view only if we are able to cite a *morally relevant difference* between humans and chimpanzees, one that illuminates in a clear, coherent, and rationally defensible way why it would be wrong to use humans, but not chimpanzees, in research like Dr. Ventricle's....

The Law

Among the difference between chimps and humans, one concerns their legal standing. It is against the law to do to human beings what Ventricle did to his chimpanzees. It is not against the law to do this to chimps. So, here we have a difference. But a morally relevant one?

The difference in the legal status of chimps and humans would be morally relevant if we had good reason to believe that what is legal and what is moral go hand in glove: where we have the former, there we have the latter (and maybe vice versa too). But a moment's reflection shows how bad the fit between legality and morality sometimes is. A century and a half ago, the legal status of black people in the United States was similar to the legal status of a house, corn, a barn: they were property, other people's property, and could legally be bought and sold without regard to their personal interests. But the legality of the slave trade did not make it moral, any more than the law against drinking, during the era of that "great experiment" of Prohibition, made it immoral to drink. Sometimes, it is true, what the law declares illegal (for example, murder and rape) is immoral, and vice versa. But there is no necessary connection, no pre-established harmony between morality and the law. So, yes, the legal status of chimps and humans differs; but that does not show that their moral status does. Their difference in legal status, in other words, is not a morally relevant difference and will not morally justify using these animals, but not humans, in Ventricle's research.

The Value of the Individual

[An] alternative vision [to utilitarian value] consists in viewing certain individuals as themselves having a distinctive kind of value, what we will call "inherent value." This kind of value is not the same as, is not reducible to, and is not commensurate either with such values as preference satisfaction or frustration (that is, mental states) or with such values as artistic or intellectual talents (that is, mental and other kinds of excellences or virtues). We cannot, that is, equate or reduce the inherent value of an individual to his or her mental states or virtues, and neither can we intelligibly compare the two. In this respect, the three kinds of value (mental states, virtues, and the inherent value of the individual) are like proverbial apples and oranges.

They are also like water and oil: they don't mix. It is not only that [a man's] inherent value is not the same as, not reducible to, and not commensurate with *his* satisfaction, pleasures, intellectual and artistic skills, etc. In addition, *his* inherent value is not the same as, is not reducible to, and is not commensurate with the valuable mental states or talents of *other* individuals, whether taken singly or collectively. Moreover, and as a corollary of the preceding, the individual's inherent value is in all ways independent both of his or her usefulness relative to the interest of others and of how others feel about the individual (for example, whether one is liked or admired, despised or merely tolerated). A prince and a pauper, a streetwalker and a nun, those who are loved and those who are forsaken, the genius and the retarded child, the artist and the philistine, the most generous philanthropist and the most unscrupulous used car salesman —all have inherent value, according to the view recommended here, and all have it equally. . . .

What Difference Does It Make?

To view the value of individuals in this way is not an empty abstraction. To the question, "What difference does it make whether we view individuals as having equal inherent value, or as utilitarians do, as lacking such value, or, as perfectionists do, as having such value but to varying degree?"—our response to this question must be, "It makes all the moral difference in the world!" Morally, we are *always* required to treat those who have inherent value in ways that display proper respect for their distinctive kind of value, and though we cannot on this occasion either articulate or defend the full range of obligations tied to this fundamental duty, we can note that we fail to show proper respect for those who have such value whenever we treat them as if they were mere receptacles of value or as if their value was dependent on, or reducible to, their possible utility relative to the interests of others. In particular, therefore, Ventricle would fail to act as duty requires—would, in other words, do what is morally wrong —if he conducted his coronary research on competent human beings, without their informed consent, on the grounds that this research just might lead to the development of drugs or surgical techniques that would benefit others. That would be to treat these human beings as mere receptacles or as mere medical resources for others, and though Ventricle might be able to do this and get away with it, and though others might benefit as a result, that would not alter the nature of the grievous wrong he would have done. And it would be wrong, not because (or only if) there were utilitarian considerations, or contractarian considerations, or perfectionist considerations against his doing his research on these human beings, but because it would mark a failure on his part to treat them with appropriate respect. To ascribe inherent value to competent human beings, then, provides us with the theoretical wherewithal to ground our moral case against using competent human beings, against their will, in research like Ventricle's.

Who Has Inherent Value?

If inherent value could nonarbitrarily be limited to competent humans, then we would have to look elsewhere to resolve the ethical issues involved in using other individuals (for example, chimpanzees) in medical research. But inherent value can only be limited to competent human beings by having the recourse to one arbitrary maneuver or another. Once we recognize that we have direct duties to competent and incompetent humans as well as to animals such as chimpanzees; once we recognize the challenge to give a sound theoretical basis for these duties in the case of these humans and animals; once we recognize the failure of indirect duty, contractarian, and utilitarian theories of obligation; once we recognize that the inherent value of competent humans precludes using them as mere resources in such research; once we recognize that perfectionist vision of morality, one that assigns degrees of inherent value on the basis of possession of favored virtues, is unacceptable because of its inegalitarian implications, and once we recognize that morality simply will not tolerate double standards, then we cannot, except arbitrarily, withhold ascribing inherent value, to an equal degree, to incompetent humans and animals such as chimpanzees. All have this value, in short, and all have it equally. All considered, this is an essential part of the most adequate total vision of morality. Morally, none of those having inherent value may be used in Ventricle-like research (research that puts them at risk of significant harm in the name of securing benefits for others, whether those benefits are realized or not). And none may be used in such research because to do so is to treat them as if their value is somehow reducible to their possible utility relative to the interests of others, or as if their value is somehow reducible to their value as "receptacles." What contractarianism, utilitarianism, and the other "isms" discussed earlier will allow is not morally tolerable.

Hurting and Harming

The prohibition against research like Ventricle's, when conducted on animals such as chimps, cannot be avoided by the use of anesthetics or other palliatives used to eliminate or reduce suffering. Other things being equal, to cause an animal to suffer is to harm that animal—is, that is, to diminish that individual animal's welfare. But these two notions—harming on the one hand and suffering on the other—differ in important ways. An individual's welfare can be diminished independently of causing her to suffer, as when, for example, a young woman is reduced to a "vegetable" by painlessly administering a debilitating drug to her while she sleeps. We mince words if we deny that harm has been done to her, though she suffers not. More generally, harms, understood as reductions in an individual's welfare, can take the form either of *inflictions* (gross physical suffering is the clearest example of a harm of this type) or *deprivations* (prolonged loss of physical freedom is a clear example of a harm of this kind). Not all harms hurt, in other words, just as not all hurts harm.

Viewed against the background of these ideas, an untimely death is seen to be the ultimate harm for both humans and animals, such as chimpanzees, and it is the ultimate harm for both because it is their ultimate deprivation or loss—their loss of life itself. Let the means used to kill chimpanzees be as "humane" (a cruel word, this) as you like. That will not erase the harm that an untimely death is for these animals. True, the use of anesthetics and other "humane" steps lessens the wrong done to these animals, when they are "sacrificed" in Ventricle-type research. But a lesser wrong is not a right. To do research that culminates in the "sacrifice" of chimpanzees or that puts these and similar animals at risk of losing their life, in the hope that we might learn something that will benefit others, is morally to be condemned, however "humane" that research may be in other respects.

The Criterion of Inherent Value

It remains to be asked, before concluding, what underlies the possession of inherent value. Some are tempted by the idea that life itself is inherently valuable. This view would authorize attributing inherent value to chimpanzees, for example, and so might find favor with some people who oppose using these animals in research. But this view would also authorize attributing inherent value to anything and everything that is alive, including, for example, crabgrass, lice, bacteria, and cancer cells. It is exceedingly unclear, to put the point as mildly as possible, either that we have a duty to treat these things with respect or that any clear sense can be given to the idea that we do.

More plausible by far is the view that those individuals have inherent value who are *the subjects of a life*—who are, that is, the experiencing subjects of a life that fares well or ill for them over time, those who have *an individual experiential welfare*, logically independent of their utility relative to the interests or welfare of others. Competent humans are subjects of a life in this sense. But so, too, are those incompetent humans who have concerned us. And so, too, and not unimportantly, are chimpanzees. Indeed, so too are the members of many species of animals: cats and dogs, monkeys and sheep, cetaceans and wolves, horses and cattle. Where one draws the line between those animals who are, and those who are not, subjects of a life is certain to be controversial. Still there is abundant reason to believe that the members of mammalian species of animals do have a psychophysical identity over time, do have an experiential life, do have an individual welfare. Common sense is on the side of viewing these animals in this way, and ordinary language is not strained in talking of them as individuals who have an experiential welfare. The behavior of these animals, moreover, is consistent with regarding them as subjects of a life, and the implications of evolutionary theory are that there are many species of animals whose members are, like the members of the species *Homo sapiens*, experiencing subjects of a life of their own, with an individual welfare. On these grounds, then, we have very strong reason to believe, even if we lack conclusive proof, that these animals meet the subject-of-a-life criterion.

If, then, those who meet this criterion have inherent value, and have it equally relative to all who meet it, chimpanzees and other animals who are subjects of a life, not just human beings, have this value *and* have neither more nor less of it than we do. (To hold that they have less than we do is to land oneself in the inegalitarian swamp of perfectionism.) Moreover, if, as has been argued, having inherent value morally bars others from treating those who have it as mere receptacles or as mere resources for others, then any and all medical research like Ventricle's, done on these animals in the name of possibly benefitting others, stands morally condemned. And it is not only cases in which the benefits for others do not materialize that are condemnable; also to be condemned are cases, such as the research done on chimps regarding hepatitis, for example, in which the benefits for others are genuine. In these cases, as in others like them in the relevant respects, the ends do not justify the means. The *many millions* of mammalian animals used each year for scientific purposes, including medical research, bear mute, tragic testimony to the narrowness of our moral vision.

Conclusions

This condemnation of such research probably is at odds with the judgment that most people would make about this issue. If we had good reason to assume that the truth always lies with what most people think, then we could look approvingly on Ventricle-like research done on animals like chimps in the name of benefits for others. But we have no good reason to believe that the truth is to be measured plausibly by majority opinion, and what we know of the history of prejudice and bigotry speaks powerfully, if painfully, against this view. Only the cumulative force of informed, fair, rigorous argument can decide where the truth lies, or most likely lies, when we examine a controversial moral question. Although openly acknowledging and, indeed, insisting on the limitations of the arguments..., these arguments make the case, in broad outline, against using animals such as chimps in medical research such as Ventricle's....

Those who oppose the use of animals such as chimps in research like Ventricle's and who accept the major themes advanced here, oppose it, then, not because they think that all such research is a waste of time and money, or because they think that it never leads to any benefits for others, or because they view those who do such research as, to use Ventricle's, words, "moral monsters," or even because they love animals. Those of us who condemn such research do so because this research is not possible except at the grave moral price of failing to show proper respect for the value of the animals who are used. Since, whatever our gains, they are ill-gotten, we must bring to an end research like Ventricle's, whatever our losses. A fair measure of our moral integrity will be the extent of our resolve to work against allowing our scientific, economic, health, and other interests to serve as a reason for the wrongful exploitation of members of species of animals other than our own.

POSTSCRIPT

Should Animal Experimentation Be Permitted?

In 1985 Congress passed the Health Research Extension Act, which directed the National Institutes of Health (NIH) to establish guidelines for the proper care of animals to be used in biomedical and behavioral research. The NIH regulations implementing the law require institutions that receive federal grants to establish Animal Care and Use Committees. The Office of Science and Technology Policies' "Principles for the Utilization and Care of Vertebrate Animals Used in Testing, Research and Training," *Federal Register* (May 20, 1985) serves as the basis for the U.S. government's policy. The NIH's *Guide for the Care and Use of Laboratory Animals,* rev. ed. (1985) offers explicit instructions.

In February 1993 a federal judge ruled that the Department of Agriculture's standards on the treatment of laboratory dogs and primates were not stringent enough and that the agency had failed to put into effect the 1985 law. Charles R. McCarthy, in "Improved Standards for Laboratory Animals?" *Kennedy Institute of Ethics* (vol. 3, no. 3, 1993), asserts that this ruling actually lowers the standard for the care of laboratory animals.

Although they do not recommend a complete ban on animal research, some authors have argued that current practices in animal research must be reevaluated and better regulated. See, for example, *Lives in the Balance: The Ethics of Using Animals in Biomedical Research* edited by Jane A. Smith and Kenneth M. Boyd (Oxford University Press, 1991) and *In the Name of Science: Issues in Responsible Animal Experimentation* by F. Barbara Orlans (Oxford University Press, 1993).

For an opposing view, see the Office of Technology Assessment's *Alternatives to Animal Use in Research, Testing, and Education* (Government Printing Office, 1986). Richard P. Vance analyzes what he believes are erroneous myths held by supporters of animal research in "An Introduction to the Philosophical Presuppositions of the Animal Liberation/Rights Movement," *Journal of the American Medical Association* (October 7, 1992). Also see F. Barbara Orlans, Tom L. Beauchamp, Rebecca Dresser, David B. Morton, and John P. Gluck, *The Human Use of Animals: Case Studies in Ethical Choice* (Oxford University Press, 1998); the Hastings Center's "Animals, Science, and Ethics," *Hastings Center Report* (May/June 1990); and the *Hastings Center Report* special supplement "The Brave New World of Animal Biotechnology" (January/February 1994).

ISSUE 16

Is Sham Surgery Ethically Acceptable in Clinical Research?

YES: Thomas B. Freeman et al., from "Use of Placebo Surgery in Controlled Trials of a Cellular-Based Therapy for Parkinson's Disease," *The New England Journal of Medicine* (September 23, 1999)

NO: Ruth Macklin, from "The Ethical Problems With Sham Surgery in Clinical Research," *The New England Journal of Medicine* (September 23, 1999)

ISSUE SUMMARY

YES: Physician Thomas B. Freeman and his colleagues contend that their study of fetal-tissue transplantation, which used imitation, or sham, surgery in one group of patients, will establish whether this treatment is beneficial or not. Furthermore, this treatment will benefit thousands of patients with Parkinson's disease if proven effective.

NO: Philosopher Ruth Macklin concludes that sham surgery is ethically unacceptable, particularly in the case of fetal-tissue transplantation, because it does not minimize harm to subjects, a fundamental principle underlying research ethics.

P*lacebo* is a Latin word that means "I shall please." In medicine, placebos are inactive substances given to "please", that is, to create the impression that something is being done to cure the disease or releive the symptoms. And, defying scientific logic, sometimes that is exactly what happens. The "placebo effect," essentially mind over matter, is powerful and mysterious. Only recently have advanced imaging techniques begun to explore the biological mechanisms that can sometimes affect the interaction between mind and body.

More commonly, however, placebos do not work for very long. In those cases, provided the patient has not been denied an effective therapy, at least he or she is no worse off. Until the mid-twentieth century, most of the nostrums doctors prescribed were placebos since there were very few scientifically proven medications. Clinical research studies involving new drugs or new uses for old drugs commonly use placebos. In these studies one group of participants is randomly assigned to receive the active agent. The other group is given a placebo that looks, smells, and tastes as much like the active drug as possible. In a "double-blind" study neither the participants nor the researchers know who is receiving the active agent. The effects are monitored so that any statistically significant differences between the two groups can be more or less reliably attributed to the active agent.

Sometimes the use of placebos in clinical drug research is controversial. For example, if there is a treatment known to be effective for the condition being studied, it is hard to justify giving subjects an inactive substance. But especially controversial is the use of placebos in surgical research. Most surgical procedures in fact have not been subjected to the same rigorous research required to introduce a new drug. An early example of placebo-controlled surgical research occurred in 1959, when Dr. Leonard Cobb of Seattle operated on 17 patients with angina, which is chest pain associated with heart disease. For eight patients he tied the arteries in a commonly used procedure known as internal mammary artery ligation. For nine patients he made the incisions but did nothing else. His results, published in *The New England Journal of Medicine,* showed that the sham surgery worked just as well as the real operation, thus effectively ending the use of that procedure. The failure to inform subjects that they might not be receiving a real treatment violated modern standards of informed consent, and sham surgery protocols were essentially put beyond the ethical pale.

However, studies of surgical interventions are once again being implemented. Now prospective subjects are told that they may or may not get the real treatment, and the risks of surgery are outlined. The most controversial studies involve implantation of fetal cell tissue into the brains of patients with Parkinson's disease, a progressive neurological disease that is ultimately fatal. Some patients given implanted fetal cells report improvement. But is it real or is it just the placebo effect? Researchers want to find out by doing real surgery on some patients, and sham surgery on others.

The following two selections debate whether such studies are ethically acceptable. Thomas B. Freeman et al. present the case in favor of sham surgery. They assert that their study design will establish conclusively whether fetal-tissue transplants are safe and effective. If they are, patients will benefit; and if they are not, patients will be spared the risks and financial burdens of an unproved operation. Ruth Macklin counters that sham surgery violates the fundamental ethical and regulatory principle that the risk of harm to subjects must be minimized. Whatever the level of risk, she maintains, surgery with no conceivable benefit to the patient should not be performed.

Thomas B. Freeman et al. 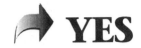 **YES**

Use of Placebo Surgery in Controlled Trials of a Cellular-Based Therapy for Parkinson's Disease

Surgical procedures are frequently introduced into general practice on the basis of uncontrolled studies that are less rigorous than those required for the approval of medical interventions.[1] The standard for the evaluation of surgical therapy is lower because of the complexity of designing and conducting scientifically valid and ethically acceptable clinical trials of surgical procedures.[2] As a result, many surgical trials fail to control for investigator bias or placebo effects.[3,4]

The list of inadequately studied invasive or surgical procedures that became part of standard medical practice only to be abandoned after closer scrutiny includes bloodletting, routine tonsillectomy, routine circumcision, repeated cesarean delivery, internal-thoracic-artery ligation, gastric freezing, jejunoilial bypass for morbid obesity, glomectomy for asthma, prophylactic portacaval shunting, laparotomy for tuberculous peritonitis or pelvic inflammatory disease, adrenalectomy for essential hypertension, and extracranial or intracranial bypass for carotid-artery occlusion. A review of coronary-artery bypass procedures showed that 38 percent of indications for the procedures are questionable.[5] Many have called for more rigorous evidence of the safety and efficacy of new surgical procedures.[1,6,7,8] In this article, we provide the scientific and ethical rationale for using an imitation operation as a placebo control in our National Institutes of Health (NIH)-sponsored double-blind trial of fetal-tissue transplantation in patients with Parkinson's disease.

Randomized, double-blind, placebo-controlled trials offer the most effective way to control for the placebo effect and investigator bias. They have become the gold standard for assessing new drug interventions.[4,9,10,11] Patients assigned to a placebo group in a pharmacologic study may incur certain risks and inconveniences, including temporarily forgoing other therapeutic options and undergoing multiple laboratory tests and clinical evaluations.[4,12,13,14,15,16] Assignment to the placebo group in a surgical study may involve greater risks.[6,17,18,19,20,21] Under what circumstances are the risks to subjects assigned to the placebo group in a medical or surgical trial justified, and what risks

From Thomas B. Freeman, Dorothy E. Vawter, Paul E. Leaverton, James H. Godbold, Robert A. Hauser, Christopher G. Goetz, and C. Warren Olanow, "Use of Placebo Surgery in Controlled Trials of a Cellular-Based Therapy for Parkinson's Disease," *The New England Journal of Medicine*, vol. 341, no. 13 (September 23, 1999). Copyright © 1999 by The Massachusetts Medical Society. All rights reserved. Reprinted by permission.

are reasonable in order to determine the benefits and adverse effects of a given intervention?[4,12,13,14,16,22] Some physicians believe that randomized, placebo-controlled surgical studies are unnecessary, cumbersome, and ethically unacceptable.[2,9,23] It has been claimed that one cannot generalize from the results of placebo-controlled surgical trials because of differences in the skills of individual surgeons and because of the confounding effect of increasing experience in performing the procedure. Finally, it has been argued that offering a subject a placebo procedure that might induce harm without offering a compensating benefit poses ethical problems[2,9,23] and that such a practice would violate the principle of doing no harm. The advent of cellular-based surgical therapies such as implantation of fetal tissues, trophic factors, and genetically altered cell lines calls for a critical examination of the methods used to evaluate these types of surgical interventions and a reconsideration of the virtual prohibition against the use of imitation surgery as a placebo control. We believe that many of these new therapies can and should be evaluated with the more rigorous methods typically used in pharmaceutical studies, an opinion shared by the Food and Drug Administration.[24]

Surgical procedures for administering cellular-based or pharmaceutical therapies tend to be less invasive, painful, burdensome, and risky than traditional surgical procedures, which may make the risks more reasonable in relation to the possible benefits. In addition, the procedures are easier to perform, standardize, and reproduce than traditional surgical procedures because they do not entail the manipulation or removal of distorted (and highly variable) tissues. Therefore, these studies are less likely to be confounded by variability in the surgeon's skill and the results are more likely to be generalizable. Finally, in many respects, the assessment of cellular therapies (which involves such variables as dose, volume of distribution, time course and magnitude of effect, toxicity, and drug interactions) has more in common with the assessment of pharmaceutical agents than with that of conventional operations.[25]

Ethics of Placebo-Controlled Trials

Researchers working in U.S. institutions that receive federal funds must comply with the federal regulations for the protection of human subjects.[26] The regulations require that the risks of a study be reasonable in relation to the anticipated benefits to the subjects, if any, and in relation to the importance of the knowledge that may reasonably be expected to be gained from the study.[26] These regulations allow for the conduct of placebo-controlled studies posing more than a minimal risk to competent adults as long as the risk is reasonable. Medical benefits do not necessarily need to accrue to all subjects.[27] Determining the reasonableness of the risks and benefits of a study is the complex task of appropriately constituted institutional review boards.

A double-blind, placebo-controlled trial should address an important research question that cannot be answered by a study with an alternative design that poses a lower risk to the subjects.[12,13,26] There must be preliminary but not conclusive evidence that the intervention is effective,[12,28] and the treatment should be sufficiently developed that it is unlikely to become obsolete before the study has been completed.[8,23,29] The risks to the subjects should be minimized whenever possible in a manner that is consistent with sound research design.[26] The study intervention should be provided in addition to standard therapy, unless there is no safe and effective standard therapy or unless the withholding of such therapy does not pose an unreasonable risk to the subjects.[4]

The study design must be sufficiently rigorous to ensure the blinding of subjects and investigators, accurate and complete data collection, and sufficient statistical power to provide a reasonable assurance that the study will answer the research question.[30] Finally, the consent process must clearly identify the risks of participation, including the risks associated with assignment to the placebo group.[12] Potential subjects must meet a high standard of comprehension, be informed about alternative medical and surgical therapies, and be advised that they will not be refused medical care if they decline to participate.[26]

A Placebo-Controlled Trial of Fetal Nigral Transplantation in Parkinson's Disease

Parkinson's disease is a disorder of motor function characterized by tremor, rigidity, bradykinesia, gait disturbance, and postural instability.[31] The main pathological features are a loss of dopaminergic neurons in the substantia nigra pars compacta and a consequent reduction in levels of striatal dopamine. Replacement therapy, with the use of the dopamine precursor levodopa combined with a decarboxylase inhibitor, is the standard medical treatment for Parkinson's disease. However, long-term treatment with levodopa may have adverse effects, and new features of the disease that are not satisfactorily controlled with available medical therapies may emerge.

Fetal-tissue transplantation for the treatment of Parkinson's disease is based on research demonstrating that implanted embryonic dopaminergic neurons can survive, reinnervate the striatum, and reverse motor abnormalities in animal models of parkinsonism.[32] At least 18 centers throughout the world have introduced clinical transplantation programs for the treatment of Parkinson's disease. The results have been variable,[32] but several centers have observed consistent and clinically meaningful benefits in open-label trials.[33,34,35,36,37] Further evidence of the potential value of this procedure comes from reports of statistically significant increases in striatal fluorodopa uptake on positron-emission tomography (PET)[32,33,34,35,36,37,38] and robust graft survival with extensive striatal reinnervation at autopsy[39,40,41]; these findings are correlated with the clinical benefits.[37,39,40]

Placebo Effects in the Treatment of Parkinson's Disease

Although we and others have demonstrated the clinical benefits of fetal nigral transplantation in open trials, we cannot exclude the possibility that these benefits are due to a placebo effect or investigator bias. Long-lasting and powerful placebo effects have been reported in Parkinson's disease. In one large, double-blind pharmacologic study, patients assigned to the placebo group had a 20 to

30 percent improvement in motor scores, which persisted throughout the six months of the trial.[4] Significant improvement and deterioration have been observed after the introduction and discontinuation, respectively, of placebo in patients with Parkinson's disease.[42,43] Placebo effects are a particular problem because of the marked variability in the magnitude and duration of responses to antiparkinsonian medication.[44] Furthermore, the magnitude of the placebo response increases with the extent of the placebo intervention,[4,6] suggesting that the response to any surgical procedure might be particularly pronounced.

It is not possible to test adequately for a placebo effect in a laboratory setting, since animals are not known to have responses to placebo.[45] Moreover, the response to implanted cells in animal models may differ from that in patients. We therefore concluded that in order to determine the safety and efficacy of fetal-tissue transplantation in patients with Parkinson's disease, it was necessary to perform a double-blind, placebo-controlled study. This study would control for placebo effects, as well as the effects of patient selection, treatment, and bias on the part of the evaluator.

The Trial Design

Thirty-six competent adults with advanced Parkinson's disease whose symptoms could not be satisfactorily controlled with medical therapy consented to be randomly assigned to undergo one of three study procedures: bilateral fetal nigral transplantation with tissue from one donor per side, bilateral transplantation with tissue from four donors per side, or bilateral placebo surgery. Calculations based on our open studies[34] indicated that a total sample of 36 subjects (12 per group) would provide the study with more than 80 percent power to detect differences between the groups with an alpha level of less than 0.05 and an independent-sample two-tailed t-test.

According to the protocol, subjects in both transplantation groups undergo two surgical procedures separated by approximately one week. Subjects randomly assigned to the control group undergo two placebo surgical procedures that are designed to provide an equivalent experience for the subjects and their family members. Each placebo procedure includes the placement of a stereotactic frame, target localization on magnetic resonance imaging, the administration of general anesthesia with a laryngeal-mask airway, and a skin incision with a partial burr hole that does not penetrate the inner cortex of the skull; there are no needle penetrations into the brain, and no fetal tissue is implanted. The duration of the surgical procedures and the perioperative care are identical in all groups. All patients receive low-dose cyclosporine for six months and continue to receive medical therapy. Subjects are evaluated in an identical manner at three-month intervals. At the conclusion of the study, if fetal-tissue transplantation is found to be safe and effective, subjects in the placebo group will be offered the better of the two transplantation procedures (with tissue from one donor per side or four donors per side).

To maintain the blinding of investigators, the surgical and evaluation sites are in separate locations. The evaluation sites identify participants, obtain informed consent, and perform all study evaluations. The same blinded evaluator carries out all clinical evaluations for each subject throughout the study. Clinical care is provided by a separate blinded investigator. PET studies are performed by a separate group of blinded investigators. The surgeon is the only member of the research team who is aware of an individual subject's group assignment. All surgical records related to the study are sequestered in a locked cabinet, and all the surgeons' communications with subjects or investigators follow a standardized script. Statistical and data-management practices are designed to maintain blinding throughout the course of the study. The study is monitored by an independent performance and safety monitoring board appointed by the NIH. To assess the integrity of the blinding, subjects and investigators complete a questionnaire at the conclusion of the study.

This study is not designed to control for any clinical changes due to the surgical lesion itself, since to do so would entail substantial additional risk for the control group. Existing data suggest that surgical trauma itself is not likely to account for the benefits we observed in our open trial. Surgical trauma or implantation of biologically inactive tissue does not result in significant improvement in primate models of parkinsonism.[45] Adrenal transplantation causes more surgical damage but does not provide lasting clinical benefits or improvement on PET.[46,47] Sprouting of endogenous dopamine neurons has never been observed in the putamen (the target of our grafts) after transplantation or surgically-induced trauma. Furthermore, we saw no evidence of host-derived sprouting in two postmortem studies of patients who had received fetal nigral transplants.[39,40,41] In our study, any differences in outcome between subjects who receive tissue from one donor per side and those who receive tissue from four donors per side can be due only to the amount of tissue implanted, not to placebo or lesion effects. Although lesion-controlled surgical trials have been conducted in other circumstances,[6,17,18,19,20,48,49,50,51,52] we do not believe that a lesion-controlled study of fetal-tissue transplantation in patients with Parkinson's disease is necessary or appropriate at this time.

Risks and Benefits of Participating in the Placebo Group

In considering a placebo-controlled trial, it is important to balance the risks to participants against the potential benefits of developing a superior therapy or determining that an unproved therapy is ineffective or harmful. The risks of participating in the placebo group in this study are not trivial; there is the remote possibility of death or harm from a study-related intervention. Risks are associated with the placement of the stereotactic equipment, the scalp incision, the burr hole (even though it does not fully penetrate the skull), general anesthesia, intravenous antibiotics, low-dose cyclosporine, and the radioisotopes used for the PET studies. Subjects also have the inconvenience of multiple clinic visits and, in some cases, long-distance travel. Their access to the study treatment, if it is beneficial, will be delayed, and they may forfeit their eligibility to participate in other clinical trials. The risks have been minimized as much as possible. For example, subjects continue to receive standard medical therapy for Parkinson's disease, a partial burr hole is used to minimize the remote risk of intracranial bleeding, renal function is monitored for cyclosporine toxicity at routine intervals, adverse events are regularly reviewed, and rules were established in the protocol for stopping the trial early.

The benefits of participating in the placebo group include contributing to advances in the treatment of a disease of great personal interest to the participants, receiving standard medical treatment at no cost, having the opportunity to obtain a fetal-tissue transplant at no cost if the procedure proves to be safe and effective, and being spared the risks associated with transplantation if it proves to be unsafe or ineffective.

In our judgment, as well as in the judgment of the institutional review boards at the institutions involved in this study, the NIH study section, the performance and safety monitoring board, and the 36 persons who agreed to participate, the risks of participating in our double-blind, placebo-controlled surgical trial of fetal-tissue transplantation are reasonable in relation to the possible benefits. In addition, we believe that we have met all the ethical conditions outlined above. The patients have a progressive neurologic disease that cannot be satisfactorily controlled with existing medical therapy. Laboratory studies and pilot clinical trials indicate that the procedure has the potential to provide a meaningful clinical benefit, and the risks of participation are reasonable and have been minimized insofar as possible. We extensively reviewed risks, benefits, procedures, and other therapeutic options with each patient and gave each an opportunity to have all questions answered. Subjects signed consent forms that were approved by the institutional review board at each institution involved in the study and by the performance and safety monitoring board appointed by the NIH to oversee it. Subjects in all groups continue to receive medical therapy, and those in the placebo group will be offered transplants if the procedure is proved safe and effective.

Conclusions

Randomized, double-blind, placebo-controlled trials are the gold standard for evaluating new interventions and are routinely used to assess new medical therapies. Surgeons have been reluctant to use imitation surgery as a placebo control in the evaluation of new procedures. It is estimated that only 7 percent of surgical investigators use a randomized study design of any type.[7] Cellular-based surgical therapies have much in common with pharmacologic treatments and lend themselves to evaluation in randomized, double-blind, placebo-controlled trials.

We elected to use this study design in our assessment of fetal-tissue transplantation before recommending its routine use. The inclusion of a placebo group in our study of 36 subjects will permit us to establish whether the benefit observed to date can be attributed to an effect of treatment apart from a placebo effect. If fetal-tissue transplants are found to be safe and effective, thousands of patients with Parkinson's disease stand to benefit, and further research will be encouraged. If the transplants are found to be unsafe or ineffective, or if they offer nothing more than a placebo effect, hundreds or even thousands of patients will be spared the risks and financial burdens of an unproved operation.

References

1. Spodick DH. Revascularization of the heart—numerators in search of denominators. Am Heart J 1971;81:149–57.
2. Love JW. Drugs and operations: some important differences. JAMA 1975;232:37–8.
3. Olanow CW, Fahn S, Muenter M, et al. A multicenter double-blind placebo-controlled trial of perogolide as an adjunct to Sinemet in Parkinson's disease. Mov Disord 1994;9:40–7.
4. Clark PI, Leaverton PE. Scientific and ethical issues in the use of placebo controls in clinical trials. Annu Rev Public Health 1994;15:19–38.
5. Leape LL, Hilborne LH, Kahan JP, et al. Coronary artery by-pass graft: a literature review and ratings of appropriateness and necessity. Santa Monica, Calif.: RAND, 1991:v–vii, 48–67. (Document no. JRA-02.)
6. Beecher HK. Surgery as placebo: a quantitative study of bias. JAMA 1961;176:1102–7.
7. Reeves B. Health-technology assessment in surgery. Lancet 1999;353:Suppl 1:SI3–SI5.
8. Baum M. Reflections on randomised controlled trials in surgery. Lancet 1999;353:Suppl 1:SI6–SI8.
9. Pocock SJ. Clinical trials: a practical approach. New York: John Wiley, 1983.
10. Hauser RA, Olanow CW. Designing clinical trials in Parkinson's disease. In: Olanow CW, Lieberman AN, eds. The scientific basis for the treatment of Parkinson's disease. Park Ridge, N.J.: Parthenon, 1992:275–93.
11. Turner JA, Deyo RA, Loeser JD, VonKorff M, Fordyce WE. The importance of placebo effects in pain treatment and research. JAMA 1994;271:1609–14.
12. Levine RJ. The use of placebos in randomized clinical trials. IRB 1985;7(2):1–4.
13. Rothman KJ, Michels KB. The continuing unethical use of placebo controls. N Engl J Med 1994;331:394–8.
14. Prentice ED, Antonson DL, Jameton A, Graber B, Sears T. Can children be enrolled in a placebo-controlled randomized clinical trial of synthetic growth hormone? IRB 1989;11(1):6–10.
15. Apfel SC, Kessler JA, Adornato BT, Litchy WJ, Sanders C, Rask CA. Recombinant human nerve growth factor in the treatment of diabetic polyneuropathy. Neurology 1998;51:695–702.
16. Freedman B, Glass KC, Weijer C. Placebo orthodoxy in clinical research. II. Ethical, legal, and regulatory myths. J Law Med Ethics 1996;24:252–9.
17. Dimond EG, Kittle CF, Crockett JE. Evaluation of internal mammary artery ligation and sham procedure in angina pectoris. Circulation 1958;18:712–3. abstract.
18. Cobb LA, Thomas GI, Dillard DH, Merendino KA, Bruce RA. An evaluation of internal-mammary-artery ligation by a double-blind technic. N Engl J Med 1959;260:1115–8.
19. Harbaugh RE, Reeder TM, Senter HJ, et al. Intracerebroventricular bethanechol chloride infusion in Alzheimer's disease: results of a collaborative double-blind study. J Neurosurg 1989;71:481–6.
20. Law PK, Goodwin TG, Fang Q, et al. Long-term improvement in muscle function, structure and biochemistry following myoblast transfer in DMD. Acta Cardiomiologica 1991;3:281–301.
21. ALS CNTF Treatment Study Group. A double-blind placebo-controlled clinical trial of subcutaneous recombinant human ciliary neurotrophic factor (rHCNTF) in amyotrophic lateral sclerosis. Neurology 1996;46:1244–9.
22. Stanley B. An integration of ethical and clinical considerations in the use of placebos. Psychopharmacol Bull 1988;24:18–20.
23. Boncheck LI. Are randomized trials appropriate for evaluating new operations? N Engl J Med 1979;301:44–5.

24. Department of Health and Human Services, Food and Drug Administration. Establishment registration and listing for manufacturers of human cellular and tissue-based products. Fed Regist 1998;63(93):26744-55.
25. Freeman TB. From transplants to gene therapy for Parkinson's disease. Exp Neurol 1997;144:47-50.
26. Department of Health and Human Services, National Institutes of Health, Office for Protection from Research Risks. Protection of human subjects. 45 CFR 46 (1991). (Appendix 4:33-49.)
27. Levine RJ. Ethics and regulation of clinical research. 2nd ed. Baltimore: Urban & Schwarzenberg, 1986.
28. Freedman B. Equipoise and the ethics of clinical research. N Engl J Med 1987;317:141-5.
29. Wagner M. IVF: out-of-date evidence, or not. Lancet 1996;348:1394.
30. Schulz KF. Subverting randomization in controlled trials. JAMA 1995;274:1456-8.
31. Olanow CW. A 61-year-old man with Parkinson's disease. JAMA 1996;275:716-22.
32. Olanow CW, Kordower JH, Freeman TB. Fetal nigral transplantation as a therapy for Parkinson's disease. Trends Neurosci 1996;19:102-9.
33. Lindvall O, Sawle G, Widner H, et al. Evidence for long-term survival and function of dopaminergic grafts in progressive Parkinson's disease. Ann Neurol 1994;35:172-80.
34. Freeman TB, Olanow CW, Hauser RA, et al. Bilateral fetal nigral transplantation into the postcommissural putamen in Parkinson's disease. Ann Neurol 1995;38:379-88.
35. Wenning GK, Odin P, Morrish P, et al. Short-and long-term survival and function of unilateral intrastriatal dopaminergic grafts in Parkinson's disease. Ann Neurol 1997;42:95-107.
36. Defer GL, Geny C, Ricolfi F, et al. Long-term outcome of unilaterally transplanted parkinsonian patients. I. Clinical approach. Brain 1996;119:41-50.
37. Hauser RA, Freeman TB, Snow BJ, et al. Long-term evaluation of bilateral fetal nigral transplantation in Parkinson's disease. Arch Neurol 1999;56:179-87.
38. Sawle GV, Bloomfield PM, Bjorklund A, et al. Transplantation of fetal dopamine neurons in Parkinson's disease: PET [18F]-6-L-fluorodopa studies in two patients with putaminal implants. Ann Neurol 1992;31:166-73.
39. Kordower JH, Freeman TB, Snow BJ, et al. Neuropathological evidence of graft survival and striatal reinnervation after the transplantation of fetal mesencephalic tissue in a patient with Parkinson's disease. N Engl J Med 1995;332:1118-24.
40. Kordower JH, Freeman TB, Chen E-Y, et al. Fetal nigral grafts survive and mediate clinical benefit in a patient with Parkinson's disease. Mov Disord 1998;13:383-93.
41. Kordower JH, Rosenstein JM, Collier TJ, et al. Functional fetal nigral grafts in a patient with Parkinson's disease: chemoanatomic, ultrastructural, and metabolic studies. J Comp Neurol 1996;370:203-30.
42. Olanow CW, Hauser RA, Gauger L, et al. The effect of deprenyl and levodopa on the progression of Parkinson's disease. Ann Neurol 1995;38:771-7.
43. Parkinson's Study Group. Effects of tocopherol and deprenyl on the progression of disability in early Parkinson's disease. N Engl J Med 1993;328:176-83.
44. Nutt JG, Holford NHG. The response to levodopa in Parkinson's disease: imposing pharmacological law and order. Ann Neurol 1996;39:561-73.
45. Taylor JR, Elsworth JD, Sladek JR Jr, Collier TJ, Roth RH, Redmond DE Jr. Sham surgery does not ameliorate MPTP-induced behavioral deficits in monkeys. Cell Transplant 1995;4:13-26.
46. Olanow CW, Koller W, Goetz CG, et al. Autologous transplantation of adrenal medulla in Parkinson's disease: 18-month results. Arch Neurol 1990;47:1286-9.
47. Guttman M, Burns RS, Martin WRW, et al. PET studies of parkinsonian patients treated with autologous adrenal implants. Can J Neurol Sci 1989;16:305-9.

48. Brem H, Piantadosi S, Burger PC, et al. Placebo-controlled trial of safety and efficacy of intraoperative controlled delivery by biodegradable polymers of chemotherapy for recurrent gliomas. Lancet 1995;345:1008–12.

49. Thomsen J, Bretlau P, Tos M, Johnson NJ. Placebo effect in surgery for Meniere's disease: a double-blind, placebo-controlled study on endolymphatic sac shunt surgery. Arch Otolaryngol 1981;107:271–7.

50. Moseley JB Jr, Wray NP, Kuykendall D, Willis K, Landon G. Arthroscopic treatment of osteoarthritis of the knee: a prospective, randomized, placebo-controlled trial: results of a pilot study. Am J Sports Med 1996;24:28–34.

51. McCarthy M. Gene therapy for rheumatoid arthritis starts clinical trials. Lancet 1996;348:323.

52. Johannes L. Sham surgery is used to test effectiveness of novel operations. Wall Street Journal. December 11, 1998:A1, A8.

NO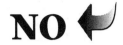

Ruth Macklin

The Ethical Problems With Sham Surgery in Clinical Research

The recent use of sham surgery in randomized, controlled trials raises three critical questions about research involving human subjects. The first question concerns the tension between the highest standard of research design and the highest standard of ethics.[1] When these two standards come into conflict and researchers cannot simultaneously meet both, which should prevail, and how should a balance be struck? The second question points to ongoing uncertainties and disagreements in assessing the risks and benefits of research protocols. When reasonable people—the members of well-established institutional review boards or the sponsors of research—disagree in their risk-benefit assessments, can one assessment or the other properly be considered the correct one? The third question concerns the relation between the risks of a protocol and the informed consent of research subjects. Does the requirement of informed consent imply that potential subjects should be permitted to decide what risks they are willing to take, in the hope of receiving some benefit? Or do research subjects require protection that may limit their choices?

Scientific and Ethical Standards

Situations in which scientific standards in research clash with ethical requirements are, fortunately, quite rare. The use of placebo controls in some types of research remains controversial despite the status of the placebo-controlled trial as the gold standard of research design.[2,3,4,5,6,7,8,9] Critics argue that it is difficult to justify the use of placebo controls when effective standard therapy exists.[3,6,10] Despite these criticisms, which typically target a particular study or class of studies, placebo controls in drug trials are widely accepted on ethical as well as scientific grounds. Commentators who consider the use of a placebo group unethical if there is a standard treatment that has been proved effective nevertheless find placebo controls ethically acceptable in research involving conditions for which there is no standard therapy or those for which standard therapy has been shown to be no more effective than placebo.[1,6]

From Ruth Macklin, "The Ethical Problems With Sham Surgery in Clinical Research," *The New England Journal of Medicine*, vol. 341, no. 13 (September 23, 1999). Copyright © 1999 by The Massachusetts Medical Society. All rights reserved. Reprinted by permission.

At first glance, the recent studies involving patients with Parkinson's disease, in which sham surgery is used as a control and real surgery is used to implant fetal cells,[11,12,13] appear to fulfill the conditions that would make the placebo controls ethically acceptable. Existing treatments for Parkinson's disease are ineffective in helping patients regain lost motor function, which is one of the hoped-for results of surgical implantation of fetal cells in the brain. The same may well be true of clinical trials that compare the effect of arthroscopic surgery for osteoarthritis with that of a sham surgical procedure.[11,13] Why should the use of sham surgery be questioned when the conditions for the ethical acceptability of a placebo-controlled study appear to be met?

The chief reason is that performing a surgical procedure that has no expected benefit other than the placebo effect violates the ethical and regulatory principle that the risk of harm to subjects must be minimized in the conduct of research.[14] In a standard, placebo-controlled drug trial, the inert substance used in the placebo group is known to have no adverse effects. The potential harm in a placebo-controlled drug trial stems from withholding or withdrawing a standard medication that has been proved effective for the treatment of the disorder being studied. The question of how great the risks of sham surgery are in any particular trial is distinct from the question of whether a surgical intervention carries risks of harm that are greater than those associated with no surgical intervention. It is undeniable that performing surgery in research subjects that has no potential therapeutic benefit fails to minimize the risk of harm. An alternative research design that did not involve sham surgery would pose a lower risk of harm to the subjects in the control group of the study. But herein lies the tension between the scientific and ethical standards: the alternative design would be less rigorous from a methodologic point of view.

Defenders of placebo-controlled surgical trials have challenged the "double standard" for drug research and surgical research. One physician asked, "If we so well accept a placebo in ... drug trials, why don't we accept it in surgery trials?"[13] The chairwoman of the National Institutes of Health committee that reviewed the proposal for the research on Parkinson's disease was quoted as saying, "Too many surgeries are done on the basis of anecdotal evidence and not put to the same sort of rigorous tests that drug therapies are."[11] Although this dichotomy in research design may be a double standard, it is based on adherence to an essential ethical standard for research: the requirement to minimize the risk of harm to subjects.

Assessing Risks and Benefits

The risk of harm in placebo-controlled surgical studies is not limited to the morbidity associated with the surgical intervention. In the studies employing sham brain surgery in patients with Parkinson's disease, general anesthesia was administered to the subjects in the placebo group. One bioethicist approved of the protocol for the sham surgery because the risks associated with sedation have dropped substantially in recent years.[13] This defense relies on the overall ethical judgment that the risks to the subjects who undergo the study procedure and those who undergo the sham procedure are outweighed by the benefits of the research—in this case, the contribution to medical science.

In a trial of a treatment for pain in patients with cancer, the investigators inserted capsules into a space at the base of the spine by means of a lumbar puncture. In some subjects, the capsules contained an inert substance, and in others it contained an analgesic that could alleviate the pain. According to one estimate, 10 percent of patients undergoing this procedure experience a severe headache that can last a day or two after the procedure. In addition, there is a risk of permanent nerve injury or paralysis.[11] These risks can hardly be considered minimal. Although the probability of nerve injury or paralysis may be low, the magnitude of the harm is great. In addition, standard treatments for cancer-related pain exist, so it is questionable whether this experiment meets the condition regarding alternative treatments that the critics of placebo controls in medical studies insist must be met.

Assessments of risks and benefits are difficult enough to make when substantial evidence of a treatment's efficacy exists and when subjects in the placebo group are not exposed to harm from the intervention. Controversies about both the magnitude of the potential harm and the risk-benefit ratio have surrounded the trials involving sham surgery in patients with Parkinson's disease. In these trials, the risk-benefit ratio is at best uncertain and at worst unfavorable. The institutional review board at Columbia-Presbyterian Medical Center would have accepted the sham surgery but stopped short at approving the administration of real antibiotics to subjects in the placebo group.[11] A group of researchers at Yale University decided to omit sham surgery from their study design on the grounds that drilling holes in a patient's head without providing treatment would require further studies in animals and humans in order to be ethically acceptable.[11] Yet one investigator who performed the sham surgery likened the risk involved to that of going to the dentist.[12] This comparison suggests that the risk is minimal, according to the definition in the federal regulations on research involving human subjects: "Minimal risk means that the probability and magnitude of harm or discomfort anticipated in the research are not greater in and of themselves than those ordinarily encountered in daily life or during the performance of routine physical or psychological examinations or tests."[14] Most people, however, would probably consider the risk associated with drilling holes in the skull greater than that associated with drilling holes in teeth.

If there were some objective way of assessing the magnitude, as well as the probability, of harm caused by these surgical interventions, the determination that there is a favorable ratio of benefits to risks in the studies involving sham surgery might be credible. However, the difficulties that institutional review boards have in making consistent, reliable assessments of benefits and risks are well documented.[15,16,17] As the National Commission for the Protection of Human Subjects of Biomedical and Behavioral Research reported:

> It is commonly said that benefits and risks must be "balanced" and shown to be "in a favorable ratio." The metaphorical character of these terms draws attention to the difficulty of making precise judgments. Only on rare occasions will quantitative techniques be available for the scrutiny of research

protocols. However, the idea of systematic, nonarbitrary analysis of risks and benefits should be emulated insofar as possible.[18]

The controversy that has arisen over the use of sham surgery in studies of Parkinson's disease demonstrates the wide variation in judgments of what sorts of "risks to subjects are reasonable in relation to anticipated benefits, if any, to subjects, and the importance of the knowledge that may reasonably be expected to result."[14]

Informed Consent in Research Involving Sham Surgery

In the era before informed consent to participate in research was an ethical and legal requirement, some researchers performed sham surgery without obtaining informed consent from subjects.[10] One article reporting the results of coronary-artery surgery in patients with angina stated, "The subjects were informed of the fact that this procedure had not been proved to be of value, and yet many were aware of the enthusiastic report published in the *Reader's Digest*. The patients were told only that they were participating in an evaluation of this operation; they were not informed of the double-blind nature of the study."[19]

Today, of course, patients entering trials that are randomized, blinded, and placebo-controlled are informed of these aspects of the research. This information does not diminish their hope that they will receive the experimental treatment rather than the placebo. A patient who underwent sham surgery in a study of Parkinson's disease said she knew there was a 50-50 chance that she had not received the real treatment, but when she was informed of that fact one year later, she said she thought she had received the real treatment. In fact, she perceived small improvements in her condition after the operation.[11] Disclosure of the research design evidently does not eliminate the known placebo effect of surgery,[20] nor does it deter patients from enrolling in the study. Yet these findings do not by themselves justify the exposure of patients to risks that would not be imposed by an alternative research design. Researchers have an obligation to minimize the risks to their subjects, and institutional review boards are charged with ensuring that the risks are reasonable in the light of the anticipated benefits. There would be no need for a system of institutional review boards to protect subjects if their informed consent were the only ethical requirement for conducting research.

Is it overly paternalistic to protect research subjects from risks they seem willing to accept? The emphasis today on respect for the autonomy of patients and research subjects creates a reluctance to question whether their choices are fully rational. In one of the studies of fetal-tissue transplantation in patients with Parkinson's disease, the subjects were told in advance that if they underwent the sham surgery, they would be eligible for the real transplantation procedure on completion of the trial, if the procedure proved to be beneficial. But because of a higher-than-anticipated incidence of death and other adverse events in the group of patients who had undergone the real surgery, the patients in the sham-surgery group were initially not offered the treatment.[11] Surprisingly, rather than being relieved that they had undergone the apparently safer, sham surgery, several subjects were outraged. They said they might not have participated in the study if they had known they would have to wait so long for the real surgery. One woman said that she and her husband, who had participated in the study, felt they had been "double shammed": first when they learned that her husband had undergone the sham procedure, and then when he was denied the real surgery on the basis of safety considerations.[11] This response exemplifies the "therapeutic misconception"[21,22]—the all-too-common assumption that research promises beneficial treatment, even in its earliest phases.

Studies of consent documents show that they sometimes overstate the benefits and understate the risks of research protocols.[23,24] But even when consent forms are accurate in describing the known risks and anticipated benefits, the expectations of research subjects may be unrealistic. In one study, people who had been research subjects told interviewers that they had trusted their doctors, believed that their physicians would do nothing to harm them, and thought that the physician-researchers had always acted in their best medical interests.[23] The misconception that research is designed to benefit the patients who are the subjects is difficult to dispel. The comments of the hopeful subjects in the studies of Parkinson's disease[11,12] suggest that the informed-consent process remains less than perfect. This observation is hardly new, and the inadequacy of informed consent is by no means unique to these trials. Yet this experience provides evidence that the protection of human subjects cannot rest solely on the ethical foundation of informed consent.

One feature of the research on Parkinson's disease prompts a different question about the quality of informed consent. Critics of the use of placebos in clinical trials claim that such use is unethical because it involves the active deception of patients. Commentators on the ethics of the use of placebos in clinical trials generally argue that it is not deception that constitutes the ethically problematic feature but rather the potential harm of withholding a treatment proved to be beneficial.[7,25]

In the studies of Parkinson's disease, although the patients were informed in advance that they had a 50-50 chance of receiving sham surgery, the researchers had to engage in active deception in performing the research maneuvers. In one study, just before the surgical procedure was performed, the surgeons asked the subjects, "Are you ready for the implant now?"[11] This was a deliberate attempt to mislead the subjects. One of the researchers was quoted as saying, "We thought it might be difficult to maintain a poker face."[11] These are words people use when they are engaged in lying. Even though the lie in this case may have been harmless, since it was uttered in a context in which the truth had previously been disclosed, it cannot be maintained that no deception was involved in the use of sham surgery. To achieve the effect that a placebo-controlled trial aims for, the researchers had to make misleading statements to the subjects in the placebo group and had to make sure their facial expressions did not reveal the true situation.

Conclusions

Sham surgery is ethically unacceptable as a placebo control in trials of fetal-cell transplantation in patients with Parkinson's disease. Sham surgery, with accompanying anesthesia, poses the risks of any surgical intervention that would not be used alone for therapeutic purposes. In trials that use antibiotics to protect subjects against infection, there are the added risks associated with antibiotic treatment. In trials that forgo the use of antibiotics in the sham-surgery group, there are the added risks of infection.

One question remains to be answered. Those who defend the use of sham surgery could argue that the possibility of a strong placebo response to surgery[20] does, in fact, confer a benefit on the subjects who are randomly assigned to the control group. Might the benefit of the placebo effect outweigh the risks of the sham surgery and therefore justify its use in research? The answer is no, unless the sham surgery would be recommended solely for therapeutic purposes outside the research context.

A related question is whether it would be ethical to conduct trials specifically designed to document the placebo effect of surgery. Three groups would be needed: an untreated control group, a group undergoing sham surgery, and a group undergoing real surgery.[20] Johnson argues that "for surgical procedures, as for drugs, the placebo effect must always be taken into account if any assessment is to be objective."[20] Yet despite the importance of the research question, Johnson contends that "none of the means of measuring placebo [effects] can be applied to surgical operations because it is unethical, for example, to make an abdominal incision and sew it up again without undertaking any procedure."[20]

Perhaps some defenders of the use of sham surgery in randomized, controlled trials would be prepared to go this far. In response to the question, "If phony operations can help people, why not just do them?" one surgeon said, "That is an important point. What to do with it, medicine is going to have to decide."[13] One cannot always predict what the medical community will decide. But one conclusion seems apparent. The placebo-controlled trial may well be the gold standard of research design, but unlike pure gold, it can be tarnished by unethical applications.

References

1. Freedman B. Placebo-controlled trials and the logic of clinical purpose. IRB 1990;12(6):1-6.
2. Lurie P, Wolfe SM. Unethical trials of interventions to reduce perinatal transmission of the human immunodeficiency virus in developing countries. N Engl J Med 1997;337:853-6.
3. Angell M. The ethics of clinical research in the Third World. N Engl J Med 1997;337:847-9.
4. Varmus H, Satcher D. Ethical complexities of conducting research in developing countries. N Engl J Med 1997;337:1003-5.
5. Clark PI, Leaverton PE. Scientific and ethical issues in the use of placebo controls in clinical trials. Annu Rev Public Health 1994;15:19-38.
6. Rothman KJ, Michels KB. The continuing unethical use of placebo controls. N Engl J Med 1994;331:394-7.

7. Freedman B, Weijer C, Glass KC. Placebo orthodoxy in clinical research. I. Empirical and methodological myths. J Law Med Ethics 1996;24:243-51.
8. Freedman B, Weijer C, Glass KC. Placebo orthodoxy in clinical research. II. Ethical, legal, and regulatory myths. J Law Med Ethics 1996;24:252-9.
9. Cohen PJ. The placebo is not dead: three historical vignettes. IRB 1998;20(2-3):6-8.
10. Orr RD. Guidelines for the use of placebo controls in clinical trials of psychopharmacologic agents. Psychiatr Serv 1996;47:1262-4.
11. Johannes L. Sham surgery is used to test effectiveness of novel operations. Wall Street Journal. December 11, 1998:A1, A8.
12. Stolberg SG. Decisive moment on Parkinson's fetal-cell transplants. New York Times. April 20, 1999:F2.
13. Stolberg SG. Sham surgery returns as a research tool. New York Times. April 25, 1999:WK3.
14. 45 CFR 46 (1991).
15. Williams PC. Success in spite of failure: why IRBs falter in reviewing risks and benefits. IRB 1984;6:1-4.
16. Martin DK, Meslin EM, Kohut N, Singer P. The incommensurability of research risks and benefits: practical help for research ethics committees. IRB 1995;17(2):8-10.
17. Meslin EM. Protecting human subjects from harm through improved risk judgments. IRB 1990;12(1):7-10.
18. National Commission for the Protection of Human Subjects of Biomedical and Behavioral Research. The Belmont Report: ethical principles and guidelines for the protection of human subjects of research. Washington, D.C.: Government Printing Office, 1978.
19. Cobb LA, Thomas GI, Dillard DH, Merendino KA, Bruce RA. An evaluation of internal-mammary-artery ligation by a double-blind technic. N Engl J Med 1959;260:1115-8.
20. Johnson AG. Surgery as a placebo. Lancet 1994;344:1140-2.
21. Appelbaum PS, Roth LH, Lidz C. The therapeutic misconception: informed consent in psychiatric research. Int J Law Psychiatry 1982;5:319-29.
22. King NMP. Experimental treatment: oxymoron or aspiration? Hastings Cent Rep 1995;25:6-15.
23. Advisory Committee on Human Radiation Experiments. Final report of the Advisory Committee on Human Radiation Experiments. New York: Oxford University Press, 1996.
24. Research involving persons with mental disorders that may affect decisionmaking capacity. Rockville, Md.: National Bioethics Advisory Commission, 1998.
25. Levine RJ. The use of placebos in randomized clinical trials. IRB 1985;7:1-4.

POSTSCRIPT

Is Sham Surgery Ethically Acceptable in Clinical Research?

In "The Placebo Is Not Dead," *IRB: A Review of Human Subjects Research* (March–June 1998), Dr. Peter Cohen presents three historical vignettes, including the cardiac surgery described in the introduction, that illustrate the scientific importance of subjecting procedures to placebo-controlled research. In each of the cases, research involving placebos shows the inadequacy of procedures "known" to be effective.

Dr. Irving Kirsch, a psychiatrist at the University of Connecticut, reviewed placebo-controlled studies of antidepressant drugs and found that placebos and active drugs worked equally well. He believes that placebos are about 50 to 60 percent as effective in controlling pain as medications like aspirin and codeine. See "Are Drug and Placebo Effects in Depression Additive?" *Biology and Psychiatry* (April 15, 2000).

See also Joel E. Frader and Donna A. Caniano, "Research and Innovation in Surgery," in Laurence B. McCullough, James W. Jones, and Baruch A. Brody, eds., *Surgical Ethics* (Oxford University Press, 1998); Anne Harrington, ed., *The Placebo Effect: An Interdisciplinary Exploration* (Harvard University Press, 1999); and Arthur K. Shapiro and Elaine Shapiro, *The Powerful Placebo* (Johns Hopkins University Press, 1997).

For journalistic accounts, see Sandra Blakeslee, "Placebos Prove So Powerful Even Experts Are Surprised," *New York Times* (October 13, 1998) describing research on the placebo effect and Dick Thompson, "Real Knife, Fake Surgery," *Time* (February 22, 1999).

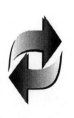

On the Internet ...

American College of Physicians–American Society of Internal Medicine Online

This Web site contains information on resources for the uninsured in the United States and is provided by the American College of Physicians–American Society of Internal Medicine (ACP–ASIM).

`http://www.acponline.org/uninsured/now.htm`

National Council on the Aging (NCOA)

The NCOA Web site includes an article entitled, "New Study Finds Seriously Ill Elderly Patients Receive Less Life-Sustaining Care Than Younger, Comparably Ill Patients: 'Over Treatment' of Young People Suspected." This article suggests that perhaps the elderly are treated appropriately while the young are over-treated. This conclusion is based on a study by the SUPPORT project, the Study to Understand Prognoses and Preferences for Outcomes and Risks of Treatments. The site also addresses other issues associated with aging.

`http://www.ncoa.org`

Organ Donation

This site provides current statistics and background information on the allocation of transplantable organs in the United States.

`http://www.organdonor.gov`

Committee of Interns and Residents

This site outlines the goals of this committee, which is the largest house staff union in the United States.

`http://www.cirdocs.org`

PART 7

Bioethics and Public Policy

*I*n its modern infancy, biomedical ethics was almost exclusively concerned with issues relating to individual doctor-patient relationships. Questions of resource allocation and public policy did occur, but mostly within the context of whether or not a patient could pay for certain kinds of care. In the past several decades, as medical care costs have skyrocketed, the issues concerning equitable distribution of scarce resources have become paramount. As medical care became more costly, it became less accessible to the uninsured and to the underinsured (people who have some health insurance but not enough to cover their own illnesses or those of their families). Managed care in many different forms is rapidly replacing the traditional fee-for-service system, and big corporations are rapidly buying up health plans, hospitals, and doctors' groups. In this new world of market-driven health care, some old problems of resource allocation and public policy take on new urgency. How can generational equity be obtained? Will physician ethics change under managed care? How far should commercialism extend? Should doctors join unions? This section takes up these issues.

- Should Health Insurance Be Based on Employment?

- Should Health Care for the Elderly Be Limited?

- Should Patient-Centered Medical Ethics Govern Managed Care?

- Should There Be a Market in Body Parts?

- Should Doctors-in-Training Be Unionized?

ISSUE 17

Should Health Insurance Be Based on Employment?

YES: William S. Custer, Charles N. Kahn III, and Thomas F. Wildsmith IV, from "Why We Should Keep the Employment-Based Health Insurance System," *Health Affairs* (November/December 1999)

NO: Uwe E. Reinhardt, from "Employer-Based Health Insurance: A Balance Sheet," *Health Affairs* (November/December 1999)

ISSUE SUMMARY

YES: Insurance and policy analysts William S. Custer, Charles N. Kahn III, and Thomas F. Wildsmith IV assert that the employment-based health care system in the United States offers a solid, proven foundation on which to base any reform, and that attempts to break the link between employment and health insurance coverage may greatly increase the number of uninsured Americans.

NO: Economist Uwe E. Reinhardt argues that, on balance, the debits of the employer-based health insurance system outweigh the credits, and that a parallel system detached from the workplace could eventually absorb the current system.

M ost Americans take it for granted that workers get health insurance through their employer. Yet employer-based insurance is something of a historical accident, having developed in the 1940s when the United States was at war. Because there was a civilian labor shortage and caps on wages, employers began to offer fringe benefits like health insurance to attract workers and to obtain business tax deductions for themselves. Before then, most Americans paid for health care out of their own pockets or joined the few existing private group plans such as Blue Cross.

Today, the American health care system is arguably the most expensive and among the most inequitable in the world. No other country spends as much —14 percent of the gross national product—on health care, including some of the most technologically advanced care possible. Yet approximately 44 million Americans, that is, one in six, have no medical insurance. Some are full-time workers whose employers do not provide health insurance as a benefit because of the cost; others are unemployed or part-time workers and ineligible for insurance; and still others are uninsurable because of current or prior health problems such as cancer, heart disease, or AIDS. Millions have medical insurance that does not pay for expensive items such as prescription drugs, mental health care, or home care. A study found that 40 percent of bankruptcies in 1999 were related to illness and medical bills, and that most of the people who declared bankruptcy had health insurance.

Public programs provide some care for some people. Medicare (for the elderly and those with end-stage kidney disease) and Medicaid (for the very poor) were enacted in the 1960s. Because these programs grew so rapidly, legislators have recently tried to curb their costs. By law, hospitals with emergency departments must treat everyone who arrives for care, but they are only required to stabilize the patient and are not required to provide ongoing care. The health care "safety net," such as it is, has many holes.

The United States is the only industrialized country other than South Africa that does not have some form of national health insurance. In some countries, such as the United Kingdom, health care is provided through a National Health Service, which employs physicians and other health care workers. In other countries, such as Germany and Canada, a national health insurance plan covers all citizens. But there can be problems with these systems. Patients often encounter long waits for elective surgery and have less access to high-tech medicine.

Until the mid-1990s most American health insurance plans used the "fee for service" model. Doctors and hospitals billed patients or their insurance companies at the going rate, and the insurance covered all or most of the costs. Because of this system's escalating and uncontrolled costs, some form of managed care has largely replaced it. Managed care comes in many varieties, but the common features are limits on hospital stays, restricted referrals to specialists, limited choice of providers, and other cost controls. Employers who offer health insurance now typically provide a choice of a few managed care plans. These plans pass on a portion of the health care costs to employees through co-pays for services, higher deductibles, and utilization limits.

Although there have been many attempts to reform health care nationwide, none have succeeded in making the system more equitable. Congress rejected the 1994 Clinton Administration's health care reform plan as too sweeping and bureaucratic. But disenchantment with many aspects of managed care has led to reconsideration of some of the fundamental premises of the American system, among them the reliance on employer-based insurance.

The following two selections address whether health insurance should be based on employment. William S. Custer, Charles N. Kahn III, and Thomas F. Wildsmith IV emphasize the strengths of workplace-based insurance and private market solutions to the problem of the uninsured. Uwe E. Reinhardt acknowledges some benefits of the current system, but finds it a poor vehicle to expand coverage to the uninsured.

William S. Custer,
Charles N. Kahn III,
and Thomas F. Wildsmith IV

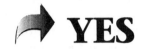 **YES**

Why We Should Keep the Employment-Based Health Insurance System

Today 168 million nonelderly Americans—old and young, wealthy and poor, healthy and sick—enjoy the security of private health insurance; the vast majority are covered through employer-sponsored health plans. Yet despite the many advantages of this system, it has come under increasing criticism.

While some see the employment-based system as limiting consumer choice, others argue that inequities within it are contributing to the growing number of uninsured Americans, estimated to rise from forty-three million to fifty-three million in the coming decade, even under favorable economic conditions.[1] But although some wish to address this problem through a health care program run by the federal government, others maintain that a health care financing structure based on individual choice would both expand private coverage and improve accountability, efficiency, and quality through a system that functions more like a "pure" free market.

This Commentary explores the benefits of the employment-based system and explains why it provides the best foundation for expanding coverage to more Americans. We note that given Americans' preference for private, voluntary health coverage, neither a government-run system nor a government-mandated individual system is a desirable option.[2]

Americans generally prefer to allocate resources using private markets, in large part because decision making is decentralized. This is especially beneficial in health care, where decisions often involve personal trade-offs. Moreover, when competition in the private market works well, it rewards innovation and punishes both low-quality and high-cost providers. Under perfect conditions, market-based systems allocate scarce resources across competing demands for those resources, thereby balancing the cost of production with consumers' preferences.

Real-world markets, however, are not always perfect, and some characteristics of our health care system limit the market's ability to allocate resources efficiently or equitably. Nevertheless, employer-sponsored health plans' ability

From William S. Custer, Charles N. Kahn III, and Thomas F. Wildsmith IV, "Why We Should Keep the Employment-Based Health Insurance System," *Health Affairs*, vol. 18, no. 6 (November/December 1999). Copyright © 1999 by The People-to-People Health Foundation, Inc. Reprinted by permission of *Health Affairs*.

to pool risks and influence both the quality and the cost of care offers significant administrative efficiencies and results in coverage that costs less than the equivalent individual coverage does. This, combined with the fact that the public benefits when each individual consumes health care services, makes the employment-based system important to national health care policy.

Tax Preference for the Employer-Based System

In 1997, 61 percent of Americans (64 percent of those under age sixty-five) were covered through an employment-based plan, as either employees or dependents. Among the nonelderly, more than 90 percent of those who have private insurance received it from an employment-based plan.[3]

The favorable tax treatment of health insurance as an employee benefit has encouraged the proliferation of employer-sponsored health plans. Since 1954 employers' contributions for employee health insurance have been excluded from income for the purpose of determining payroll taxes and federal and state income taxes. This exclusion is essentially a subsidy for the purchase of health insurance for those who receive coverage through the workplace.

Most employers that offer health coverage contribute to its cost; in larger firms this contribution typically represents about 75 percent of the cost of individual coverage and about 65 percent of the cost of family coverage.[4] This means that there is little benefit from not participating in a health plan, even for those who perceive their health risk as low. Participation rates are consequently very high, and persons generally considered to be good health risks remain in the employer's risk pool, which effectively reduces the premium and makes employment-based health insurance more cost-effective than the alternatives.[5] . . .

Employment-based insurance spreads risk more broadly and therefore more efficiently than individual health insurance, and, consequently, is less affected by adverse selection. The problems created for the individual health insurance market by consumers' particular health care needs, which shape the purchasing decision, are well documented.[6] In contrast, employer-sponsored health plans are offered to employees and their dependents as part of a compensation package—and a person's self-assessment of risk is only one of many factors leading to acceptance or rejection of a job offer.[7]

The tax subsidy promotes participation in health plans by those who otherwise would experience large net losses from participation. Some evidence exists that without tax subsidies, low-risk persons might leave pools at a higher rate than high-risk persons do because the cost of coverage would exceed its value.[8] If enough employees chose not to participate, employers might simply terminate their health plans, especially if those who dropped out tended to be better risks.[9]

If the tax subsidy were removed with no other changes in the tax code, twenty million adults would no longer have employment-based health insurance.[10] About 3.5 million more adults would purchase individual health insurance policies. But those in poor health—according to self-reported measures of health status—would be hit hard: The number of employer-insured adults with at least one family member in poor health would fall from 47 percent to 31 percent, a drop of sixteen percentage points.

Even more telling, the percentage of good risks with private coverage outside the employment-based system would increase by three percentage points, while the percentage of poor risks with other private coverage would fall slightly. Even the percentage of employer-insured adults with healthy families would fall twelve percentage points if the exclusion were repealed. These results further support the notion that the tax subsidy reinforces the risk pooling inherent in employment-based health insurance, thereby increasing the number of Americans with coverage.

In short, an inherent economic dynamic favors employment-based group coverage over individual coverage. Employers' decisions to offer health insurance depend on the demand for coverage by the workforce they wish to attract and retain. Although good risks have a lower demand for health insurance than poorer risks have, the tax preference for employer-sponsored coverage in effect lowers its price. This induces more good risks to demand insurance; as the demand rises, more employers offer coverage. And when coverage is offered as a part of compensation, the vast majority of employees participate, thereby reducing the effects of adverse selection. Thus, the group purchase of health insurance through the workplace makes that coverage affordable to poorer risks —the more vulnerable members of society. Individual purchase of insurance would not achieve this societal good.

Finally, some economists have argued that the tax preference provides an incentive for the purchase of too much insurance, resulting in a distorted market for health services, inefficient allocation of scarce resources, and increased health care cost inflation.[11] This argument ignores the social benefit provided by a person's access to health care services. Clearly, the current public policy debate centers on increasing health insurance coverage, not limiting it. . . .

The Employer-Based System: Basis for Reform

The employment-based health insurance system is not a historical accident. Its characteristics flow directly from our society's desire to maximize access to health care, our commitment to voluntary private markets, and the market advantages of employer-sponsored health insurance.

The inherent structural advantages of the employment-based private health insurance market, coupled with complementary tax and public policies, have allowed employers to help control health care costs, improve quality, and maximize health benefits for a wide range of Americans from diverse economic and social backgrounds. The success of these efforts, during the past decade in particular, shows that the employer-based system harnesses the unique risk factors and other attributes of the health insurance market, for the benefit of the public. These advantages simply are impossible to replicate in any alternative based on a voluntary system.

Voluntary markets will continue for the foreseeable future, markets in which each purchaser must compare the value of the coverage received with the cost of the premiums and decide whether or not coverage makes sense.

With a voluntary market, any implicit subsidy that requires some people to pay more for health insurance so that others can pay less is, in effect, a "tax" that can be avoided simply by not buying health insurance.

Continued reliance on the employment-based health insurance system, with its ability to attract a broad range of individuals, in conjunction with targeted subsidies for specific population segments who are not eligible for, or cannot afford, employer coverage, would seem to be the best strategy for increasing access in a voluntary market. Access to affordable coverage needs to be extended to far more Americans, but such efforts should supplement and strengthen the current employment-based system, not replace it.

e◆ﾟ

Our society continues to face important challenges in moving toward a more efficient, cost-effective, and universal health care system. Perhaps the most difficult challenge is to maintain the balance between private and public coverage to maximize access to health care services, control costs, and reward innovation. As long as we continue to rely on the voluntary purchase of health insurance, the natural tendency of consumers to make financial decisions that are in their own economic best interest will limit the size of the implicit subsidies that can be generated, particularly in the individual market, without greatly reducing the number of persons who choose to purchase coverage. The employment-based health care system offers a solid, proven foundation upon which to build any reform, and it should be preserved. On the other hand, reforms based on attempts to break the link between employment and health insurance coverage are unlikely to be successful and have the potential to greatly increase the number of Americans who lack health insurance.

Notes

1. W. Custer, *Health Insurance Coverage and the Uninsured* (Washington: Health Insurance Association of America, January 1999).
2. An exhaustive literature exists on the disadvantages of a government system and the antipathy of Americans to such a system. See, for example, R. Blendon et al., "Voters and Health Care in the 1998 Election," *Journal of the American Medical Association* (14 July 1999): 189–194; M. Walker and M. Zelder, *Waiting Your Turn: Hospital Waiting Lists in Canada (9th Edition)*, Critical Issues Bulletin (Vancouver, B.C.: Fraser Institute, September 1999); S. Hall, "For British Health System, Bleak Prognosis," *New York Times*, 30 January 1997, A1; K. Donelan et al., "The Cost of Health System Change: Public Discontent in Five Nations." *Health Affairs* (May/June 1999): 206–216; T. Jost, "German Health Care Reform: The Next Steps," *Journal of Health Politics, Policy and Law* (August 1998): 697–711; and C. Dargie, S. Dawson, and P. Garside, *Policy Futures for UK Health: Pathfinder* (Draft) (London: Nuffield Trust for Research and Policy Studies in Health Services, September 1999).
3. Custer, *Health Insurance Coverage and the Uninsured*.
4. *National Survey of Employer-Sponsored Health Plans, 1997* (New York: William M. Mercer, 1998).
5. A. Monheit et al., "How Are Net Health Insurance Benefits Distributed in the Employment-Related Insurance Market?" *Inquiry* (Winter 1995/96): 372–391.

6. A consumer's choice of health insurance coverage in an individual market is determined by a self-assessment of his or her own risk and income. Those with the greatest demand for health insurance are thus most likely to use health care services. Premiums in the individual market therefore are higher, to cover the costs of the greater risks. *Providing Universal Access in a Voluntary Private-Sector Market,* Public Policy Monograph (Washington: American Academy of Actuaries, February 1996); L. Nichols, "Regulating Non-Group Health Insurance Markets: What Have We Learned So Far?" (Paper presented at the Robert Wood Johnson Foundation/ Alpha Center meeting, The Evolution of the Individual Insurance Market: Now and in the Future, Washington, D.C., 20 January 1999); S. Zuckerman and S. Rajan, "An Alternative Approach to Measuring the Effects of Insurance Market Reforms," *Inquiry* (Spring 1999): 44–56; L.J. Blumberg and L.M. Nichols, "First, Do No Harm: Developing Health Insurance Market Reform Packages," *Health Affairs* (Fall 1996): 35–53; and L. Blumberg and L. Nichols, *Health Insurance Market Reforms: What They Can and Cannot Do* (Washington: Urban Institute, 1995).
7. Although employment itself may act as a health screen, given employment-based coverage's favorable selection, just under half of Americans with employment-based coverage are dependents of workers. P. Fronstin, *Features Of Employment-Based Health Insurance,* EBRI Issue Brief no. 201 (Washington: Employee Benefit Research Institute, 1998).
8. Monheit et al., "How Are Net Health Insurance Benefits Distributed?"
9. *Tax Reform and the Impact on Employee Benefits,* Public Policy Monograph (Washington: American Academy of Actuaries, Spring 1997).
10. This estimate is based on variations in state marginal income tax rates. See W. Custer and P. Ketsche, "The Tax Preference for Employment-Based Health Insurance Coverage," Working Paper (Center for Risk Management and Insurance Research, Georgia State University, April 1999).
11. M. Feldstein, "The Welfare Loss of Excess Health Insurance," *Journal of Political Economy* (March/April 1973): 251–280; M. Feldstein and B. Freidman, "Tax Subsidies, the Rational Demand for Insurance, and the Health Care Crisis," *Journal of Public Economics* (April 1977):155–178; and M. Pauly, "Taxation, Health Insurance, and Market Failure in the Medical Economy," *Journal of Economic Literature* 24, no. 2 (1986): 629–675.

NO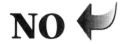

Uwe E. Reinhardt

Employer-Based Health Insurance: A Balance Sheet

As the United States faces the dynamic global economy of the next millennium, many policy analysts and even some members of Congress have begun to wonder whether employment-based health insurance can remain a cornerstone of the U.S. health care system.

The employer-based system traces its origins to World War II, when Congress illogically allowed employers to use fringe benefits as a means of evading the wage caps that it had imposed at the time. The system thrived in the postwar years, when the U.S. economy ruled the world and American workers enjoyed virtually tenured jobs. Its growth has been further abetted by a tax preference that allows employers to treat the group-insurance premiums paid on behalf of employees as tax-deductible expenses without requiring employees to pay income taxes on this part of their compensation. In effect, this tax preference allows employed Americans to purchase health insurance out of pretax income, a privilege not extended to self-employed or unemployed Americans.

Although the employer-based insurance system covers about two-thirds of the U.S. population, it accounts for less than one-third of total national health spending. This is because public insurance programs have become the catch basins for relatively high cost Americans—the elderly, the poor, and the disabled. Government's relative importance as a payer for health care is likely to grow in the next century, as the population ages.

Doubts about the employer-based health insurance system's future have grown during the 1990s, because the system actually shrank as the economy and total employment expanded apace. About 18 percent of working adults are not now offered any health insurance by their employer.[1] The more nonelderly Americans are eclipsed and left uninsured by the employer-based system, the more compelling is the search for a robust alternative to that system....

From Uwe E. Reinhardt, "Employer-Based Health Insurance: A Balance Sheet," *Health Affairs*, vol. 18, no. 6 (November/December 1999). Copyright © 1999 by The People-to-People Health Foundation, Inc. Reprinted by permission of *Health Affairs*.

The System's Debits

"Unsurance"   Unquestionably the worst shortcoming of the employer-based system is that the health insurance protection of entire families, including children, is tied to a particular job and lost with that job. By international standards, privately insured Americans cannot really be considered "insured." They are "temporarily insured," or "unsured" for short.

In virtually all other industrialized nations, young people know that, come what may, they will have permanent, fully portable health insurance. The United States has never been able to afford its citizens that luxury. Would any private health insurer today be able to offer a young American a life-cycle health insurance contract, akin to the whole-life insurance policies that are available to young Americans? The job-based system has been a major roadblock to the development of fully portable, life-cycle health insurance contracts.

Job lock   Because the employer-based system ties health insurance to a particular job, it can induce employees to remain indentured in a detested job simply because it is the sole source of affordable health coverage. As Jonathan Gruber and Maria Hanratty have shown empirically, relative to the U.S. health system, the fully portable health insurance provided by the Canadian provinces actually facilitates greater labor mobility.[2] Fully portable health insurance, of course, is not contingent on government provision. Within a proper statutory framework, it should be possible to develop fully portable private health insurance that is detached from the workplace.[3]

Inequity   The tax preference enjoyed by the employer-based system is inequitable for two reasons. First, it has never been fully extended to self-employed and unemployed Americans, which is unfair on its face. Second, even among employed Americans with employer coverage, those with high incomes benefit proportionately more from the tax preference than do low-income employees in lower marginal tax brackets.

This inequity is most glaring in connection with the flexible spending accounts available only through the employer-based system. At the beginning of the year employed Americans may deposit into these accounts, out of pretax income, specified amounts to cover out-of-pocket health spending. With this set-aside, well-to-do families can purchase a dollar's worth of, say, orthodontic work or plastic surgery at an after-tax cost of only about fifty cents, whereas low-income families would pay eighty-five cents or more after taxes for the same work. Furthermore, the law includes the inflationary provision that unspent year-end balances in the accounts accrue to the employer. One suspects that Congress enacted this inequitable, inflationary provision at the behest of private employers, which found the arrangement helpful in their quest to make their workers accept more overt cost sharing for their health care.

Lack of choice   Whatever benefits employees derive from the current paternalistic system, one price they pay is limits on their choices in the health insurance market. As Stan Jones, Lynn Etheredge, and Larry Lewin reported in

1996, close to half of American employees are offered only one health plan by their employers.[4] They are in what one may call a private single-payer system. Another quarter or so of employees are offered a choice of only two health plans. A more recent Kaiser/Commonwealth national survey of health insurance corroborates these estimates.[5] This lack of choice makes a mockery of the idea of "managed competition."

Lack of privacy In many instances, the employer-based system gives private employers access to their employees' medical records.[6] It is one thing to know that a private insurance carrier has information on the most intimate details of one's life. It is quite another to think that the personnel department of one's employer can get access to that information as well. Whatever one may think about health systems abroad, patients in those countries do not worry about this invasion of privacy.

Administrative complexity The defenders of employer-based health insurance tend to view it as more "efficient" than alternative arrangements. That proposition is incredible, given the current system's administrative complexity. [As a result] of a multiyear study by McKinsey and Company of the American and German health systems, the latter of which is based on private, not-for-profit sickness funds that operate within a tight statutory framework,[7] [t]he McKinsey research team concluded that the U.S. system is more productively efficient than Germany's system is. It based that conclusion on the finding that in 1990 Germans actually spent $390 more per capita on strictly medical inputs (hospital days, physician visits, drugs, and the like) than did Americans. [H]owever, the U.S. system burned up more than the entire savings from its allegedly superior clinical productivity on higher administrative expenses ($360 per capita) and on higher outlays on the catch-all category "other" ($259). Because Medicare and Medicaid are known to spend relatively little on administration, the higher U.S. figure must reflect mainly private insurance. Given that the U.S. system outranks no other system in the industrialized world in either measured health status indicators or patient satisfaction, it can fairly be asked: In what sense is employer-based health insurance "efficient"?

Lack of transparency Standard economic theory and empirical research have convinced economists that the premiums paid by employers on behalf of employees are merely part of the total price of labor and, over the longer run, are shifted back to employees collectively through commensurate reductions in take-home pay. Unfortunately, it is not known precisely how employers do this. That may be why employees typically assume that their employer fully absorbs the part of the premium that is not explicitly deducted from their paycheck. Unaware of how much their health insurance actually costs them in terms of forgone take-home pay, employed Americans have never showed nearly enough self-interest in health care cost containment. This may explain why over the long run the employer-based system has so frequently acted as the inflationary locomotive in American health care....

Although different evaluators may come up with different debits, credits, and account balances for the employer-based health insurance system, I conclude from the exercise that the debits outweigh the credits. This conclusion does not call for the outright abolition of the current system, but it does suggest the need for a parallel system that would be detached from the workplace and that might, over time, absorb the bulk of the current system. With a proper regulatory framework, such a parallel system need not be public; it could rely on private insurance as well.

Notes

1. Kaiser/Commonwealth 1997 National Survey of Health Insurance, "Working Families at Risk: Coverage, Access, Costs, and Worries" (8 December 1997), 40.
2. J. Gruber and M. Hanratty, "The Labor Market Effects of Introducing National Health Insurance," *Journal of Business and Economic Statistics* (April 1995):163–174.
3. M.V. Pauly et al., "A Plan for 'Responsible National Health Insurance'," *Health Affairs* (Spring 1991): 5–25; and U.E. Reinhardt, "An 'All-American' Health Reform Proposal," *Journal of American Health Policy* (May/June 1993):11–17.
4. L. Etheredge, S.B. Jones, and L. Lewin, "What Is Driving Health System Change?" *Health Affairs* (Winter 1996): 94.
5. Kaiser/Commonwealth 1997 National Survey of Health Insurance.
6. E.E. Schultz, "Medical Data Gathered by Firms Can Prove Less Than Confidential," *Wall Street Journal,* 18 May 1994, A1, A5.
7. McKinsey Global Institute, *Health Care Productivity* (Los Angeles: McKinsey and Company, October 1996).

POSTSCRIPT

Should Health Insurance Be Based on Employment?

As the number of uninsured Americans continues to grow, some efforts are being made to expand employer-based coverage through governmental subsidies. Small businesses and those that employ low-income workers in particular need assistance. For example, Healthy New York is a new, state-run program geared toward firms with low-income workers. A state fund will reimburse insurers if an employee incurs particularly high medical costs during a single year. For a firm to be eligible for the program, at least 30 percent of its workers must earn less than $30,000 annually. Businesses that participate must pay at least half of the insurance premium and must offer coverage to all of their low-wage workers, even those who work part-time. Employees who join the program pay half of the insurance premium and substantial copayments for services.

Other efforts to expand coverage, particularly for children, are based on Medicaid eligibility. Changes in federal welfare policy that separated eligibility for welfare from eligibility for Medicaid reduced the number of people on Medicaid, even though the people were still eligible.

Medicare has become one of the most popular public programs, but it too has many limitations. Public pressure has focused on Medicare's failure to pay for prescription drugs, and several competing plans have been offered to add this benefit.

For other views on employer-based health insurance, see the articles by David A. Rochfort (pro) and Nancy S. Jecker (con), in *The Politics of Health Care Reform: Lessons From the Past, Prospects for the Future* (Duke University Press, 1994). In "How Large Employers Are Shaping the Health Care Marketplace (Second of Two Parts)," *The New England Journal of Medicine* (April 9, 1998), Thomas Bodenheimer and Kip Sullivan discuss the influence of employers on health care services. They assert that employers have largely succeeded in their first cost-cutting strategy—channeling employees into managed care plans. However, the success of their second strategy—bringing employers together in large regional plans and contracting directly with health care providers—is still in doubt. See also John D. Banja, "The Improbable Future of Employment-Based Insurance," *Hastings Center Report* (May–June 2000) and R. Kuttner, "The American Health Care System: Employer-Sponsored Health Coverage," *The New England Journal of Medicine* (January 21, 1999).

ISSUE 18

Should Health Care for the Elderly Be Limited?

YES: Daniel Callahan, from "Limiting Health Care for the Old?" *The Nation* (August 15, 1987)

NO: Amitai Etzioni, from "Spare the Old, Save the Young," *The Nation* (June 11, 1988)

ISSUE SUMMARY

YES: Philosopher Daniel Callahan maintains that since health care resources are scarce, people who have lived a full natural life span should be offered care that relieves suffering but not expensive life-prolonging technologies.

NO: Sociologist Amitai Etzioni argues that rationing health care for the elderly would encourage conflict between generations and would invite restrictions on health care for other groups.

America is aging. In 1965 the 18.5 million people over the age of 65 accounted for only 9.5 percent of the population. By 1987 the number had climbed to 29 million, or 12 percent of the population. The number of people over 85—the "old old"—is the fastest-growing age group in the United States. By the year 2040 the elderly will represent 21 percent of the population.

Older people are more likely to need health care than the young. In 1980 people over 65 accounted for 29 percent of the total American health care expenditures of $219.4 billion. By 1986 the bill had risen to $450 billion, and the share devoted to the elderly to 31 percent. The costs of Medicare—the federal program that supports the health care of people over 65—are expected to rise dramatically in the future. The American population over 65 will increase by 70 percent between 2010 and 2030.

Although Medicare coverage of nursing homes and home care remains inadequate to meet the need, organ transplants are now covered. The typical cost of such an operation is $200,000.

Many (but not all) elderly people do not want to have their lives prolonged through the use of expensive technology such as kidney dialysis, respirators, and intensive care. They fear losing control of their medical care and dying "hooked up to tubes."

There are many competing interests vying for the increasingly scarce health care dollar. Groups representing patients suffering from particular diseases—cancer, AIDS, diabetes, and heart disease, to name just a few—advocate increased spending on research and care. Those who speak for the poor, especially poor children, point out that the poor often do not have access to the most basic medical care, such as immunizations. The costs of treating premature, low-birth-weight infants are extremely high; yet programs that provide prenatal care and adequate nutrition to mothers at risk, which might prevent many such births, are inadequately funded.

In such a complex web of competing claims, when not all interests can be met, how should decisions to ration care be determined? Should age be one criterion? In Great Britain, which has a National Health Service and centralized planning, patients over the age of 55 have been routinely denied kidney dialysis ostensibly on "medical" grounds, even though the procedure is performed in the United States on very old patients.

Should this pattern be followed in the United States? The following selections present the contrasting views. Daniel Callahan says that we must confront realities: in the interest of ensuring adequate health care for the younger generation, we must limit the kinds of care that will be available to those who have lived a full natural life span. Amitai Etzioni objects to this call to ration health care to the elderly on the grounds that it will lead to denying care to people of younger ages and other groups deemed less productive to society.

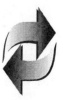

Daniel Callahan 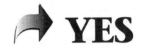 **YES**

Limiting Health Care for the Old?

$\mathbf{I}$s it sensible, in the face of the rapidly increasing burden of health care costs for the elderly, to press forward with new and expensive ways of extending their lives? Is it possible even to hope to control costs while simultaneously supporting innovative research, which generates new ways to spend money? Those are now unavoidable questions....

Anyone who works closely with the elderly recognizes that the present Medicare and Medicaid programs are grossly inadequate in meeting their real and full needs. The system fails most notably in providing decent long-term care and medical care that does not constitute a heavy out-of-pocket drain. Members of minority groups and single or widowed women are particularly disadvantaged. How will it be possible, then, to provide the growing number of elderly with even present levels of care, much less to rid the system of its inadequacies and inequities, and at the same time add expensive new technologies?

The straight answer is that it will be impossible to do all those things and, worse still, it may be harmful even to try. It may be so because of the economic burdens that would impose on younger age groups, and because of the requisite skewing of national social priorities too heavily toward health care. But that suggests to both young and old that the key to a happy old age is good health care, which may not be true.

In the past few years three additional concerns about health care for the aged have surfaced. First, an increasingly large share of health care is going to the elderly rather than to youth. The Federal government, for instance, spends six times as much providing health benefits and other social services to those over 65 as it does to those under 18. And, as the demographer Samuel Preston observed in a provocative address to the Population Association of America in 1984, "Transfers from the working-age population to the elderly are also transfers away from children, since the working ages bear far more responsibility for childrearing than do the elderly."

Preston's address had an immediate impact. The mainline senior-citizen advocacy groups accused Preston of fomenting a war between the generations. But the speech also stimulated Minnesota Senator David Durenberger and others to found Americans for Generational Equity (AGE) to promote debate about

From Daniel Callahan, "Limiting Health Care for the Old?" *The Nation* (August 15, 1987). Adapted from Daniel Callahan, *Setting Limits: Medical Goals in an Aging Society* (Simon & Schuster, 1987). Copyright © 1987 by Daniel Callahan. Reprinted by permission.

the burden on future generations, particularly the Baby Boom cohort, of "our major social insurance programs." Preston's speech and the founding of AGE signaled the outbreak of a struggle over what has come to be called "intergenerational equity," which is now gaining momentum.

The second concern is that the elderly, in dying, consume a disproportionate share of health care costs. "At present," notes Stanford University economist Victor Fuchs, "the United States spends about 1 percent of the gross national product on health care for elderly persons who are in their last year of life.... One of the biggest challenges facing policy makers for the rest of this century will be how to strike an appropriate balance between care for the [elderly] dying and health services for the rest of the population."

The third issue is summed up in an observation by Dr. Jerome Avorn of the Harvard Medical School, who wrote in *Daedalus,* "With the exception of the birth-control pill, [most] of the medical-technology interventions developed since the 1950s have their most widespread impact on people who are past their fifties—the further past their fifties, the greater the impact." Many of the techniques in question were not intended for use on the elderly. Kidney dialysis, for example, was developed for those between the ages of 15 and 45. Now some 30 percent of its recipients are over 65.

The validity of those concerns has been vigorously challenged, as has the more general assertion that some form of rationing of health care for the elderly might become necessary. To the charge that old people receive a disproportionate share of resources, the response has been that assistance to them helps every age group: It relieves the young of the burden of care they would otherwise have to bear for elderly parents and, since those young will eventually become old, promises them similar care when they need it. There is no guarantee, moreover, that any cutback in health care for the elderly would result in a transfer of the savings directly to the young. And, some ask, Why should we contemplate restricting care for the elderly when we wastefully spend hundreds of millions on an inflated defense budget?

The assertion that too large a share of funds goes to extending the lives of elderly people who are terminally ill hardly proves that it is an unjust or unreasonable amount. They are, after all, the most in need. As some important studies have shown, it is exceedingly difficult to know that someone is dying; the most expensive patients, it turns out, are those who were expected to live but died. That most new technologies benefit the old more than the young is logical; most of the killer diseases of the young have now been conquered.

There is little incentive for politicians to think about, much less talk about, limits on health care for the aged. As John Rother, director of legislation for the American Association of Retired Persons, has observed, "I think anyone who wasn't a champion of the aged is no longer in Congress." Perhaps also, as Guido Calabresi, dean of the Yale Law School, and his colleague Philip Bobbitt observed in their thoughtful 1978 book *Tragic Choices,* when we are forced to make painful allocation choices, "Evasion, disguise, temporizing... [and] averting our eyes enables us to save some lives even when we will not save all."

I believe that we must face this highly troubling issue. Rationing of health care under Medicare is already a fact of life, though rarely labeled as such. The requirement that Medicare recipients pay the first $520 of hospital care costs, the cutoff of reimbursement for care after 60 days and the failure to cover long-term care are nothing other than allocation and cost-saving devices. As sensitive as it is to the senior-citizen vote, the Reagan Administration agreed only grudgingly to support catastrophic health care coverage for the elderly (a benefit that will not help very many of them), and it has already expressed its opposition to the recently passed House version of the bill. It is bound to be far more resistant to long-term health care coverage, as will any administration.

But there are reasons other than the economics to think about health care for the elderly. The coming economic crisis provides a much-needed opportunity to ask some deeper questions. Just what is it that we want medicine to do for us as we age? Other cultures have believed that aging should be accepted, and that it should be in part a time of preparation for death. Our culture seems increasingly to dispute that view, preferring instead, it often seems, to think of aging as hardly more than another disease, to be fought and rejected. Which view is correct?

Let me interject my own opinion. The future goal of medical science should be to improve the quality of old people's lives, not to lengthen them. In its longstanding ambition to forestall death, medicine has reached its last frontier in the care of the aged. Of course children and young adults still die of maladies that are open to potential cure; but the highest proportion of the dying (70 percent) are over 65. If death is ever to be humbled, that is where endless work remains to be done. But however tempting the challenge of that last frontier, medicine should restrain itself. To do otherwise would mean neglecting the needs of other age groups and of the old themselves.

Our culture has worked hard to redefine old age as a time of liberation, not decline, a time of travel, of new ventures in education and self-discovery, of the ever-accessible tennis court or golf course and of delightfully periodic but thankfully brief visits from well-behaved grandchildren. That is, to be sure, an idealized picture, but it arouses hopes that spur medicine to wage an aggressive war against the infirmities of old age. As we have seen, the costs of such a war would be prohibitive. No matter how much is spent the ultimate problem will still remain: people will grow old and die. Worse still, by pretending that old age can be turned into a kind of endless middle age, we rob it of meaning and significance for the elderly.

There is a plausible alternative: a fresh vision of what it means to live a decently long and adequate life, what might be called a "natural life span." Earlier generations accepted the idea that there was a natural life span—the biblical norm of three score and ten captures that notion (even though in fact that was a much longer life span than was typical in ancient times). It is an idea well worth reconsidering and would provide us with a meaningful and realizable goal. Modern medicine and biology have done much, however, to wean us from that kind of thinking. They have insinuated the belief that the average life span is not a natural fact at all, but instead one that is strictly dependent on the state of medical knowledge and skill. And there is much to that belief as a statistical fact: The average life expectancy continues to increase with no end in sight.

But that is not what I think we ought to mean by a natural life span. We need a notion of a full life that is based on some deeper understanding of human needs and possibilities, not on the state of medical technology or its potential. We should think of a natural life span as the achievement of a life that is sufficiently long to take advantage of those opportunities life typically offers and that we ordinarily regard as its prime benefits—loving and "living," raising a family, engaging in work that is satisfying, reading, thinking, cherishing our friends and families. People differ on what might be a full natural life span; my view is that it can be achieved by the late 70s or early 80s.

A longer life does not guarantee a better life. No matter how long medicine enables people to live, death at any time—at age 90 or 100 or 110—would frustrate some possibility, some as-yet-unrealized goal. The easily preventable death of a young child is an outrage. Death from an incurable disease of someone in the prime of young adulthood is a tragedy. But death at an old age, after a long and full life, is simply sad, a part of life itself.

As it confronts aging, medicine should have as its specific goals the averting of premature death, that is, death prior to the completion of a natural life span, and thereafter, the relief of suffering. It should pursue those goals so that the elderly can finish out their years with as little needless pain as possible—and with as much vitality as can be generated in contributing to the welfare of younger age groups and to the community of which they are a part. Above all, the elderly need to have a sense of the meaning and significance of their stage in life, one that is not dependent on economic productivity or physical vigor.

What would medicine oriented toward the relief of suffering rather than the deliberate extension of life be like? We do not have a clear answer to that question, so longstanding, central and persistent has been medicine's preoccupation with the struggle against death. But the hospice movement is providing us with much guidance. It has learned how to distinguish between the relief of suffering and the lengthening of life. Greater control by elderly persons over their own dying—and particularly an enforceable right to refuse aggressive life-extending treatment—is a minimal goal.

What does this have to do with the rising cost of health care for the elderly? Everything. The indefinite extension of life combined with an insatiable ambition to improve the health of the elderly is a recipe for monomania and bottomless spending. It fails to put health in its proper place as only one among many human goods. It fails to accept aging and death as part of the human condition. It fails to present to younger generations a model of wise stewardship.

How might we devise a plan to limit the costs of health care for the aged under public entitlement programs that is fair, humane and sensitive to their special requirements and dignity? Let me suggest three principles to undergird a quest for limits. First, government has a duty, based on our collective social obligations, to help people live out a natural life span but not to help medically extend life beyond that point. Second, government is obliged to develop under its research subsidies, and to pay for under its entitlement programs, only the kind and degree of life-extending technology necessary for medicine to achieve and serve the aim of a natural life span. Third, beyond the point of a natural life span, government should provide only the means necessary for the relief of suffering, not those for life-extending technology.

A system based on those principles would not immediately bring down the cost of care of the elderly; it would add cost. But it would set in place the beginning of a new understanding of old age, one that would admit of eventual stabilization and limits. The elderly will not be served by a belief that only a lack of resources, better financing mechanisms or political power stands between them and the limitations of their bodies. The good of younger age groups will not be served by inspiring in them a desire to live to an old age that maintains the vitality of youth indefinitely, as if old age were nothing but a sign that medicine has failed in its mission. The future of our society will not be served by allowing expenditures on health care for the elderly to escalate endlessly and uncontrollably, fueled by the false altruistic belief that anything less is to deny the elderly their dignity. Nor will it be aided by the pervasive kind of self-serving argument that urges the young to support such a crusade because they will eventually benefit from it also.

We require instead an understanding of the process of aging and death that looks to our obligation to the young and to the future, that recognizes the necessity of limits and the acceptance of decline and death, and that values the old for their age and not for their continuing youthful vitality. In the name of accepting the elderly and repudiating discrimination against them, we have succeeded mainly in pretending that, with enough will and money, the unpleasant part of old age can be abolished. In the name of medical progress we have carried out a relentless war against death and decline, failing to ask in any probing way if that will give us a better society for all.

NO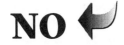

Amitai Etzioni

Spare the Old, Save the Young

In the coming years, Daniel Callahan's call to ration health care for the elderly, put forth in his book *Setting Limits,* is likely to have a growing appeal. Practically all economic observers expect the United States to go through a difficult time as it attempts to work its way out of its domestic (budgetary) and international (trade) deficits. Practically every serious analyst realizes that such an endeavor will initially entail slower growth, if not an outright cut in our standard of living, in order to release resources to these priorities. When the national economic "pie" grows more slowly, let alone contracts, the fight over how to divide it up intensifies. The elderly make an especially inviting target because they have been taking a growing slice of the resources (at least those dedicated to health care) and are expected to take even more in the future. Old people are widely held to be "nonproductive" and to constitute a growing "burden" on an ever smaller proportion of society that is young and working. Also, the elderly are viewed as politically well-organized and powerful; hence "their" programs, especially Social Security and Medicare, have largely escaped the Reagan attempts to scale back social expenditures, while those aimed at other groups—especially the young, but even more so future generations—have been generally curtailed. There are now some signs that a backlash may be forming.

If a war between the generations, like that between the races and between the genders, does break out, historians may accord former Governor Richard Lamm of Colorado the dubious honor of having fired the opening shot in his statement that the elderly ill have "got a duty to die and get out of the way." Phillip Longman, in his book *Born to Pay,* sounded an early alarm. However, the historians may well say, it was left to Daniel Callahan, a social philosopher and ethicist, to provide a detailed rationale and blueprint for limiting the care to the elderly, explicitly in order to free resources for the young. Callahan's thesis deserves close examination because he attempts to deal with the numerous objections his approach raises. If his thesis does not hold, the champions of limiting funds available to the old may have a long wait before they will find a new set of arguments on their behalf.

In order to free up economic resources for the young, Callahan offers the older generation a deal: Trade quantity for quality; the elderly should

From Amitai Etzioni, "Spare the Old, Save the Young," *The Nation* (June 11, 1988). Copyright © 1988 by The Nation Company, Inc. Reprinted by permission.

not be given life-*extending* services but better years while alive. Instead of the relentless attempt to push death to an older age, Callahan would stop all development of life-extending technologies and prohibit the use of ones at hand for those who outlive their "natural" life span, say, the age of 75. At the same time, the old would be granted more palliative medicine (e.g., pain killers) and more nursing-home and home-health care, to make their natural years more comfortable.

Callahan's call to break an existing ethical taboo and replace it with another raises the problem known among ethicists and sociologists as the "slippery slope." Once the precept that one should do "all one can" to avert death is given up, and attempts are made to fix a specific age for a full life, why stop there? If, for instance, the American economy experiences hard times in the 1990s, should the "maximum" age be reduced to 72, 65—or lower? And should the care for other so-called unproductive groups be cut off, even if they are even younger? Should countries that are economically worse off than the United States set their limit, say, at 55?

This is not an idle thought, because the idea of limiting the care the elderly receive in itself represents a partial slide down such a slope. Originally, Callahan, the Hastings Center (which he directs) and other think tanks played an important role in redefining the concept of death. Death used to be seen by the public at large as occurring when the lungs stopped functioning and, above all, the heart stopped beating. In numerous old movies and novels, those attending the dying would hold a mirror to their faces to see if it fogged over, or put an ear to their chests to see if the heart had stopped. However, high technology made these criteria obsolete by mechanically ventilating people and keeping their hearts pumping. Hastings et al. led the way to provide a new technological definition of death: brain death. Increasingly this has been accepted, both in the medical community and by the public at large, as the point of demise, the point at which care should stop even if it means turning off life-extending machines, because people who are brain dead do not regain consciousness. At the same time, most doctors and a majority of the public as well continue strongly to oppose terminating care to people who are conscious, even if there is little prospect for recovery, despite considerable debate about certain special cases.

Callahan now suggests turning off life-extending technology for all those above a certain age, even if they could recover their full human capacity if treated. It is instructive to look at the list of technologies he would withhold: mechanical ventilation, artificial resuscitation, antibiotics and artificial nutrition and hydration. Note that while several of these are used to maintain brain-dead bodies, they are also used for individuals who are temporarily incapacitated but able to recover fully; indeed, they are used to save young lives, say, after a car accident. But there is no way to stop the development of such new technologies and the improvement of existing ones without depriving the young of benefit as well. (Antibiotics are on the list because of an imminent "high cost" technological advance—administering them with a pump implanted in the body, which makes their introduction more reliable and better distributes dosages.)

One may say that this is Callahan's particular list; other lists may well be drawn. But any of them would start us down the slope, because the savings that are achieved by turning off the machines that keep brain-dead people alive are minimal compared with those that would result from the measures sought by the people calling for new equity between the generations. And any significant foray into deliberately withholding medical care for those who can recover does raise the question, Once society has embarked on such a slope, where will it stop?

Those opposed to Callahan, Lamm and the other advocates of limiting care to the old, but who also favor extending the frontier of life, must answer the question, Where will the resources come from? One answer is found in the realization that defining people as old at the age of 65 is obsolescent. That age limit was set generations ago, before changes in life styles and medicines much extended not only life but also the number and quality of productive years. One might recognize that many of the "elderly" can contribute to society not merely by providing love, companionship and wisdom to the young but also by continuing to work, in the traditional sense of the term. Indeed, many already work in the underground economy because of the large penalty—a cut in Social Security benefits—exacted from them if they hold a job "on the books."

Allowing elderly people to retain their Social Security benefits while working, typically part-time, would immediately raise significant tax revenues, dramatically change the much-feared dependency-to-dependent ratio, provide a much-needed source of child-care workers and increase contributions to Social Security (under the assumption that anybody who will continue to work will continue to contribute to the program). There is also evidence that people who continue to have meaningful work will live longer and healthier lives, without requiring more health care, because psychic well-being in our society is so deeply associated with meaningful work. Other policy changes, such as deferring retirement, modifying Social Security benefits by a small, gradual stretching out of the age of full-benefit entitlement, plus some other shifts under way, could be used readily to gain more resources. Such changes might be justified prima facie because as we extend life and its quality, the payouts to the old may also be stretched out.

Beyond the question of whether to cut care or stretch out Social Security payouts, policies that seek to promote intergenerational equity must be assessed as to how they deal with another matter of equity: that between the poor and the rich. A policy that would stop Federal support for certain kinds of care, as Callahan and others propose, would halt treatment for the aged, poor, the near-poor and even the less-well-off segment of the middle class (although for the latter at a later point), while the rich would continue to buy all the care they wished to. Callahan's suggestion that a consensus of doctors would stop certain kinds of care for all elderly people is quite impractical; for it to work, most if not all doctors would have to agree to participate. Even if this somehow happened, the rich would buy their services overseas either by going there or by importing the services. There is little enough we can do to significantly enhance economic equality. Do we want to exacerbate the inequalities that already exist by completely eliminating access to major categories of health care services for those who cannot afford to pay for them?

In addition to concern about slipping down the slope of less (and less) care, the *way* the limitations are to be introduced raises a serious question. The advocates of changing the intergenerational allocation of resources favor rationing health care for the elderly but nothing else. This is a major intellectual weakness of their argument. There are other major targets to consider within health care, as well as other areas, which seem, at least by some criteria, much more inviting than terminating care to those above a certain age. Within the medical sector, for example, why not stop all interventions for which there is no hard evidence that they are beneficial? Say, public financing of psychotherapy and coronary bypass operations? Why not take the $2 billion or so from plastic surgery dedicated to face lifts, reducing behinds and the like? Or require that all burials be done by low-cost cremations rather than using high-cost coffins?

Once we extend our reach beyond medical care to health care, if we cannot stop people from blowing $25 billion per year on cigarettes and convince them to use the money to serve the young, shouldn't we at least cut out public subsidies to tobacco growers before we save funds by denying antibiotics to old people? And there is the matter of profits. The high-technology medicine Callahan targets for savings is actually a minor cause of the increase in health care costs for the elderly or for anyone—about 4 percent. A major factor is the very high standard of living American doctors have, compared to those of many other nations. Indeed, many doctors tell interviewers that they love their work and would do it for half their current income as long as the incomes of their fellow practitioners were also cut. Another important area of saving is the exorbitant profits made by the nondoctor owners of dialysis units and nursing homes. If we dare ask how many years of life are enough, should we not also be able to ask how much profit is "enough"? This profit, by the way, is largely set not by the market but by public policy.

Last but not least, as the United States enters a time of economic constraints, should we draw new lines of conflict or should we focus on matters that sustain our societal fabric? During the 1960s numerous groups gained in political consciousness and actively sought to address injustices done to them. The result has been some redress and an increase in the level of societal stress (witness the deeply troubled relationships between the genders). But these conflicts occurred in an affluent society and redressed deeply felt grievances. Are the young like blacks and women, except that they have not yet discovered their oppressors—a group whose consciousness should be raised, so it will rally and gain its due share?

The answer is in the eye of the beholder. There are no objective criteria that can be used here the way they can be used between the races or between the genders. While women and minorities have the same rights to the same jobs at the same pay as white males, the needs of the young and the aged are so different that no simple criteria of equity come to mind. Thus, no one would argue that the teen-agers and those above 75 have the same need for schooling or nursing homes.

At the same time, it is easy to see that those who try to mobilize the young —led by a new Washington research group, Americans for Generational Equity (AGE), formed to fight for the needs of the younger generation—offer many arguments that do not hold. For instance, they often argue that today's young, age 35 or less, will pay for old people's Social Security, but by the time that they come of age they will not be able to collect, because Social Security will be bankrupt. However, this argument is based on extremely farfetched assumptions about the future. In effect, Social Security is now and for the foreseeable future overprovided, and its surplus is used to reduce deficits caused by other expenditures, such as Star Wars, in what is still an integrated budget. And, if Social Security runs into the red again somewhere after the year 2020, relatively small adjustments in premiums and payouts would restore it to financial health.

Above all, it is a dubious sociological achievement to foment conflict between the generations, because, unlike the minorities and the white majority, or men and women, many millions of Americans are neither young nor old but of intermediate ages. We should not avoid issues just because we face stressing times in an already strained society; but maybe we should declare a moratorium on raising new conflicts until more compelling arguments can be found in their favor, and more evidence that this particular line of divisiveness is called for.

POSTSCRIPT

Should Health Care for the Elderly Be Limited?

Callahan's views are amplified in his book *Setting Limits: Medical Goals in an Aging Society* (Simon & Schuster, 1987). See Paul Homer and Martha Holstein, eds., *A Good Old Age: The Paradox of Setting Limits* (Touchstone, 1990) for responses to Callahan's arguments. Also see Robert L. Barry and Gerard V. Bradley, eds., *Set No Limits: A Rebuttal to Daniel Callahan's Proposal to Limit Health Care for the Elderly* (University of Illinois Press, 1991). In "Elder Choice," *American Journal of Law and Medicine* (vol. 19, no. 3, 1993), Alfred F. Conard argues that artificial prolongation of life is usually undesirable and that health care for the aged should include information about advance directives.

A study of critically ill elderly patients concluded that age alone is not an adequate predictor of long-term survival and quality of life. See L. Chelluri et al., "Long-Term Outcome of Critically Ill Elderly Patients Requiring Intensive Care," *Journal of the American Medical Association* (June 23/30, 1993).

For contrasting views on age as a criterion for medical care, see David C. Thomasma, "Functional Status Care Categories and National Health Policy," *Journal of the American Geriatrics Society* (April 1993); Mark Siegler, "Should Age Be a Criterion for Health Care?" and James F. Childress, "Ensuring Care, Respect, and Fairness for the Elderly," both in the *Hastings Center Report* (October 1984); and Nancy S. Jecker and Robert A. Pearlman, "Ethical Constraints on Rationing Medical Care by Age," *Journal of the American Geriatrics Society* (November 1989). Marshall B. Kapp opposes Callahan's view in "Rationing Health Care: Will It Be Necessary? Can It Be Done Without Age or Disability Discrimination?" *Issues in Law and Medicine* (Winter 1989). Pat Milmoe McCarrick's *The Aged and the Allocation of Health Care Resources* (Scope Note No. 13, Kennedy Institute of Ethics, 1990) offers a good bibliography.

See Edward L. Schneider and Jack M. Guralnik, "The Aging of America: Impact on Health Care Costs," *Journal of the American Medical Association* (May 2, 1990) for a discussion of how the rapid increase in the elderly population will affect health care costs.

An international perspective is taken in Daniel Callahan, Ruud H. T. Ter Meulen, and Eva Topinkova, eds., *A World Growing Old: The Coming Health Care Challenges* (Georgetown University Press, 1995). See also Richard Posner, *Aging and Old Age* (University of Chicago Press, 1995). Callahan's most recent book is *False Hopes: Why America's Quest for Perfect Health Is a Recipe for Failure* (Simon and Schuster, 1998).

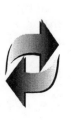

ISSUE 19

Should Patient-Centered Medical Ethics Govern Managed Care?

YES: Ezekiel J. Emanuel and Nancy Neveloff Dubler, from "Preserving the Physician-Patient Relationship in the Era of Managed Care," *Journal of the American Medical Association* (January 25, 1995)

NO: Brendan Minogue, from "The *Two* Fundamental Duties of the Physician," *Academic Medicine* (May 2000)

ISSUE SUMMARY

YES: Physician Ezekiel J. Emanuel and attorney Nancy Neveloff Dubler argue that the expansion of managed care and the imposition of significant cost controls could undermine critical aspects of the physician-patient relationship, including freedom of choice, careful assessments of physician competence, time available for communication, and continuity of care.

NO: Philosopher Brendan Minogue asserts that physicians must balance the interests and wishes of the patient with the welfare of the health care system in which they practice and must stop viewing the case manager as the unavoidable but unwanted child within the family of medicine.

Health care in the United States is going through a profound period of economic and structural change. In the past, providers of health care (hospitals, physicians, suppliers of technology and other services) dictated prices and terms. In this system, provider income increased with greater numbers of patients, more procedures, and longer stays. As a result, health care costs grew at a rate that many considered unacceptable, especially since it was not accompanied by significantly broadened access to care. In order to restrain this trend, major purchasers of medical services (large employers and government programs such as the Veterans Administration, Medicare, and Medicaid) began to aggressively seek the best deal at the best price. In this system, fewer patients, fewer procedures, and shorter hospital stays mean lowered costs.

The generic term for this system is *managed care,* a term that covers a variety of organizational structures and practices, some with long histories and some that are quite new. Some do not even provide health care directly but are "packagers" of a specific group of services. Corporate, for-profit control of health care, in which organizational decisions must consider profit to shareholders as a prime goal, has become an increasingly prominent feature of the system. The presumed benefit is that increased competition, along with tough business practices, will reduce costs without reducing quality.

By the end of 1995 more than 56 million Americans were enrolled in some type of health maintenance organization (HMO). In 1994 publicly traded HMOs completed acquisitions worth more than $4 billion. Hospital mergers are occurring widely, often resulting in the closure of or reduction of services in one of the hospitals. Publicly traded physician practice companies are doing well, as evidenced by a *Wall Street Journal* article predicting that 10 companies would be competing for a potential $200 billion market. In short, health care is a big, profitable business with a growing consolidation of power in a few large corporations.

"Capitation" is a key concept in the new systems. Under the traditional "fee-for-service" approach, patients pay a fee for each visit to the doctor (some or all of which might be reimbursed by insurance) and also for the diagnostic or therapeutic interventions that the doctor recommends. Providers have an economic incentive to do more because each intervention means additional income. Under a capitated system, by contrast, the provider is paid a fixed, or capitated, fee for each person (per head, literally) each year. If the person rarely becomes ill and does not require expensive interventions, the provider realized a profit at the end of the year. If, however, a great deal of costly medical care is required, the patient is a financial loss to the system. In this framework, the economic incentive is to do less because each intervention reduces profit. Less intervention may mean less unnecessary surgery and fewer expensive and marginally useful procedures, medications, and visits. It may also mean postponing needed care or failing to provide appropriate follow-up.

While most attention has been focused on whether or not managed care actually saves money and whether or not others besides corporate executives and investors are reaping any benefits from the savings, the impact on medical ethics is equally important. The following selections look at managed care from that broad perspective. Ezekiel J. Emanuel and Nancy Neveloff Dubler contend that the physician-patient relationship remains the cornerstone for achieving, maintaining, and improving health. Although they acknowledge that the current system fails many in this regard, they worry that imposing significant cost controls in an environment where financial pressures are intense and omnipresent may restrict patient choice, reduce the time available for communication, and create conflicts of interest between patient and physician. Brendan Minogue rejects what he calls the "single-stewardship model" of medicine that prevailed until recently. In this model the physician's ethical responsibilities are defined exclusively in terms of the individual patient. He advocates a "dual-stewardship model" in which the physician must balance the duty to the patient with the duty to other stakeholders in the health care system, such as other patients in the organization.

Ezekiel J. Emanuel and
Nancy Neveloff Dubler

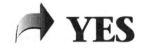 **YES**

Preserving the Physician-Patient Relationship in the Era of Managed Care

The Ideal Physician-Patient Relationship

To evaluate the effects of managed care, we need to delineate an ideal conception of the physician-patient relationship. This ideal establishes the normative standard for assessing the effect of the current health care system as well as changes in the system. Although patients receive health care from a diverse number of providers, and the use of nonphysician providers, such as nurse practitioners, physician assistants, and nurse midwives, is likely to increase with more emphasis on primary care and managed care, we chose to concentrate on the physician-patient relationship. The reasons for this focus are many: physicians outnumber nonphysician providers; most Americans continue to receive their health care from physicians rather than nonphysician providers; there have been many more years, indeed, centuries, for reflection on the elements that constitute the ideal physician-patient relationship, while the ethical guidelines and legal rulings on nonphysician provider-patient relationships are more recent and have not been as exhaustively developed; and there is substantially more empirical research on the physician-patient relationship with which to formulate educated projections....

We suggest that the fundamental elements of the ideal physician-patient relationship that are embodied in our intuitions and common to ethical analyses and legal standards can be expressed as six C's: choice, competence, communication, compassion, continuity, and (no) conflict of interest. While many people emphasize the importance of trust in the physician-patient relationship, we believe trust is the culmination of realizing these six C's, not an independent element....

The Physician-Patient Relationship in the Era of Managed Care

Despite the lack of comprehensive health care system reform legislation, significant changes are occurring without legislative and governmental regulation,

From Ezekiel J. Emanuel and Nancy Neveloff Dubler, "Preserving the Physician-Patient Relationship in the Era of Managed Care," *Journal of the American Medical Association*, vol. 273, no. 4 (January 25, 1995), pp. 323–324, 326–328. Copyright © 1995 by The American Medical Association. Reprinted by permission. Some references omitted.

driven predominantly by the increased efforts of employers to reduce health care costs. These changes include more managed care, increased use of primary care physicians and generalists rather than specialists, increased use of non-physician providers, emphasis on preventive measures, greater commitment to the care of children, and intensive quality assessment.[1,2] Although it is impossible to predict the precise concrete manifestations and effects of all these changes, it is possible to provide some educated reflections on their probable implications for the physician-patient relationship (Table 1). Because the health care system is so complex, the changes may not always tend in a coherent direction; some aspects may enhance a particular element of the physician-patient relationship while others undermine it. It is often difficult to know which tendency will dominate in practice, and so we try to outline the potential trends in both directions.

Admittedly, these predictions are speculative. But they are no more speculative than projections on the cost of certain changes or on the economic consequences of particular managed care programs.[3] And just as economic projections, with uncertainty, are essential in evaluating health care proposals, so too we hope these predictions will provide a basis for planning and promoting those parts of the trend toward managed care that enhance the ideal physician-patient relationship, anticipating threats to the ideal posed by managed care, and acting to mitigate the ill effects.

Potential Improvements

With some expansion of managed care, the range of choice for many insured Americans could also increase. Americans who live in regions without significant managed care penetration, such as the South, will soon have the option of care in a managed care setting. In addition, other Americans could now have several managed care plans as well as fee-for-service options to choose from. However, if managed care expands too much, it may threaten to eliminate fee-for-service practitioners in a region altogether, as it appears to be doing in northern California and Minnesota. Under such circumstances, patients' choice of practice setting, even for well-insured Americans, could be effectively reduced.

Managed care may also provide the insured with a wider range of treatment alternatives. For example, by removing financial barriers, managed care plans should give enrollees more effective choice over utilizing preventive interventions, such as screening tests. Indeed, studies consistently demonstrate greater use of preventive tests and procedures among managed care enrollees.[4-6] In addition, many managed care plans contain benefits packages that include services not currently covered by many insurance programs. Indeed, pediatric patients may significantly benefit from the coverage of vaccinations, small co-payments for well-child visits, and coverage of dental and visual services for children.

Managed care plans are increasingly attempting to develop quality measures; they are trying to use these quality measures for routine assessments of performance and to provide the public with the performance results based on

Table 1

The Effects of Managed Care on the Physician-Patient Relationship

Potential Improvements	Potential Threats
Choice	
. Expanded choice of managed care plans, particularly in areas with low managed care penetration	. "Cherry picking" increasing the number of uninsured Americans
. Expanded choice of preventive and pediatric services	. Employers restricting patients' choice of managed care plans and physicians
	. Price competition forcing patients to choose between continuing with their current physicians or switching to a cheaper plan
	. Financial failures of managed care plans forcing change in managed care plan without choice
	. Restrictions by managed care plans of choice of specialists and particular services
Competence	
. Development and use of measures to assess quality of physicians and managed care plans	. Underutilization of specialists and specialized facilities
. Greater use of preventive medical care	. Unreliable and non–risk-adjusted quality measures providing a distorted view of competence
Communication	
. Increased number of generalists and primary care providers	. Productivity requirements creating shorter office visits, reduced telephone access, and other access barriers to physicians
. Creation of physician–nonphysician provider teams to provide a broader range of providers knowledgeable about the patient's condition	. Adversiting creating inflated patient expectations
Compassion	
	. Less time for interaction with patients during stressful decisions
Continuity	
	. Price competition forcing patient choice of continuity at a higher price vs the cheapest plan
	. "Deselection" of physicians disrupting existing physician-patient relations
	. Frequent changes by employer of managed care plans forcing changes of physician
(No) Conflict of Interest	
	. Linking physician salary incentives and bonuses to reduced used of tests and procedures for patients

these quality indicators. While such extensive efforts at quality assessment in medicine have never before been undertaken and there is skepticism that these measures will be reliable and valid, if this effort is successful, many Americans will have a rigorous and systematic mechanism to evaluate the competence of their health plans and physicians.[7,8]

Besides closer monitoring of quality, other changes could improve physicians' competence and their communication with patients. The pressure created by cost controls, the resource-based relative value scale, and managed care has resulted in trends to improve reimbursement for primary care and to train more generalists. Although these initiatives are untested, they could increase the number of generalists, prompt the retraining of specialists in general medicine, and decrease the excessive reliance on specialists with their tendency toward higher use of diagnostic tests and technical interventions without notable effect on traditional health status measures.[9,10] In addition, managed care's increased emphasis on primary care will accelerate the trend toward greater use of nurse practitioners, physician assistants, and midwives and teams composed of physicians and nonphysician providers. While the transition to such a team approach could not be accomplished instantaneously, and while it would require changing habits and increased communications among health care providers, research demonstrates that, when it is well implemented, it can improve patient care, communication, and satisfaction.[11-13] With such multidisciplinary teams, several providers are knowledgeable about the patient's condition and available to the patient, enhancing communication and continuity of care.[11-12] By increasing the number of providers for a patient, this team approach may increase the chances that patients with different cultural backgrounds might establish rapport and understanding with a provider.[11,12]

Potential Threats

There are aspects of managed care, especially under significant cost controls and price competition, with the potential to undermine, or preclude the realization of, the ideal physician-patient relationship. The spread of managed care is being promoted by big employers and corporations; it is closely linked to price competition—if not outright managed competition—which has ramifications for almost every facet of the ideal physician-patient interaction.

First, to hold down costs, many insurance companies and managed care organizations may try to select enrollees who are likely to use fewer and cheaper services ("cherry pick") through selective marketing, increased use of exclusions, modifications of benefits offered, and other techniques. In the absence of significant health insurance regulatory reform legislation or universal coverage, such techniques could mean that more Americans will be unable to afford health insurance or effectively barred from coverage. Indeed, recent statistics suggest that the ranks of the uninsured are growing.[14] In turn, this deprives more Americans of the ideal physician-patient relationship. In addition, without insurance reform legislation to ensure transportability of health coverage when people change jobs, a significant number of Americans could be forced either to forgo coverage for periods of time or to change managed care plans with each job change. Given that 7 million Americans change jobs or become employed each month, there could be significant disruption of choice, communication, and continuity.

Second, to restrain costs, a growing number of employers are restricting patient choice in all its facets.[15–19] An increasing number of employers are offering only one health care plan; other employers are requiring their workers to enroll in a particular managed care plan or select a physician from a pre-certified list; still others are requiring their workers to pay substantially more for the opportunity to see a physician of their choosing outside their managed care panel; and still others are discouraging workers from selecting higher priced health plans. Some employers are even reverting to an old practice of hiring their own "company" physicians.[19] Through these and other techniques, a growing, albeit unknown, number of insured Americans are having their choice limited mainly by employers.[15] These practices may seriously disrupt, or require patients to abandon, long-standing relationships with physicians. In addition, in some instances, especially in managed care settings, patient choice of specialists, specialty facilities, and particular treatments is being eroded.[20]

Increasingly, managed care plans will compete for employers' contracts and subscribers on the basis of price. Yet there is no guarantee that the cheapest plan this year will be the cheapest plan during the next enrollment period. Indeed, if price competition is effective, the cheapest plan should change from year to year.[21] In such a price-competitive marketplace, employers may switch health care plans from year to year and patients may be forced to choose between continuing with their current physician and managed care plan at a higher price or switching to the cheaper plan. While patients may appear to opt for discontinuous care rather than pay more, the cost pressures—which fall disproportionately on those with lower incomes—hardly make such choices voluntary.[22–24] A recent study demonstrates a direct linear relationship between a lower family income and willingness to switch to cheaper health care plans.[15] The importance of such decisions lies in the reason for change of physician.[21] Change is harmful if it is imposed on patients explicitly or implicitly by financial incentives and interrupts continuity. When the patient, however, decides to switch physicians, continuity of care has been outweighed in the patient's mind by other factors, such as competence or communication. Consequently, significant price competition, while not engendered by managed care, is certainly exacerbated by it and could have an adverse effect on both patient choice of practice type and physician and continuity of care.[15,21]

A third threat to choice in the physician-patient relationship comes from the potential financial failure of managed care plans. If price competition is effective, inefficient plans will lose in the marketplace and close. Plan failure could pose a serious threat to patient choice and continuity of care, especially if the collapse happens between enrollment periods. Under such conditions, patients may be randomly assigned to other managed care plans. Or, their former physician may become affiliated with a plan that they are unable to join. Another threat to the physician-patient relationship may occur when managed care plans "deselect" a physician. In such circumstances, patients cannot choose that physician unless they are willing to go out of the plan. More important, patients who have been receiving care from that physician may be forced to switch to another physician in the managed care panel, again undermining patient choice and continuity of care.

Managed care also poses potential threats to competence. Its greater emphasis on the provision of primary care could adversely affect competence. Since specialists are more expensive than generalists, cost considerations foster a tendency to have generalists or even nonphysicians manage conditions that are best handled by specialists. For example, follow-up of cancer patients may be shifted from oncologists to primary care physicians. And there is some suggestion that these changes lead to fewer follow-up visits and less monitoring of the progress of disease in the managed care setting.[25] In addition, since time spent with specialists is expensive, there may be a tendency to use medications or other less expensive interventions in place of consultations with specialists.[26] Similarly, given the current shortage of generalists, there is already a movement to retrain specialist physicians as generalists. Since there are no standards for the amount and type of education needed for retraining, these retrained specialists may lack the breadth of knowledge, skills, and experience necessary to be competent primary care providers. Assessments of quality outcomes may be insensitive to these threats to competence.[27]

There are worries about the development of quality indicators. We lack quality indicators for most aspects of medical care. In addition, many quality indicators require risk adjustments for severity of illness that cannot be, or currently are not being, performed.[27,28] It will take significant time and resources to develop reliable and validated quality indicators and risk adjusters for medical procedures. Yet the demand for these indicators could result in a rush to implementation without proper pretesting and validation. Mistakes related to the imperative to release of Medicare hospital mortality data as a quality measure before they were properly adjusted may be repeated on an even larger scale.[29-32] Use of faulty quality information could damage attempts to improve the competence of physicians, undermine patient trust, and cause patients to switch physicians unnecessarily.

Communication in the physician-patient relationship could be undermined by practice efficiencies necessitated by intensified price competition and financial pressures on managed care plans. Productivity requirements may translate into pressure on physicians to see more patients in shorter time periods, reducing the time to discuss patient values, alternative treatments, or the impact of a therapy on the patient's overall life.[33,34] Such changes have been tried by managed care plans in the competitive Boston, Mass, health care market.[35] Compressing physician-patient interactions into short time periods in the name of productivity could curtail, if not eliminate, productive communication and compassion. A recent survey of patients in managed care plans showed that the physician spent less time with the patient and offered less explanation of care compared with those in traditional fee-for-service settings.[20] Similarly, to reduce costs, managed care plans might restrict telephone calls to the patient's primary care physician. Currently some plans limit patients' calls to their physicians to 1-hour time periods in the day. In addition, incentives might be put into place to encourage patients to talk with or see physicians or nonphysician providers with whom they are unfamiliar or who are not of their choosing.[26] All of these cost-saving mechanisms could easily inhibit physician-patient communication and continuity of care.

A further problem may arise in the competition among managed care plans to lure subscribers. They are likely to use advertising with implicit if not explicit promises of higher quality or more wide-ranging services. Such advertisements could easily create high expectations on the part of patients.[36–38] Simultaneously, however, to control costs plans will require physicians to be efficient in their personal time allocation as well as in their ordering of tests and use of other services. This could easily create a conflict between patient expectations and physician restrictions, undermining good communication, compassion, and trust.

Finally, while there has been significant attention on conflict of interest in fee-for-service practice,[39] there has been much less effort to investigate and address conflict of interest in managed care. Physician decision making may account for as much as 75% of health care costs. In the setting of significant price competition, managed care plans trying to reduce costs will therefore try to influence physician decision making, especially to reduce the use of medical services.[33] Managed care plans have already tried various mechanisms to try to reduce physician use of health care resources for their patients, including providing bonuses to physicians who order few tests and basing a percentage of physicians' salaries on volume and test ordering standards.[33,39,40] Such conflicts of interest may proliferate with increased price competition, the need for managed care plans to reduce costs, and the absence of governmental regulation.

Conclusions

The physician-patient relationship is the cornerstone for achieving, maintaining, and improving health. The structure of financing and regulation should be designed to foster and support an ideal relationship between the physician and the patient. Clearly, the current system incompletely realizes this ideal even for many well-insured Americans, and trends within the current system threaten to make this ideal even more elusive.

Managed care offers some advantages in realizing the ideal physician-patient relationship. For many Americans, increased use of managed care may secure choice, especially for preventive services, possibly expand continuity in their relationship with physicians, and implement a systematic assessment of quality and competence. But the expansion of managed care, in an environment that encourages competition and makes financial pressures intense and omnipresent, could promote serious impediments to realizing the ideal physician-patient relationship. Some practical steps that might diminish these impediments include (1) using global budgets instead of price competition among managed care plans for cost control; (2) prohibiting all schemes that use salary incentives or bonuses tied to physician test ordering patterns; (3) restricting expensive advertising by managed care plans by capping their promotion budgets; (4) requiring managed care plans to have a board of patients and physicians to approve policies regarding length of office visits and telephone calls: (5) creating an independent review board to assess the reliability and validity of all quality indicators before they are approved or required for use by managed care plans; (6) implementing insurance reform legislation to ensure mobility of insurance with job changes and purchasing of coverage by individuals; and (7) providing universal coverage to enable otherwise uninsured patients to have an opportunity for an ideal physician-patient relationship. As changes in our health care system develop, we must find ways, such as these, to encourage fiscal prudence without undermining the fundamental elements of the ideal physician-patient relationship.

References

1. Igelhart JK. The struggle between managed care and fee for service practice. *N Engl J Med.* 1994;331:63–67.
2. *Effects of Managed Care: An Update.* Washington, DC: Congressional Budget Office; 1994.
3. *Managed Health Care: Effects on Employers' Costs Difficult to Measure.* Washington, DC: US General Accounting Office; 1993.
4. Bernstein AB, Thompson GB, Harlan LC. Differences in rates of cancer screening by usual source of medical care: data from the 1987 National Health Interview Survey. *Med Care.* 1991;29:196–209.
5. Retchin SM, Brown B. The quality of ambulatory care in Medicare health maintenance organizations. *Am J Public Health.* 1990;80:411–415.
6. Udvarhelyi IS, Jennison K, Phillips RS, Epstein AM. Comparison of the quality of ambulatory care for fee-for-service and prepaid patients. *Ann Intern Med.* 1991;327:424–429.
7. Laffel G, Berwick DM. Quality in health care. *JAMA.* 1992;268:407–409.
8. Kritchevsky SB, Simmons BP. Continuous quality improvement: concepts and applications for physician care. *JAMA.* 1991;266:1817–1823.
9. Greenfield S, Nelson EC, Zubkoff M, et al. Variations in resource utilization among medical specialties and systems of care. *JAMA.* 1992;267:1624–1630.
10. Schroeder SA, Sandy LG. Specialty distribution of U.S. physicians—the invisible driver of health care costs. *N Engl J Med.* 1993; 328:961–963.
11. *Nurse Practitioners, Physicians' Assistants, and Certified Nurse Midwives: Policy Analysis.* Washington, DC: Office of Technology Assessment; 1986.
12. Freund C. Research in support of nurse practitioners. In: Mezey M, McGivern D, eds. *Nurses and Nurse Practitioners: The Evolution to Advanced Practice.* New York, NY: Springer Publishing Co Inc; 1993.
13. Kavesh W. Physician and nurse-practitioner relationships. In: Mezey M, McGivern D, eds. *Nurses and Nurse Practitioners: The Evolution to Advanced Practice.* New York, NY: Springer Publishing Co Inc; 1993.
14. Pear R. Health insurance percentage is lowest in four Sun Belt states. *New York Times.* October 6, 1994:A16.
15. The Kaiser/Commonwealth Fund Second National Health Insurance Survey. November 10, 1993.
16. Lewis DE. Coping without coverage. *Boston Globe.* May 5, 1993:53.
17. Lewis DE. Union oks Boston gas accord. *Boston Globe.* May 5, 1993:53.
18. Seitz R. The political tea leaves point to medical networks. *New York Times.* December 20, 1992: D10.
19. Pasternak J. In-house doctors give some firms a health care remedy. *Los Angeles Times.* July 11, 1993:A1.

20. Blendon RJ, Knox RA, Brodie M, Benson JM, Chervinsky G. Americans compare managed care, Medicare, and fee for service. *J Am Health Policy.* 1994;4:42–47.
21. Emanuel EJ, Brett AS. Managed competition and the patient-physician relationship. *N Engl J Med.* 1993;329;879–882.
22. Travis MR, Russell G, Cronin S. Determinants of voluntary disenrollment. *J Health Care Marketing.* 1989;9:75–76.
23. Hennelly VD, Boxerman SB. Out-of-plan use and disenrollment: outgrowths of dissatisfaction with a prepaid group plan. *Med Care.* 1983;21:348–359.
24. Sorenson AA, Wersinger RP. Factors influencing disenrollment from an HMO. *Med Care.* 1981;19:766–773.
25. Clement DG, Retchin SM, Brown RS, Stegall MH. Access and outcomes of elderly patients enrolled in managed care. *JAMA.* 1994;271:1487–1492.
26. Henneberger M. Managed care changing practice of psychotherapy. *New York Times.* October 9, 1994:A1, A50.
27. Salem-Schatz S, Moore G, Rucker M, Pearson SD. The case for case-mix adjustment in practice profiling: when good apples look bad. *JAMA.* 1994;272:871–874.
28. McNeil BJ, Pederson SH, Gatsonis C. Current issues in profiling quality of care. *Inquiry.* 1992;29:298–307.
29. Green J, Passman LJ, Wintfield N. Analyzing hospital mortality: the consequences of diversity in patient mix. *JAMA.* 1991;265:1849–1853.
30. Burke M. HCFA's Medicare mortality data: the controversy continues. *Hospitals.* 1992:118, 120, 122.
31. Greenfield S, Aronow HU, Elashoff RM, Wantanabe D. Flaws in mortality data: the hazards of ignoring comorbid disease. *JAMA.* 1988;260:2253–2255.
32. Robinson ML. Limitations of mortality data confirmed: studies. *Hospitals.* 1988;62:23–24.
33. Baker LC, Cantor JC. Physician satisfaction under managed care. *Health AFF* (Millwood). 1993;12(suppl):258–270.
34. Jellinek MS, Nurcombe B. Two wrongs don't make a right: managed care, mental health, and the marketplace. *JAMA.* 1993;270:1737–1739.
35. Knox RA, Stein C. HMO doctors want boss out in dispute on patient load. *Boston Globe.* November 21, 1991:1, 27.
36. Freidson E. Prepaid group practice and the new 'demanding patients.' *Milbank Mem Fund Q.* 1973;51:473–488.
37. Schroeder JL, Clarke JT, Webster JR. Prepaid entitlements: a new challenge for physician-patient relationships. *JAMA.* 1985;254:3080–3082.
38. Brett AS. The case against persuasive advertising by health maintenance organizations. *N Engl J Med.* 1992;326:1253–1257.
39. Rodwin M. *Medicine, Money, and Morals.* New York, NY: Oxford University Press Inc; 1993.
40. Hillman AL, Pauly MV, Kerstein JJ. How do financial incentives affect physicians' clinical decisions and the financial performance of health maintenance organizations? *N Engl J Med.* 1989;321:86–92.

NO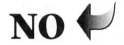

Brendan Minogue

The *Two* Fundamental Duties of the Physician

The Single-Stewardship Model

Until the late 1960s the traditional role of the physician was to secure the medical welfare of his or her patient. The modern notion that the physician's stewardship extends not only to the medical welfare but also to the wishes of the patient is very new. During the long history that preceded the advent of the modern bioethical movement, patients' wishes were treated as secondary to their medical welfare. But this ancient view crashed into the wall of the contemporary bioethics movement. The core of that movement is the notion that the doctor has a deep commitment to secure the wishes and rights of the patient. Patients' autonomy is portrayed not only as valuable in itself but also as necessary for determining what is in the best interests of the individual.[1] However, what is crucial to recognize is that from this perspective, wishes are relevant to the actions of a faithful physician whether they are consistent with the patient's welfare or not. In short, the autonomous individual has a legitimate claim to define what is best for himself or herself as a patient even if the doctor disagrees.

It was difficult for the medical practitioners of the 1960s to admit this criterion into their everyday practice. Nevertheless, it is now common to acknowledge that both clinical science and the autonomy of the individual patient are relevant to the duty of the physician. I refer to this approach as the single-stewardship model because in this view, the individual patient represents the intrinsic value or the highest good of the medical steward. Using this model, the ethical responsibilities of the good physician—and the basis for his or her decision making—are defined exclusively in terms of one consideration: the individual patient. This is at odds with nearly all other areas of life, where individuals—patients and non-patients alike—are recognized as having a variety of considerations influencing their decision making. Should we as a society continue with this single-focus, individual-centered ideal?

The answer is No! Good physicians have an additional obligation. They must balance their duty to the patient with their duty to other stakeholders in

From Brendan Minogue, "The *Two* Fundamental Duties of the Physician," *Academic Medicine*, vol. 75, no. 5 (May 2000). Copyright © 2000 by The Association of American Medical Colleges. Reprinted by permission of *Academic Medicine* and The Association of American Medical Colleges.

the health care system. Physicians, as a matter of fact, *already* follow the dual-stewardship model I am proposing, but many feel guilty about it, and this needs to stop. The argument begins by recognizing a fundamental contradiction between managed health care, in which over 75% of U.S. physicians practice, and the single-stewardship model. Most managed care organizations admit that they do not offer the highest-quality packages of health care services. They do not pretend to offer the best. They do not promise to meet all the wishes of all patients. Rather, most offer decent levels of quality, and *decent* is not equivalent to *the best* or to *all that is wished*. The contradiction emerges here. For if the physician who follows the single-stewardship model must seek only the best or what the patient desires, then it would follow that the majority of physicians are intrinsically unethical. This is a tough pill to swallow. When the ethic of an organization implies that the overwhelming number of practitioners are immoral, then either the ethic of the organization must go or practitioners must be eliminated from the profession. In this article I propose a way to revise the ethic.

One possible revision involves changing the physician's duty into a promise to provide what is best for the patient within the limits of the system. In this revised version the system clearly sets the limits for what is a decent level of health care, and the doctor merely administers these limits. The doctor is innocent of any violation of his or her stewardship if the limits of the health care system do not maximize the health interests of the patient. He or she is, after all, a mere administrator of limits that are set by others.

However, this retreat to defining the physician as an administrative bureaucrat is catastrophic. For example, if a patient needs itraconozole for a fungal infection, and if that medication is not part of the preferred drug formulary, then the physician's duty is discharged merely by writing the prescription and informing the patient that it is not covered. In this scenario, the doctor is a mere administrator of the managed care formulary, not a patient advocate.[2]

What is troublesome about this revised view of the physician as administrator is that it is exactly like the single-stewardship model. In both models the physician is *unidimensional*. In the first model, all the physician needs to know is the latest from the clinical journals that can help the patient; questions of cost are treated as ethically irrelevant. In the second model, all the physician needs to know is clinical science plus information regarding coverage. In this view, the doctor is nothing but an administrator.

The Dual-Stewardship Model

The dual-stewardship model I advocate rejects both of the above models not only because they are unidimensional but also because they too narrowly define the courage, commitment, and trustworthiness that are essential to medicine. To be an effective advocate of the patient who needs itraconozole involves being a trustworthy agent of both the patient and the managed care system. Both the patient and the managed care system must trust that the physician will not prescribe itraconozole without necessity. Single-stewardship physicians are not and never have been *organizationally* trustworthy, and consequently patients suffer because they often need the organization to pay for medically necessary but expensive treatment. Organizations have duties to hosts of patients, and these duties need to be discharged by individual physicians who are organizationally trustworthy. (On the other hand, physicians singly devoted to being mere administrators are not trustworthy agents of patients.) A thought experiment can clarify the need to include organizational trust within the identity of the doctor. Imagine that physicians were to generally "game the system"[3,4] to secure all the medical wishes and the absolute best care for their patients. The result of such "gaming" would be that the health care system becomes economically unstable. That result would, in turn, harm the patients. In this scenario, the ideal or perfect doctor (practicing single-stewardship medicine) becomes the enemy of the truly good doctor (practicing dual-stewardship medicine).

Practicing dual-stewardship medicine involves a shift away from seeking to fulfill the patient's interests and wishes at any cost toward *seeking the best health-care value for the patient.*[5] The argument for practicing cost-effective medicine is grounded in the notion that a physician should neither try to secure the *absolute* best care for the patient nor try to satisfy all the wishes of the patient. These goals are too high to be meaningful, and when goals are meaningless they are ignored. Rather, as just stated, the duty of the physician is to secure the best value for the patient. By *best value* I mean something that is a function of both cost and quality. A generic antibiotic may have the same outcome as the newest antibiotic off the research tables. But if they differ in cost, they differ in value. If the generic is much less expensive while therapeutically equivalent to the new antibiotic, then it has a greater value for the patient. Of course, if the generic is less expensive but is also less effective, then it also falls in value. Focusing on the best value for the patient rather than on the patient's absolute best interest and autonomy is to transform the health care system into something that inflates normally because it is bounded by limits rather than mistakenly being considered limitless.

This dual-stewardship model replaces the idea that doctors must treat their patients as their only concern with the idea that there are *two* equally high duties of the physician. The physician has a duty to secure both his or her patient's welfare and his or her organization's welfare. The two values compete, and balancing them requires as much artistic skill as that required by the surgeon. This balancing skill is not novel for the physician. When a patient's best interest is at odds with that patient's wishes, physicians sometimes resort to medical art to balance these opposing considerations in order to secure an overall good outcome. Similarly, the physician's duties to the health care system are not always commensurable with the maximum well-being or preferences of the patient. Patients often autonomously wish for things that are incompatible with the best interests of the system as a whole. The easy examples are the cosmetic surgeries or the unnecessary diagnostic procedures that may psychologically benefit the patient but threaten the health care system. Harder examples involve last-chance therapies and experimental protocols.

Two Criticisms

We can further explore this idea of dual stewardship by addressing two criticisms of it. The first criticism is that such a change will undermine patients' confidence in physicians. That is, if we as a society permit physicians to take the system into consideration when making health care decisions, then patients will lose trust in their physicians. One can imagine a patient responding to his or her doctor's prescription for an antibiotic with the following question: "Doctor, is this the cheapest or the best antibiotic?"

This criticism contains a hidden assumption. It assumes that any increase in distrust would harm overall patient outcomes. But there is a growing body of evidence that indicates that a little more distrust may have had an overall beneficial result on patient outcomes. For example, one report[6] indicates that nearly 30% of the surgeries carried out in fee-for-service health care were unnecessary. A little increase in patient distrust might have diminished the appalling harm that flowed from these unnecessary and often iatrogenic services. Furthermore, physicians often ignore the large number of unnecessary, expensive diagnostic procedures[7] because they hurt only *payers.*

Surely trust in the physician is the most effective placebo in the arsenal of medicine, but a reasonable level of trust is compatible with a reasonable level of distrust. Trust is not like pregnancy. It comes in degrees, and patients understand this. Patients' expectations of the physician are simply not as childlike as the single-stewardship model presumes. Many health care services are beneficial but too expensive, and refusing to cover these services is permissible so long as one has not promised otherwise. Health maintenance organizations (HMOs) create formularies to clarify their promises. These indicate that they will not pay for some pharmaceutical products even though they may offer clinical advantages. Single-stewardship physicians are deeply troubled by this, since they are ethically forbidden to do anything but what is best for their patients.

For physicians who have this patient-only focus, it is not surprising that payers' needs are not even on their radar screens. But it is precisely this attitude of treating the individual patient as more valuable than the health care system that has brought the fee-for-service health care system to the end of its institutional life. When payers feel that their legitimate needs for resources to sustain their institutions must be sacrificed to the needs of the health care provider, then reason requires revolution. In short, what is most troubling about the single-stewardship model is that it perfectly justifies spending unlimited amounts of resources to eliminate even the smallest risk. This follows because the physician, the central figure in medicine, is structurally forbidden by his or her ethics to be concerned about the health of the system.

In response to this reluctance on the part of single-stewardship physicians to take costs seriously and play the role of rational distributors of scarce resources, the health care system has expanded to include an entirely new health profession, the case manager. This new and expensive profession does not provide any patient care and adds to the cost of the system. Its only job is to resist the single-stewardship physicians! Because physicians, who logically should play the case-manager role, have steadfastly balked at playing it, the bureaucracy of medicine has grown into a nightmare of inefficiency and often delayed necessary treatment. Acceptance of the dual-stewardship model will lead to the elimination of these administratively needed but medically unnecessary professions. To be a doctor is to serve two inextricably related masters. The case manager's role should be incorporated into the very identity of the physician.

The second criticism of the dual-stewardship model is that once it is accepted, the scope of the physician's commitment will be so extensive that it will permit and justify gag clauses to inhibit free and open communication between patients and physicians. Physicians' contracts with HMOs have often contained these gag clauses, which prohibit the physician from engaging in conversation that may economically harm the HMO. Here is an actual example of such a clause: "The physician shall not say anything to the enrollees that could weaken the confidence of the enrollees in the managed care plan."[8] *From the perspective of the plan,* the goal of these clauses is to protect the economic interests and proprietary information of the plan.

Both public and private managed care plans tend to view themselves as businesses, and as such they claim the traditional right to expect that their employees or other agents will be loyal to the economic interests of stakeholders (the citizenry, if public; the investors, if private). *From the perspective of the patient and the provider,* such clauses often increase nondisclosure, thereby undermining patients' understanding of their options, and may weaken the capacity of physicians to secure the medical welfare and wishes of their patients. Because gag clauses inhibit free and informed consent, they undermine the patient's welfare and autonomy.[9]

Shifting from a single- to a dual-stewardship model does not, however, require that we support the gag clause. The central theme of the dual-stewardship model is that the physician will value the health system as well as the patient. With such an approach, the physician will not feel he has a right to "game the system" to satisfy the wishes or interests of the patient. The tendency to "massage" a diagnosis in order to accomplish what the patient wants is something that weakens the power of the HMO to accomplish its fundamental goal. That goal, as stated in much of the managed care legislation of the 1970s and 1980s, was to maximize distribution of a decent level of health care by reducing medical inflation. The physician who is a dual steward understands and supports that goal, and while the dual-stewardship role prohibits the massaging of diagnoses and other such deceptions, this does not require that the physician deliberately withhold relevant information. Alternative treatments may not be covered or fully covered by an HMO, and learning this may indeed disappoint the patient. Furthermore, this limitation on types of treatments may diminish a patient's satisfaction, but that is common whenever treatments, their costs, and their availability are being weighed. Few patients believe that signing an HMO contract involves a promise to fund everything. Patients are consumers, and as such they select among competing HMOs. Such tradeoffs are compatible with free communication among physicians and patients.

A Difficult Question

Now we come to the difficult question of what it means to say that the duty of the physician is to secure the best value for a patient within a third-party payer system such as an HMO. HMOs come in a variety of forms. Some are "for-profit," some are private "not-for-profit," while others are "government sponsored." Often critics believe that it is only the "for-profit" HMOs that need to be opposed, as if profit were something unethical that soils everything that it touches. What is important to recognize is that the dual-stewardship model does not aim to defend "for-profit" managed care. Rather, in this model the question of profit is irrelevant, since the determination of best value is the central goal of the physician. This is something to be determined by multiplying the quality of the medical service by its cost. It does not matter whether the HMO is a for-profit or a not-for-profit or a government agency. What matters is to increase value for the patient. This is a function not only of the physician's taking dual-stewardship duties seriously to achieve the best value, but also a function of how well the particular HMO strives for the best value. If stockholders can produce the best value, then dual-stewardship physicians should side with them. If "not-for-profit" approaches secure maximum value, then they win the value war. If the government can best decrease costs and increase quality, then it is the best means of securing value. My own bias is that a mixture of all three types of HMOs will yield maximum medical value over time. The jury is still out on the solution to this challenging problem. But in all of these scenarios, physicians have a dual rather than a single stewardship role.

Of course, patients do often want their physicians to treat them as if money were irrelevant. What is comforting to recognize is that all three HMO types refuse to accommodate this desire. All three reject the adolescent idea that the doctor's role is to secure the absolute best interests and wishes of the patient, period. All three hold that achieving the best value for the patient is the duty of the physician.

Are the hundreds of thousands of physicians who interact with HMOs immoral for taking HMO costs seriously? If we accept the single-stewardship view of the physician, then answer is yes! But if we reject that view and accept the new vision of the physician's duty, then the common behavior of hundreds of thousands of physicians becomes consistent with our image of the good physician. The good physician is not someone for whom cost of care is irrelevant, but neither is he or she unconcerned about the practices of the HMO. Reasonable medicine is often sacrificed for short-term benefits to the HMO, and this is why physicians' commitment to patients requires that they constantly monitor their HMOs to determine that their practice guidelines and drug formularies secure a reasonably decent level of health care. For while such physicians are legitimate agents of the HMO, they are also agents of the patients they serve, and this dual relationship means that they both support and resist the HMOs in which they practice. Ideally, they would seek to transform a problem HMO into one where both it and the physician could find optimal ways to achieve best value for their patients.

The dual-stewardship role is consistent with the idea that conflicts among the HMO, the physician, and the patient are inevitable. What are the duties of the physician in such conflicts? The first duty is avoid "gaming the system" by distorting the medical facts to secure additional services for their patients. That is the physician's primary commitment to the HMO. The second duty is to share with patients information about the full range of procedures, medications, and services available within and without the HMO. A physician who allows himself or herself to be gagged by the HMO and thus prevented from sharing medically relevant information with the patient has given up the ideal of balancing one's duty to the patient with one's duty to the HMO and instead treats the commitment to the patient as little more than a commitment to the financial integrity of the HMO. A gagged physician becomes the exclusive agent of the HMO rather than someone who faces the more daunting challenge of balancing the good of the patient with the good of the HMO. If a physician believes that an HMO could offer a better value to a patient, then he is obligated to advocate this better value. If an experimental protocol, for example, offers the best chance for life to a patient, and the HMO does not cover this protocol, then there is a clear duty on the part of the physician to inform the patient of this alternative. But there should be no attempt on the part of the physician to secure this protocol by any form of deceptive interpretation of the disease.

. . . [L]et me state what dual-stewardship physicians cannot do. They cannot guarantee that a decent minimum of health care will be available to everyone. Because a plumber is efficiently offering plumbing services for sale, he or she does not guarantee that plumbing will be available to everyone. All the plumber promises are values to those who can afford his or her services. HMOs and the demands that they make on physicians to practice dual-stewardship medicine have not provided a decent level of health care to all U.S. citizens. Forty-five million people in our nation still have no access to medical coverage. As of now, the United States has not decided to treat health care as a right. However, what the dual-stewardship model makes possible is an opportunity to provide a reasonable level of medical care at a cost that does not irrationally inflate the health care system beyond the inflation occurring within other typical sectors of the economy. If the government ever decides to extend coverage to the uninsured, then this extension will not involve offering to everyone the kind of entitlement that could dangerously hyper-inflate the health care system.

References

1. Beauchamp TL, Childress JF. Principles of Biomedical Ethics. 4th ed. New York: Oxford University Press,1994 .
2. Brodell R. Ethics and managed care. Arch Dermatol.1996; 132:1013.
3. Morreim EH. Gaming the system, dodging the rules, ruling the dodgers. Arch Intern Med.1991; 151:443-7.
4. Morreim EH. Balancing Act: The New Medical Ethics of Medicine's New Economies. Washington, DC: Georgetown University Press, 1995.
5. Buchanan A. Managed care: rationing without justice, but not unjustly. J Health Politics, Policy, and Law. 1998; 23:617-33.

6. Chassin MR, Kosecoff JK, Park RE. Does inappropriate use explain geographic variations in the use of health care services. JAMA. 1987; 258:2533–7.
7. Hillman BJ, Joseph CA, Mabry MR. Frequency and cost of diagnostic imaging in office practice: a comparison of self-referring and radiologist-referring physicians. N Engl J Med.1990; 323:1604–8.
8. American Medical News. February 19,1996; 39:15 .
9. American Medical Association, Council on Ethical and Judicial Affairs. Ethical issues in managed care. JAMA. 1995; 273:300–5.

POSTSCRIPT

Should Patient-Centered Medical Ethics Govern Managed Care?

In June 2000 the U.S. Supreme Court ruled that HMOs that offer financial incentives to doctors to hold down costs are not liable in federal courts for violating a duty to put patients first. The case at issue involved a patient who suffered a burst appendix when her HMO made her wait eight days for tests to diagnose her abdominal pain. The Court's ruling left such lawsuits in the jurisdiction of state courts, while referring to Congress a political decision on patients' rights. Both political parties have offered versions of patients' rights bills, but none has passed.

Donald W. Light provides an overview of the American health care system, beginning with early corporate practices in the late nineteenth century and ending with the rise of managed care, in "The Restructuring of the American Health Care System," in Theodore Litman, ed., *Health Politics and Policy,* 3rd ed. (Delmare, 1997). A historical perspective is also part of a comprehensive analysis of managed care by John C. Fletcher and Carolyn L. Engelhard in "Ethical Issues in Managed Care: A Report of the University of Virginia Study Group of Managed Care," *Virginia Medical Quarterly* (vol. 122, no. 3, 1995).

An entire issue of *American Journal of Law and Medicine* (vol. 22, nos. 2 and 3, 1996) is devoted to "Health Care Capitated Systems." See also Mark A. Hall, "Rationing Health Care at the Bedside," *New York University Law Review* (October–November 1994). To assess patient response to the changing health care environment, Karen Davis et al. surveyed patient satisfaction with managed care. They report their findings in "Choice Matters: Enrollees' Views of Their Health Plans," *Health Affairs* (Summer 1995). In an editorial entitled "Managing Care—Should We Adopt a New Ethic?" *The New England Journal of Medicine* (August 6, 1998), editor Jerome P. Kassirer warns against "capitulating to an ethic of the group rather than the individual . . . and allow[ing] market forces to distort our ethical standards." Another physician, Eric J. Cassell, believes that putting "payer" between "doctor" and "patient" distorts the process of care. See "The Future of the Doctor-Payer-Patient Relationship," *Journal of the American Geriatrics Society* (March 1998). A survey of physicians conducted in 1997 found that only 17 percent believed that financial incentives to limit services are ethically acceptable, and 80 percent believed that changes in the health care system have diminished physicians' undivided loyalty to patients. See Daniel P. Sulmasy, et al., "Physicians' Ethical Beliefs About Cost-Control Arrangements," *Archives of Internal Medicine* (March 13, 2000).

ISSUE 20

Should There Be a Market in Body Parts?

YES: J. Radcliffe-Richards et al., from "The Case for Allowing Kidney Sales," *The Lancet* (June 27, 1998)

NO: David J. Rothman, from "The International Organ Traffic," *The New York Review of Books* (March 26, 1998)

ISSUE SUMMARY

YES: Philosopher J. Radcliff-Richards and colleagues of the International Forum for Transplant Ethics contend that bans on selling organs remove the only hope of the destitute and the dying. Arguments against selling organs are weak attempts to justify the repugnance felt by people who are rich or healthy.

NO: Historian David J. Rothman asserts that trafficking in organs for transplantation is motivated by greed and subverts the ethical principles of the medical profession.

Human organ transplantation, unachievable at mid-century and still experimental a few decades ago, has now become routine. Dr. Joseph E. Murray of Brigham and Women's Hospital in Boston performed the first successful kidney transplant in 1954. By the 1980s livers, hearts, pancreases, lungs, and heart-lungs had also been successfully transplanted. Surgical techniques, as well as methods for preserving and transporting organs, had improved over the years. But the most significant advance came from a single drug, cyclosporine, discovered by Jean Borel in the mid-1970s and approved by the Food and Drug Administration in 1983. Cyclosporine suppresses the immune system so that the organ recipient's body does not reject the transplanted organ. However, the drug does not suppress the body's ability to fight infection from other sources.

This achievement has its darker side in that there is a shortage of transplantable organs and many seriously ill people wait for months to receive one. Some die before one becomes available. In 1996 almost 4,000 people on waiting lists died while waiting to receive an organ. According to the United Network of Organ Sharing (UNOS), the national agency responsible for allocating organs, on January 6, 1999, there were 60,656 patients waiting for transplants. Over 40,000 of these patients were waiting for kidney transplants, and over 11,000 for liver transplants. The next highest categories were heart transplants (over 4,000) and lung transplants (over 3,000).

By contrast, the UNOS data show that in 1997 only 10,045 transplants were performed, with kidney alone transplants leading the list. (Double kidney, lung, and heart-lung transplants were counted as one transplant.) Of the 11,470 kidney alone transplants, 3,700 came from living donors, and the rest were from the recently deceased. Living donors are almost always relatives of the recipient. Like any surgery, transplantation presents risks to the donor but these are usually not grave. A person can live with one kidney, although should that kidney fail, the donor would require regular dialysis (cleansing the blood of toxic substances through a machine) or a transplant.

The shortage of transplantable organs in the U.S. is attributed to many factors: the reluctance of families to approve donation after death, even if the donor has indicated the desire to do so; the reluctance of medical personnel to approach families at a time of crisis; religious objections; and mistrust of the medical system. Despite many educational programs and publicity about donation, Americans seem unwilling either to move to a system of required request (mandated in a few states) or to presume that potential donors would agree to having their organs used for transplantation, unless they had explicitly consented in advance.

The shortage of organs is acute in the United States, but is even more acute in other parts of the world, where cultural or religious objections to removing organs from the deceased remain strong. Organ transplantation is one area in which "technology transfer"—the export of the science and training for the procedure—has been particularly strong. Organ transplant centers have grown rapidly in areas of the world that lack even basic public health measures. However, although some countries have the technology for transplantation, they do not have enough organs to meet the demand.

Thus the question of selling organs arises mostly in the international context. In the United States, the National Organ Transplant Act (Public Law 98-507), passed in 1984, made it illegal to buy and sell organs. Violators are subject to fines and imprisonment. Congress passed this law because it was concerned that traffic in organs might lead to inequitable access to donor organs with the wealthy having an unfair advantage. (Even with the ban, the wealthy have an advantage in being able to pay for the transplant and the necessary post-transplant supportive services, and thus are more likely to be accepted for a waiting list.)

Although many countries and international medical organizations officially ban the sale of organs as well, the practice goes on. The following selections present opposing views on whether the ban should be reexamined or more aggressively implemented. J. Radcliff-Richards and other members of the International Forum for Transplant Ethics favor reexamining the arguments against the commercialization of organ transplantation. They maintain that the ban unfairly punishes both the destitute (whose only hope is selling an organ) and the dying (whose only hope is obtaining one). David J. Rothman sees the burgeoning traffic in human organs as evidence not only of the exploitation of the poor but of greed and a subversion of medical ethics.

J. Radcliffe-Richards et al.

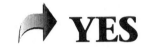
YES

The Case for Allowing Kidney Sales

When the practice of buying kidneys from live vendors first came to light some years ago, it aroused such horror that all professional associations denounced it[1,2] and nearly all countries have now made it illegal.[3] Such political and professional unanimity may seem to leave no room for further debate, but we nevertheless think it important to reopen the discussion.

The well-known shortage of kidneys for transplantation causes much suffering and death.[4] Dialysis is a wretched experience for most patients, and is anyway rationed in most places and simply unavailable to the majority of patients in most developing countries.[5] Since most potential kidney vendors will never become unpaid donors, either during life or posthumously, the prohibition of sales must be presumed to exclude kidneys that would otherwise be available. It is therefore essential to make sure that there is adequate justification for the resulting harm.

Most people will recognise in themselves the feelings of outrage and disgust that led to an outright ban on kidney sales, and such feelings typically have a force that seems to their possessors to need no further justification. Nevertheless, if we are to deny treatment to the suffering and dying we need better reasons than our own feelings of disgust.

In this [selection] we outline our reasons for thinking that the arguments commonly offered for prohibiting organ sales do not work, and therefore that the debate should be reopened.[6,7] Here we consider only the selling of kidneys by living vendors, but our arguments have wider implications.

The commonest objection to kidney selling is expressed on behalf of the vendors: the exploited poor, who need to be protected against the greedy rich. However, the vendors are themselves anxious to sell,[8] and see this practice as the best option open to them. The worse we think the selling of a kidney, therefore, the worse should seem the position of the vendors when that option is removed. Unless this appearance is illusory, the prohibition of sales does even more harm than first seemed, in harming vendors as well as recipients. To this argument it is replied that the vendors' apparent choice is not genuine. It is said that they are likely to be too uneducated to understand the risks, and that this precludes informed consent. It is also claimed that, since they are coerced by their economic circumstances, their consent cannot count as genuine.[9]

From J. Radcliffe-Richards, A. S. Daar, R. D. Guttmann, R. Hoffenberg, I. Kennedy, M. Lock, R. A. Sells, and N. Tilney, "The Case for Allowing Kidney Sales," *The Lancet,* vol. 351 (June 27, 1998), pp. 1950–1952. Copyright © 1998 by The Lancet, Ltd. Reprinted by permission.

Although both these arguments appeal to the importance of autonomous choice, they are quite different. The first claim is that the vendors are not competent to make a genuine choice within a given range of options. The second, by contrast, is that poverty has so restricted the range of options that organ selling has become the best, and therefore, in effect, that the range is too small. Once this distinction is drawn, it can be seen that neither argument works as a justification of prohibition.[7]

If our ground for concern is that the range of choices is too small, we cannot improve matters by removing the best option that poverty has left, and making the range smaller still. To do so is to make subsequent choices, by this criterion, even less autonomous. The only way to improve matters is to lessen the poverty until organ selling no longer seems the best option; and if that could be achieved, prohibition would be irrelevant because nobody would want to sell.

The other line of argument may seem more promising, since ignorance does preclude informed consent. However, the likely ignorance of the subjects is not a reason for banning altogether a procedure for which consent is required. In other contexts, the value we place on autonomy leads us to insist on information and counselling, and that is what it should suggest in the case of organ selling as well. It may be said that this approach is impracticable, because the educational level of potential vendors is too limited to make explanation feasible, or because no system could reliably counteract the misinformation of nefarious middlemen and profiteering clinics. But even if we accepted that no possible vendor could be competent to consent, that would justify only putting the decision in the hands of competent guardians. To justify total prohibition it would also be necessary to show that organ selling must always be against the interests of potential vendors, and it is most unlikely that this would be done.

The risk involved in nephrectomy is not in itself high, and most people regard it as acceptable for living related donors.[10] Since the procedure is, in principle, the same for vendors as for unpaid donors, any systematic difference between the worthwhileness of the risk for vendors and donors presumably lies on the other side of the calculation, in the expected benefit. Nevertheless the exchange of money cannot in itself turn an acceptable risk into an unacceptable one from the vendor's point of view. It depends entirely on what the money is wanted for.

In general, furthermore, the poorer a potential vendor, the more likely it is that the sale of a kidney will be worth whatever risk there is. If the rich are free to engage in dangerous sports for pleasure, or dangerous jobs for high pay, it is difficult to see why the poor who take the lesser risk of kidney selling for greater rewards—perhaps saving relatives' lives,[11] or extricating themselves from poverty and debt—should be thought so misguided as to need saving from themselves.

It will be said that this does not take account of the reality of the vendors' circumstances: that risks are likely to be greater than for unpaid donors because poverty is detrimental to health, and vendors are often not given proper care. They may also be underpaid or cheated, or may waste their money through inexperience. However, once again, these arguments apply far more strongly to many other activities by which the poor try to earn money, and which we do not forbid. The best way to address such problems would be by regulation and perhaps a central purchasing system, to provide screening, counselling, reliable payment, insurance, and financial advice.[12]

To this it will be replied that no system of screening and control could be complete, and that both vendors and recipients would always be at risk of exploitation and poor treatment. But all the evidence we have shows that there is much more scope for exploitation and abuse when a supply of desperately wanted goods is made illegal. It is, furthermore, not clear why it should be thought harder to police a legal trade than the present complete ban.

Furthermore, even if vendors and recipients would always be at risk of exploitation, that does not alter the fact that if they choose this option, all alternatives must seem worse to them. Trying to end exploitation by prohibition is rather like ending slum dwelling by bulldozing slums: it ends the evil in that form, but only by making things worse for the victims. If we want to protect the exploited, we can do it only by removing the poverty that makes them vulnerable, or, failing that, by controlling the trade.

Another familiar objection is that it is unfair for the rich to have privileges not available to the poor. This argument, however, is irrelevant to the issue of organ selling as such. If organ selling is wrong for this reason, so are all benefits available to the rich, including all private medicine, and, for that matter, all public provision of medicine in rich countries (including transplantation of donated organs) that is unavailable in poor ones. Furthermore, all purchasing could be done by a central organisation responsible for fair distribution.[12]

It is frequently asserted that organ donation must be altruistic to be acceptable,[13] and that this rules out payment. However, there are two problems with this claim. First, altruism does not distinguish donors from vendors. If a father who saves his daughter's life by giving her a kidney is altruistic, it is difficult to see why his selling a kidney to pay for some other operation to save her life should be thought less so. Second, nobody believes in general that unless some useful action is altruistic it is better to forbid it altogether.

It is said that the practice would undermine confidence in the medical profession, because of the association of doctors with money-making practices. That, however, would be a reason for objecting to all private practice; and in this case the objection could easily be met by the separation of purchasing and treatment. There could, for instance, be independent trusts[12] to fix charges and handle accounts, as well as to ensure fair play and high standards. It is alleged that allowing the trade would lessen the supply of donated cadaveric kidneys.[14] But although some possible donors might decide to sell instead, their organs would be available, so there would be no loss in the total. And in the meantime, many people will agree to sell who would not otherwise donate.

It is said that in parts of the world where women and children are essentially chattels there would be a danger of their being coerced into becoming vendors. This argument, however, would work as strongly against unpaid living kidney donation, and even more strongly against many far more harmful practices which do not attract calls for their prohibition. Again, regulation would provide the most reliable means of protection.

It is said that selling kidneys would set us on a slippery slope to selling vital organs such as hearts. But that argument would apply equally to the case of the unpaid kidney donation, and nobody is afraid that that will result in the donation of hearts. It is entirely feasible to have laws and professional practices that allow the giving or selling only of non-vital organs. Another objection is that allowing organ sales is impossible because it would outrage public opinion. But this claim is about western public opinion: in many potential vendor communities, organ selling is more acceptable than cadaveric donation, and this argument amounts to a claim that other people should follow western cultural preferences rather than their own. There is, anyway, evidence that the western public is far less opposed to the idea, than are medical and political professionals.[15]

It must be stressed that we are not arguing for the positive conclusion that organ sales must always be acceptable, let alone that there should be an unfettered market. Our claim is only that none of the familiar arguments against organ selling works, and this allows for the possibility that better arguments may yet be found.

Nevertheless, we claim that the burden of proof remains against the defenders of prohibition, and that until good arguments appear, the presumption must be that the trade should be regulated rather than banned altogether. Furthermore, even when there are good objections at particular times or in particular places, that should be regarded as a reason for trying to remove the objections, rather than as an excuse for permanent prohibition.

The weakness of the familiar arguments suggests that they are attempts to justify the deep feelings of repugnance which are the real driving force of prohibition, and feelings of repugnance among the rich and healthy, no matter how strongly felt, cannot justify removing the only hope of the destitute and dying. This is why we conclude that the issue should be considered again, and with scrupulous impartiality.

References

1. British Transplantation Society Working Party. Guidelines on living organ donation. *BMJ* 1986; 293: 257–58.
2. The Council of the Transplantation Society. Organ sales. *Lancet* 1985; 2: 715–16.
3. World Health Organization. A report on developments under the auspices of WHO (1987–1991). WHO 1992 Geneva. 12–28.
4. Hauptman PJ, O'Connor KJ. Procurement and allocation of solid organs for transplantation. *N Engl J Med* 1997; 336: 422–31.
5. Barsoum RS. Ethical problems in dialysis and transplantation: Africa. In: Kjellstrand CM, Dossetor JB, eds. Ethical problems in dialysis and transplantation. Kluwer Academic Publishers, Netherlands. 1992: 169–82.
6. Radcliffe-Richards J. Nephrarious goings on: kidney sales and moral arguments. *J Med Philosph.* Netherlands: Kluwer Academic Publishers, 1996; 21: 375–416.
7. Radcliffe-Richards J. From him that hath not. In: Kjellstrand CM, Dossetor JB, eds. Ethical problems in dialysis and transplantation. Netherlands: Kluwer Academic Publishers, 1992: 53–60.
8. Mani MK. The argument against the unrelated live donor, ibid. 164.
9. Sells RA. The case against buying organs and a futures market in transplants. *Trans Proc* 1992; 24: 2198–202.

10. Daar AD, Land W, Yahya TM, Schneewind K, Gutmann T, Jakobsen A. Living-donor renal transplantation: evidence-based justification for an ethical option. *Trans Reviews* (in press) 1997.
11. Dossetor JB, Manickavel V. Commercialisation: the buying and selling of kidneys. In: Kjellstrand CM, Dossetor JB, eds. Ethical problems in dialysis and transplantation. Netherlands: Kluwer Academic Publishers, 1992: 61–71.
12. Sells RA. Some ethical issues in organ retrieval 1982–1992. *Trans Proc* 1992; **24**: 2401–03.
13. Sheil R. Policy statement from the ethics committee of the Transplantation Society. *Trans Soc Bull* 1995; **3**: 3.
14. Altshuler JS, Evanisko MJ. *JAMA* 1992; **267**: 2037.
15. Guttmann RD, Guttmann A. Organ transplantation: duty reconsidered. *Trans Proc* 1992; **24**: 2179–80.

NO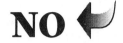

David J. Rothman

The International Organ Traffic

Over the past fifteen years, transplanting human organs has become a standard and remarkably successful medical procedure, giving new life to thousands of people with failing hearts, kidneys, livers, and lungs. But very few countries have sufficient organs to meet patients' needs....

This lack of available organs arouses desperation and rewards greed.... The international commerce in organs is unregulated, indeed anarchic. We know a good deal about trafficking in women and children for sex. We are just beginning to learn about the trafficking in organs for transplantation.

1.

The routes that would-be organ recipients follow are well known to both doctors and patients. Italians (who have the lowest rate of organ donation in Europe) travel to Belgium to obtain their transplants; so do Israelis, who lately have also been going to rural Turkey and bringing their surgeon along with them. Residents of the Gulf States, Egyptians, Malaysians, and Bangladeshis mainly go to India for organs. In the Pacific, Koreans, Japanese, and Taiwanese, along with the residents of Hong Kong and Singapore, fly to China. Less frequently, South Americans go to Cuba and citizens of the former Soviet Union go to Russia. Americans for the most part stay home, but well-to-do foreigners come to the United States for transplants, and some centers allot up to 10 percent of their organs to them.

All of these people are responding to the shortages of organs that followed on the discovery of cyclosporine in the early 1980s. Until then, transplantation had been a risky and experimental procedure, typically a last-ditch effort to stave off death; the problem was not the complexity of the surgery but the body's immune system, which attacked and rejected the new organ as though it were a foreign object. Cyclosporine moderated the response while not suppressing the immune system's reactions to truly infectious agents. As a result, in countries with sophisticated medical programs, kidney and heart transplantation became widely used and highly successful procedures....

Transplantation spread quickly from developed to less developed countries. By 1990, kidneys were being transplanted in nine Middle Eastern, six

From David J. Rothman, "The International Organ Traffic," *The New York Review of Books* (March 26, 1998), pp. 14–17. Copyright © 1998 by NYREV, Inc. Reprinted by permission of *The New York Review of Books*.

South American, two North African, and two sub-Saharan African countries. Kidney transplants are by far the most common, since kidney donors can live normal lives with one kidney, while kidneys are subject to disease from a variety of causes, including persistent high blood pressure, adult diabetes, nephritis (inflammation of vessels that filter blood), and infections, which are more usually found in poor countries. (It is true that the donor runs the risk that his remaining kidney will become diseased, but in developed countries, at least, this risk is small.) The transplant techniques, moreover, are relatively simple. Replacing one heart with another, for example, is made easier by the fact that the blood-carrying vessels that must be detached from the one organ and reattached to the other are large and relatively easy to handle. (A transplant surgeon told me that if you can tie your shoes, you can transplant a heart.)

Fellowships in American surgical programs have enabled surgeons from throughout the world to master the techniques and bring them home. Countries such as India and Brazil built transplant centers when they might have been better advised to invest their medical resources in public health and primary care. For them the centers are a means for enhancing national prestige, for persuading their surgeons not to leave the country, and for meeting the needs of their own middle-class citizens.

In China, more than fifty medical centers report they perform kidney transplants, and in India hundreds of clinics are doing so. Reliable information on the success of these operations is hard to obtain, and there are reports that hepatitis and even AIDS have followed transplant operations. But according to physicians I have talked to whose patients have traveled to India or China for a transplant, and from published reports within these countries, some 70 to 75 percent of the transplants seem to have been successful.[1]

With patient demand for transplantation so strong and the medical capacity to satisfy it so widespread, shortages of organs were bound to occur. Most of the doctors and others involved in early transplants expected that organs would be readily donated as a gift of life from the dead, an exchange that cost the donor nothing and brought the recipient obvious benefits. However, it turns out that powerful cultural and religious taboos discourage donation, not only in countries with strong religious establishments but in more secular ones as well. The issue has recently attracted the attention of anthropologists, theologians, and literary scholars, and some of their findings are brought together in the fascinating collection of essays, *Organ Transplantation: Meanings and Realities*.[2]

In the Middle East, it is rare to obtain organs from cadavers. Islamic teachings emphasize the need to maintain the integrity of the body after death, and although some prominent religious leaders make an exception for transplants, others refuse. An intense debate occurred... in Egypt when the government-appointed leader of the most important Sunni Muslim theological faculty endorsed transplantation as an act of altruism, saying that permitting it was to accept a small harm in order to avoid a greater harm—the same rationale that allows a Muslim to eat pork if he risks starvation. But other clerics immediately objected, and there is no agreement in favor of donation.

In Israel, Orthodox Jewish precepts define death exclusively as the failure of the heart to function, not the cessation of brain activity, a standard that makes it almost impossible to retrieve organs. The primary purpose of statutes defining death as the absence of brain activity is to ensure that organs to be transplanted are continuously supplied with oxygen and nutrients; in effect, the patient is declared dead, and a respirator keeps the heart pumping and the circulatory system working until the organs have been removed, whereupon the respirator is disconnected. Some rabbis give precedence to saving a life and would therefore accept the standard of brain death for transplantation. But overall rates of donation in Israel are very low. The major exceptions are kibbutz members, who tend to be community-minded, as well as other secular Jews.

In much of Asia, cultural antipathy to the idea of brain death and, even more important, conceptions of the respect due elders, have practically eliminated organ transplantation. For all its interest in new technology and its traditions of gift-giving, Japan has only a minuscule program, devoted almost exclusively to transplanting kidneys from living related donors. As the anthropologist Margaret Lock writes: "The idea of having a deceased relative whose body is not complete prior to burial or cremation is associated with misfortune, because in this situation suffering in the other world never terminates."[3] For tradition-minded Japanese, moreover, death does not take place at a specific moment. The process of dying involves not only the heart and brain but the soul, and it is not complete until services have been held on the seventh and forty-ninth days after bodily death. It takes even longer to convert a deceased relative into an ancestor, all of which makes violating the integrity of the body for the sake of transplantation unacceptable.

Americans say they favor transplantation but turn out to be very reluctant to donate organs. Despite countless public education campaigns, organ donation checkoffs on drivers' licenses, and laws requiring health professionals to ask families to donate the organs of a deceased relative, the rates of donation have not risen during the past five years and are wholly inadequate to the need.... One recent study found that when families were asked by hospitals for permission to take an organ from a deceased relative, 53 percent flatly refused....

2.

If organs are in such short supply, how do some countries manage to fill the needs of foreigners? The answers vary. Belgium has a surplus of organs because it relies upon a "presumed consent" statute that probably would be rejected in every American state. Under its provisions, you must formally register your unwillingness to serve as a donor; otherwise, upon your death, physicians are free to transplant your organs. To object you must go to the town hall, make your preference known, and have your name registered on a national computer roster; when a death occurs, the hospital checks the computer base, and unless your name appears on it, surgeons may use your organs, notwithstanding your family's objections. I was told by heath professionals in Belgium that many citizens privately fear that if they should ever need an organ, and another patient simultaneously needs one as well, the surgeons will check the computer and give the organ to the one who did not refuse to be a donor. There is no evidence that surgeons actually do this; still many people feel it is better to be safe than sorry, and so they do not register any objections.

One group of Belgian citizens, Antwerp's Orthodox Jews, have nonetheless announced they will not serve as donors, only as recipients, since they reject the concept of brain death. An intense, unresolved rabbinic debate has been taking place over the ethics of accepting but not giving organs. Should the Jewish community forswear accepting organs? Should Jews ask to be placed at the bottom of the waiting list? Or should the Jewish community change its position so as to reduce the prospect of fierce hostility or even persecution?

Because its system of presumed consent has worked so well, Belgium has a surplus of organs and will provide them to foreigners. However, it will not export them, say, to Milan or Tel Aviv, which would be entirely feasible. Instead, it requires that patients in need of a transplant come to Belgium, which then benefits from the surgical fees paid to doctors and hospitals.

Not surprisingly, money counts even more in India, which has an abundant supply of kidneys because physicians and brokers bring together the desperately poor with the desperately ill. The sellers include impoverished villagers, slum dwellers, power-loom operators, manual laborers, and daughters-in-law with small dowries. The buyers come from Egypt, Kuwait, Oman, and other Gulf States, and from India's enormous middle class (which numbers at least 200 million). They readily pay between $2,500 and $4,000 for a kidney (of which the donor, if he is not cheated, will receive between $1,000 and $1,500) and perhaps two times that for the surgery. From the perspective of patients with end-stage renal disease, there is no other choice. For largely cultural reasons, hardly any organs are available from cadavers; dialysis centers are scarce and often a source of infection, and only a few people are able to administer dialysis to themselves at home (as is also the case in the US). Thus it is not surprising that a flourishing transplant business has emerged in such cities as Bangalore, Bombay, and Madras.

꧁◦◦꧂

The market in organs has its defenders. To refuse the sellers a chance to make the money they need, it is said, would be an unjustifiable form of paternalism. Moreover, the sellers may not be at greater risk living with one kidney, at least according to US research. A University of Minnesota transplant team compared seventy-eight kidney donors with their siblings twenty years or more after the surgery took place, and found no significant differences between them in health; indeed, risk-conscious insurance companies do not raise their rates for kidney donors.[4] And why ban the sale of kidneys when the sale of other body parts, including semen, female eggs, hair, and blood, is allowed in many countries? The argument that these are renewable body parts is not persuasive if life without a kidney does not compromise health. Finally, transplant surgeons, nurses, and social workers, as well as transplant retrieval teams and the hospitals, are all paid for their work. Why should only the donor and the donor's family go without compensation?

But because some body parts have already been turned into commodities does not mean that an increasing trade in kidneys and other organs is desirable. To poor Indians, as Margaret Radin, professor of law at Stanford, observes, "Commodification worries may seem like a luxury. Yet, taking a slightly longer view, commodification threatens the personhood of everyone, not just those who can now afford to concern themselves about it." Many of the poor Indians who sell their organs clearly feel they have had to submit to a degrading practice in order to get badly needed sums of money. They would rather not have parts of their body cut out, an unpleasant experience at best, and one that is probably more risky in Bombay than in Minnesota. Radin concludes: "Desperation is the social problem that we should be looking at, rather than the market ban.... We must rethink the larger social context in which this dilemma is embedded."[5]

In 1994, perhaps for reasons of principle or because of public embarrassment—every world medical organization opposes the sale of organs—a number of Indian states, including the regions of Bombay, Madras, and Bangalore, outlawed the practice, which until then had been entirely legal. But the laws have an egregious loophole so that sales continue almost uninterrupted. A detailed and persuasive report in the December 26, 1997, issue of *Frontline*, one of India's leading news magazines, explains how the new system works.[6] The legislation permits donations from persons unrelated to the recipient if the donations are for reasons of "affection or attachment," and if they are approved by "authorization committees." These conditions are easily met. Brokers and buyers coach the "donors" on what to say to the committee—that he is, for example, a cousin and that he has a (staged) photograph of a family gathering to prove it, or that he is a close friend and bears great affection for the potential recipient. Exposing these fictions would be simple enough, but many committees immediately approve them, unwilling to block transactions that bring large sums to hospitals, surgeons, and brokers.

Accurate statistics on kidney transplantation in India are not available, but *Frontline* estimates that about one third of transplants come from living, unrelated donors; four years after the new law went into effect, the rate of transplantation has returned to its earlier levels. It is true that not every hospital participates in the charade, that the market in kidneys is less visible than it was, and it may well be that fewer foreigners are coming to India for a transplant. But the lower classes and castes in India, already vulnerable to so many other abuses, continue to sell their organs. As *Frontline* reports, many donors who sell their organs do so because they are badly in debt; and before long they are again in debt.

3.

China is at the center of the Pacific routes to organ transplantation because it has adopted the tactic of harvesting the organs of executed prisoners. In 1984, immediately after cyclosporine became available, the government issued a document entitled "Rules Concerning the Utilization of Corpses or Organs from the Corpses of Executed Prisoners." Kept confidential, the new law provided that organs from executed prisoners could be used for transplants if the prisoner agreed, if the family agreed, or if no one came to claim the body. (Robin Munro of Human Rights Watch/Asia brought the law to light.) That the law lacks an ethical basis according to China's own values is apparent from its stipulations. "The use of corpses or organs of executed prisoners must be kept strictly secret," it stated, "and attention must be paid to avoiding negative repercussions." The cars used to retrieve organs from the execution grounds cannot bear health department insignia; the people involved in obtaining organs are not permitted to wear white uniforms. In my own interviews with Chinese transplant surgeons, none would admit to the practice; when I showed them copies of the law, they shrugged and said it was news to them.

But not to other Asian doctors. Physicians in Japan, Hong Kong, Singapore, and Taiwan, among other countries, serve as travel agents, directing their patients to hospitals in Wuhan, Beijing, and Shanghai. The system is relatively efficient. Foreigners do not have to wait days or weeks for an organ to be made available; executions can be timed to meet market needs and the supply is more than adequate. China keeps the exact number of executions secret but Amnesty International calculates on the basis of executions reported in newspapers that there are at least 4,500 a year, and perhaps three to four times as many. Several years ago a heart transplant surgeon told me that he had just been invited to China to perform a transplant; accustomed to long waiting periods in America, he asked how he could be certain that a heart would be available when he arrived. His would-be hosts told him they would schedule an execution to fit with his travel schedule. He turned down the invitation. In February [1998] the FBI arrested two Chinese nationals living in New York for allegedly soliciting payment for organs from executed prisoners to be transplanted in China.

China's system also has its defenders. Why waste the organs? Why deprive prisoners of the opportunity to do a final act of goodness? But once again, the objections should be obvious. The idea that prisoners on death row—which in China is a miserable hovel in a local jail—can give informed consent to their donations is absurd. Moreover, there is no way of ensuring that the need for organs might not influence courtroom verdicts. A defendant's guilt may be unclear, but if he has a long criminal record, why not condemn him so that a worthy citizen might live?

To have physicians retrieve human organs at an execution, moreover, subverts the ethical integrity of the medical profession. There are almost no reliable eyewitness accounts of Chinese practices, but until 1994, Taiwan also authorized transplants of organs from executed prisoners, and its procedures are probably duplicated in China. Immediately before the execution, the physician sedates the prisoner and then inserts both a breathing tube in his lungs and a catheter in one of his veins. The prisoner is then executed with a bullet to his head; the physician immediately moves to stem the blood flow, attach a respirator to the breathing tube, and inject drugs into the catheter so as to increase blood pressure and cardiac output. With the organs thus maintained, the body is transported to a hospital where the donor is waiting and the surgery is performed. The physicians have become intimate participants in the executions; instead of protecting life, they are manipulating the consequences of death.

The motive for all such practices is money. The Europeans, Middle Easterners, and Asians who travel to China, India, Belgium, and other countries pay handsomely for their new organs and in hard currencies. Depending on the organization of the particular health care system and the level of corruption, their fees will enrich surgeons or medical centers, or both. Many of the surgeons I interviewed were quite frank about how important the income from transplants was to their hospitals, but they were far more reluctant to say how much of it they kept for themselves. Still, a leading transplant surgeon in Russia is well known for his vast estate and passion for horses. His peers in India and China may be less ostentatious but not necessarily less rich. They will all claim to be doing good, rescuing patients from near death.

4.

The international trade in organs has convinced many of the poor, particularly in South America, that they or their children are at risk of being mutilated and murdered. Stories are often told of foreigners who arrive in a village, survey the scene, kidnap and murder several children, remove their organs for sale abroad, and leave the dissected corpses exposed in the graveyard. In Guatemala in 1993 precisely such fears were responsible for one innocent American woman tourist being jailed for a month, and another being beaten to death.

Villagers' anxieties are shared by a number of outside observers who believe that people are being murdered for their organs. The author of the report of a transplant committee of the European Parliament unequivocally asserted that

> Organized trafficking in organs exists in the same way as trafficking in drugs. It involved killing people to remove organs which can be sold at a profit. To deny the existence of such trafficking is comparable to denying the existence of ovens and gas chambers during the last war.[7]

So, too, the rapporteur of a UN committee on child welfare circulated a questionnaire asserting that "the sale of children is mainly carried out for the purpose of organ transplantation." It then asked: "To what extent and in what ways and forms do these violations of children's rights exist in your country? Please describe."[8]

The stories of organ snatching have an American version. I have heard it from my students, read about it on e-mail, been told about it with great conviction by a Moscow surgeon, and been asked about it by more than a dozen journalists. According to the standard account, a young man meets an attractive woman in a neighborhood bar; they have a few drinks, go back to her place, whereupon he passes out and then wakes up the next morning to find a sewn-up wound on his side. When he seeks medical attention, he learns that he is missing a kidney.

Although there have been sporadically reported stories of robberies of kidneys from people in India, I have not found a single documented case of abduction, mutilation, or murder for organs, whether in North or South America. I was in Guatemala in 1993 when the atrocities are alleged to have occurred, and heard seemingly reliable people say there was convincing evidence for them. I stayed long enough to see every claim against the two American women tourists proven false. Nevertheless, as the anthropologist Nancy Scheper-Hughes argues, the villagers' fears and accusations are understandable in the light of their everyday experience. The bodies of the poor are ordinarily treated so contemptuously that organ snatching does not seem out of character. In Guatemala, babies are regularly kidnapped for sale abroad in the adoption market. Local doctors and health workers admitted to me that "fattening houses" have been set up so that kidnapped babies would be more attractive for adoption.

But it is extremely dangerous to investigate the adoption racket, since highly placed officials in the government and military take a cut of the large sums of money involved. Moreover, Scheper-Hughes continues, if street children in Brazil can be brazenly murdered without recrimination, it is not farfetched for slum dwellers to believe that the organs of the poor are being removed for sale abroad. And since girls and boys can be kidnapped with impunity to satisfy an international market in sex, why not believe they are also kidnapped to satisfy an international market for organs?[9]

In truth, medical realities make such kidnappings and murder highly unlikely. The rural villages and the urban apartments in which transplants are alleged to secretly take place do not have the sterile environment necessary to remove or implant an organ. Organs from children are too small to be used in adults. And however rapacious health care workers may seem, highly trained and medically sophisticated teams of surgeons, operating room nurses, anesthesiologists, technicians, and blood transfusers are not likely to conspire to murder for organs or accept them off the street. Had they done so, at least one incident would have come to light during the past fifteen years.

5.

The well-documented abuses are bad enough. Is there some way of diminishing them? The Bellagio Task Force, an international group including transplant surgeons, human rights activists, and social scientists, has made several proposals that might be effective if they could be carried out.[10]

Almost all major national and international medical bodies have opposed the sale of organs and the transplantation of organs from executed prisoners; but none of the medical organizations has been willing to take action to enforce their views. The World Medical Association in 1984, 1987, and 1994 condemned "the purchase and sale of human organs for transplantation." But it asks "governments of all countries to take effective steps," and has adopted no measures of its own. It has also criticized the practice of using organs from executed prisoners without their consent; but it fails to ask whether consent on death row can be meaningful. The association leaves it to national medical societies to "severely discipline the physicians involved." Neither it nor any other medical organization has imposed sanctions on violators.

The Bellagio Task Force has posed several challenges to the international medical societies. What would happen if they took their proclaimed principles seriously, established a permanent monitoring body, and kept close surveillance on organ donation practices? What if they threatened to withhold training fellowships from countries which tolerated exploitative practices? What if they refused to hold international meetings in those countries, and, as was the case with South Africa under apartheid, did not allow physicians from those countries to attend their meetings? Why, moreover, couldn't the Novartis company, the manufacturer of cyclosporine, insist that it would sell its product only to doctors and hospitals that meet strict standards in obtaining organs? Such measures would be likely to have a serious effect, certainly in India, probably even in China. But as with the organs themselves, the willingness of doctors to use the moral authority of medicine as a force for change has, so far, been in short supply.

Notes

1. Xia Sui-sheng, "Organ Transplantation in China: Retrospect and Prospect," *Chinese Medical Journal,* 105 (1992), pp. 430–432.

2. Edited by Stuart J. Youngner, Renée C. Fox, and Laurence J. O'Connell (University of Wisconsin Press, 1996).

3. "Deadly Disputes: Ideologies and Brain Death in Japan," in Youngner et al., *Organ Transplantation,* pp. 142–167.

4. John S. Najarian, Blanche M. Chavers, Lois E. McHugh, and Arthur J. Matas, "20 Years or More of Follow-Up of Living Kidney Donors," *Lancet,* 340 (October 3, 1992), pp. 807–809.

5. Margaret Jane Radin, *Contested Commodities* (Harvard University Press, 1996), p. 125.

6. "Kidneys Still for Sale," *Frontline,* 14 (December 13–26, 1997), pp. 64–79.

7. This and other examples of lending credence to the rumors may be found in the United States Information Agency Report of December 1994, "The Child Organ Trafficking Rumor," written by Todd Leventhal.

8. Vitit Muntarbhorn, "Sale of Children," Report of the Special Rapporteur to the United Nations Commission on Human Rights, January 12, 1993.

9. Nancy Scheper-Hughes, "Theft of Life: The Globalization of Organ Stealing Rumours," *Anthropology Today,* 12 (June 1996), pp. 3–11.

10. D.J. Rothman, E. Rose, et al., "The Bellagio Task Force Report on Transplantation, Bodily Integrity, and the International Traffic in Organs," *Transplantation Proceedings,* 29 (1997), pp. 2739–2745. I am currently serving as chair of the Bellagio group.

POSTSCRIPT

Should There Be a Market in Body Parts?

In September 2000 the Department of Health and Human Servies announced that the number of organ donors increased nearly four percent during the first half of the year compared to the same period in 1999. The increase is attibuted to greater outreach and education efforts.

The most controversial consideration in the allocation of transplantable organs in the United States is whether the organs should be allocated nationally or locally. The Department of Health and Human Services (DHHS) proposed in March 1998 that current geographic disparities in the allocation of scarce organs should be addressed by creating national uniform criteria for determining a patient's medical status and eligibility for placement on a waiting list. Under the current system, local centers have first chance at organs in their region, even though patients in other areas may have greater medical need or have been on the waiting list longer. This disparity gained public attention when baseball star Mickey Mantle received a liver transplant very quickly because he led the waiting list in Texas.

This proposal was received enthusiastically by the large transplant centers, which attract the most ill and most affluent recipients, who can travel to the center and remain for months. However, it was criticized by smaller transplant centers, which rely on local recipients and the value of being able to tell potential donors or their families that the organs will be given to a local resident. Congress placed a one-year moratorium on implementing DHHS's proposal and asked the Institute of Medicine (IOM), an independent agency, to study the impact of the rule, with particular attention to the impact on racial minorities and low-income patients, waiting times, cost of transplantation services, and other factors. The IOM's report, issued in July 1999, agreed that organs should be allocated on the basis of medical need across wider geographical areas.

For more information on organ transplantation, see Courtney S. Campell, "The Selling of Organs, the Sharing of Self," *Second Opinion* (vol. 19, no. 2, 1993); Stuart J. Youngner, Renee C. Fox, and Laurence J. O'Connell, eds., *Organ Transplantation: Meanings and Realities* (University of Wisconsin Press, 1996); and the title essay in Arthur Caplan, *If I Were a Rich Man, Could I Buy a Pancreas?* (Indiana University Press, 1992).

ISSUE 21

Should Doctors-in-Training Be Unionized?

YES: Andrew C. Yacht, from "Collective Bargaining Is the Right Step," *The New England Journal of Medicine* (February 10, 2000)

NO: Jordan J. Cohen, from "White Coats Should Not Have Union Labels," *The New England Journal of Medicine* (February 10, 2000)

ISSUE SUMMARY

YES: Physician Andrew C. Yacht argues that doctors-in-training, like other workers, should have the right to organize and to bargain collectively for better working conditions in hospitals so that they can provide enhanced care for their patients.

NO: Physician and medical educator Jordan J. Cohen asserts that doctors-in-training are primarily students, not employees, and that union activities would negatively affect the educational experience.

After four years of college and three more grueling years of medical school, successful students reach their goal of an M.D. degree. But that is hardly the end of the process. They must then apply to and be matched with an educational and clinical facility that will provide the additional years of supervision and training they need to go on to specialize in a branch of medicine, such as surgery or psychiatry, or to enter general practice. Although these graduates can now legally be called a doctor, they begin at the lowest rung of the hospital chain of command. They are called, variously, interns, residents, housestaff, house officers, or PGYs (Postgraduate Years) 1, 2, or 3.

If medical school was hard, the residency experience is more so. Residents are expected to provide patient care with the supervision of an "attending" doctor. Housestaff are paid a salary beginning at around $25,000 a year and are offered some benefits as well. Particularly in public hospitals, where most patients do not have their own doctor in the community, residents may be the only doctors patients see. Residents work long hours with little sleep, and are expected to be able to respond to all kinds of situations. For many years the exhausting regimen was considered a rite of passage into the medical profession.

More recently, staffing cutbacks and the complex level of care many patients require have added to the burden.

Under such conditions, it is not surprising that doctors-in-training sometimes make mistakes. In 1984 in New York City, for example, Libby Zion, the 18-year-old daughter of a well-known attorney and journalist, died unexpectedly within hours after being hospitalized for fever and pain. Her father stated that she had received inadequate care from overworked and undersupervised medical housestaff. A grand jury did not indict the physicians involved in the case, but recommended several changes in residency training. The New York State Department of Health convened a special committee, popularly known as the Bell Committee, to design new working rules. These rules primarily limited the number of hours a resident could spend on duty during a shift and over the course of a week.

Shorter working hours and better working conditions are, of course, standard union goals. Medical residents have formed unions since the late 1950s. The Committee of Interns and Residents, for example, represents 10,000 house officers in more than 50 public and private hospitals in California, Florida, Massachusetts, New Jersey, New York, and the District of Columbia. In 1997 this committee became affiliated with the Service Employees International Union, creating a national organization within its health care division. Residents at public institutions such as municipal hospitals, covered by different laws from those applying to private institutions, have been negotiating contracts for forty years.

Residents at private institutions have had a harder time unionizing. In a 1976 decision discussed in the following selections, the National Labor Relations Board (NLRB) ruled that interns and residents were not "employees within the meaning of the . . . [National Labor Relations] Act." They were students, the Board stated, participating in these programs to "pursue the graduate medical education that is a requirement for the practice of medicine."

This decision was challenged in 1997 when the Boston City Hospital, a public institution, and Boston University Medical Center Hospital, a private institution, merged. Residents at the Boston Medical Center stood to lose their unionized status. On January 29, 1998, the Board reversed its 1976 decision.

The following selections present opposing viewpoints on whether doctors-in-training should be unionized. Andrew C. Yacht argues that for fifty years the ability to bargain collectively has given strength to those on the front lines of patient care, and that unions are needed more than ever at a time when patient needs have been dangerously obscured by financial considerations. Jordan J. Cohen contends that the NLRB ruling was correct in 1976 and should not have been reversed in 1998. Cohen asserts that residents have other avenues to redress problems.

Andrew C. Yacht 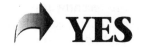 **YES**

Collective Bargaining Is the Right Step

On November 26, the National Labor Relations Board (NLRB) ruled that interns and residents [doctors-in-training or house staff] in private hospitals are considered under federal law to be employees, rather than students, and therefore have the right to form unions and engage in collective bargaining. This ruling overturned a controversial 1976 decision by the NLRB that blocked the house staff at Cedars-Sinai Medical Center in Los Angeles from organizing a union.[1]

After the 1976 ruling, several private hospitals that had previously recognized collective-bargaining rights of their residents withdrew their recognition of house-staff unions. At the same time, however, residents at public institutions, who were covered by a separate set of laws, were allowed to form unions. At these primarily municipal hospitals, residents' salaries, employee benefits, and improvements in working conditions have now been guaranteed under contract for more than 40 years.

Unionization of House Officers: The Experience at One Medical Center

Residents at Boston City Hospital in Boston were granted union recognition in 1969 under Massachusetts General Laws chapter 150E, the state's public-employee collective-bargaining act, administered by the Massachusetts Labor Relations Commission. A binding contract was negotiated at that time, with terms mutually agreed on by the hospital's residents and administration. When Boston City Hospital and Boston University Medical Center Hospital made plans to merge into a private, nonprofit hospital in 1996, the city of Boston and the management of Boston University Medical Center Hospital indicated that the new hospital would not continue to recognize the house officers' union because they were not required to do so under the 1976 NLRB ruling. In last-minute negotiations that held up the necessary City Council vote on the merger by several hours, the management of the new Boston Medical Center, formed by the merger of the two hospitals, agreed to recognize the union "voluntarily."

Since the original contract recognizing the union was signed in 1969, residents at Boston City Hospital and now Boston Medical Center have been

From Andrew C. Yacht, "Collective Bargaining Is the Right Step," *The New England Journal of Medicine*, vol. 342, no. 6 (February 10, 2000). Copyright © 2000 by The Massachusetts Medical Society. All rights reserved. Reprinted by permission.

guaranteed adequate salaries; health, malpractice, and disability insurance; sufficient provision for ancillary services; a cap on hours of work; and due process under binding legal contracts negotiated every two to three years. Over the past three decades, the contracts have been mutually respected and enforced, with only a handful of grievances requiring resolution through arbitration.

Despite the good working relationship between the residents at Boston Medical Center and the hospital administration, there was no guarantee that the hospital would continue its "voluntary" recognition of the House Officers' Association, the bargaining unit that represents the house staff, at the time of the next contract negotiation. Although the residents at Boston Medical Center worked an average of 80 to 100 hours per week on busy rotations, received salaries, paid taxes, and contributed to retirement savings accounts, they were still considered students under the 1976 Cedars-Sinai decision. For this reason, the private hospital was not obligated to negotiate with the residents, who, under federal case law, were not guaranteed collective-bargaining rights.

The NLRB Ruling

In 1997, the Committee of Interns and Residents filed a petition for certification with the NLRB for the 430 house officers at Boston Medical Center, seeking to overturn the 1976 Cedars-Sinai decision. The House Officers' Association at Boston Medical Center had become affiliated with the Committee of Interns and Residents in 1993. Formed in 1957, the committee represents 10,000 house-staff members in more than 50 public and private hospitals across the country. In 1997, it became affiliated with the Service Employees International Union (SEIU) to form a national organization of physicians within SEIU's health care division. Twenty-one days of hearings took place at the Boston office of the NLRB between March and July 1997, with five house officers and numerous members of the hospital administration and faculty testifying. The testimony was presented to the regional director of the NLRB, and then ultimately to the five members of the NLRB in Washington, D.C.

In its November 1999 ruling, the NLRB stated, "We are convinced by normal statutory and legal analysis, including resort to legislative history, experience, and the overwhelming weight of judicial and scholarly opinion, that the Board reached an erroneous result in *Cedars-Sinai.* Accordingly, we overrule that decision and its offspring, conclude that house staff are employees as defined by the Act, and find that such individuals are therefore entitled to all statutory rights and obligations that flow from our conclusion."[2] With this decision, house officers in all public and private institutions are granted collective-bargaining rights under federal law and may form unions.

After the Decision

Before and since the announcement of the decision, there has been much speculation about the potential consequences for house-staff members, hospitals, patient care, and medical education. For the more than 50,000 residents in private hospitals throughout the country, collective bargaining will mean a stronger voice in improving their working conditions. In the current climate of sweeping federal cuts in health care funding, widespread hospital mergers, and local budgetary constraints, residents have found themselves increasingly employed to provide basic services, such as phlebotomy, placement of intravenous lines, and transportation of patients, as the numbers of workers who have traditionally provided these services have been thinned. Although these tasks are necessary for patient care and should continue to be an important component of residency training, relying on residents to perform such services routinely in the name of training takes time away from more valuable doctor-patient interactions. With collective bargaining on such matters, residents may be better able to focus on skills in patient care that will remain important through all stages of their careers.

Residents have always worked long hours, often one to two days straight with only brief periods of sleep. At this time, however, only the state of New York, in large part because of the efforts of the Committee of Interns and Residents, regulates the number of hours residents can work; they are limited to no more than 24 continuous hours or a total of 80 hours per week. It is unknown how many errors in patient care are made by exhausted house-staff members toward the end of a 36-hour working period. Appropriate supervision and other safeguards are currently in place in many residency-training programs, but the future of these measures is not ensured; other programs do not have adequate safeguards.

Collective bargaining by house staff across the country has added important contractual guarantees to help limit residents' hours of work. Common examples include providing one day off in every seven days, averaged over each month, limiting the frequency of nights on call to one in three, and rescheduling "post-call" clinics rather than having residents care for outpatients after having worked for 30 continuous hours. These negotiated guarantees include a process for handling violations and offer more timely resolution than accreditation site visits, which may occur only every three to five years.

Residency-training programs have always been and will continue to be arduous, since many skills and much knowledge need to be acquired during a short period. At the same time, though, our patients deserve doctors who are able to perform their duties well, without clouded judgment or diminished compassion brought on by extreme fatigue.

Advantages for Education

Many fear that the NLRB decision will destroy medical education by interfering with the time-honored relationship between teacher and learner and by allowing nonmedical arbitrators to determine educational requirements and methods for the evaluation of clinical competency. On the basis of the experience at Boston Medical Center, this fear is unfounded. During the NLRB hearings, the director of graduate medical education at Boston Medical Center referred to her participation in 50 to 60 residency and institutional reviews for accreditation. In her testimony, she stated that the Accreditation Council for Graduate Medical Education "never indicated in any of those reviews that collective bargaining was detrimental to graduate medical education."[2] When referring to the separation between the employment and educational aspects of residency-training programs, the associate director of the Committee of Interns and Residents testified that "certification is a separate procedure, i.e., arbitrators never mandate a department chairman to issue a letter certifying that a resident has satisfactorily completed the program . . . or should be eligible to sit for the requisite board exam."[2]

Furthermore, the management-rights section of the contract between Boston Medical Center and the House Officers' Association explicitly states that "the Hospital retains the exclusive right to establish educational policy; to establish the standards and qualifications for hiring and advancement through the residency program; to determine training methods and curricula; to establish residency programs and to determine the number and qualifications of persons admitted to such programs."[3] The collective-bargaining agreement guarantees due process in reviews of training competency and access to residents' files. In no way are the contents of training programs' curriculum, criteria for evaluation, or requirements for promotion determined during contract negotiations or at the time of arbitration.

The Boston City Hospital case showed that over a 30-year period during which a union contract was in place, medical education was actually improved. In fact, during the merger between Boston City Hospital and Boston University Medical Center Hospital, the Boston City Hospital medical and dental staff voted unanimously to "express its support for the house staff of the newly-created Boston Medical Center to have the option of organizing themselves for the purposes of collective bargaining."[4] Because the agreement guarantees critical patient care services, provides funding for educational resources, and contributes to a safe and secure working environment, residents have been better able to focus on the care of their patients—the primary and most important source of learning.

Preserving a Sacred Trust

The biggest concern among critics is the possibility of work actions by house officers. In 1980, Boston City Hospital wanted to remove ancillary-service guarantees that the union had won through arbitration, potentially compromising patient care. The Boston City Hospital house staff went on a modified "strike" for six days, though ensuring that a sufficient number of residents remained in place to care for patients in the hospital. The dispute was soon resolved through mediation by the Massachusetts Labor Relations Commission, leaving patient care guarantees in place. This was the last time a job action was taken by the house staff, and it was done as a last resort to ensure good patient care. There has never been a strike by house staff over salary issues at Boston Medical Center or elsewhere. Regular negotiations and legally enforceable, collectively bargained agreements may actually prevent strikes. They provide open communication and processes for the resolution of problems before a crisis is reached.

With the strength and privilege of collective bargaining, however, comes collective responsibility. The needs of our patients must always come before our own desires and other responsibilities. No action, large or small, should ever be taken without full comprehension of potential short- and long-term consequences for our patients and our profession. Unions of residents have always been run by physicians for physicians, despite any affiliation with larger nonphysician organizations, and they must continue to reflect residents' professionalism and dedication.

Given the dramatic and often negative effects of the general restructuring of our health care system—in particular, as a consequence of the financial shortfall created by the Balanced Budget Act of 1997—concern has been expressed about the future stability and mission of academic medical centers.[5] At this critical time, residents across the country need an organized voice to ensure them of reasonable working conditions and to enhance their ability to care for patients. For nearly half a century, the ability to bargain collectively has given strength to those on the front lines of patient care. At a time when the needs of patients have become dangerously obscured by financial considerations, we need to do what we can to protect those for whom we have sworn to care.

References

1. Cedars-Sinai Medical Center, 223 NLRB 251, 91 LRRM 1398 (1976).
2. Boston Medical Center, 330 NLRB No. 30 (1999).
3. Agreement between Boston Medical Center and House Officers' Association (1997). Boston: Boston Medical Center.
4. Boston City Hospital Medical and Dental Staff Resolution (1996). Boston: Boston Medical Center.
5. Iglehart JK. Support for academic medical centers—revisiting the 1997 Balanced Budget Act. N Engl J Med 1999;341:299–304.

NO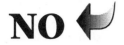

Jordan J. Cohen

White Coats Should Not Have Union Labels

Medicine has been subjected to more changes in the past several years than in any other period in the history of our profession. Now comes the decision by the National Labor Relations Board (NLRB) to change its long-standing view about the nature of residents in training. No longer primarily students, says the NLRB, residents are henceforth to be considered primarily employees under the provisions of the National Labor Relations Act.[1] Is this change for the better or for the worse?

Change, whether for better or worse, is always difficult. Resistance to change seems hard-wired into our nature as human beings. And when changes come with such speed and ferocity as they do today, it is easy to reject all changes reflexively, without examining their individual merits. This raises a question: Are those of us who wish to resist medicine's present trend toward commercialization, and its seeming tilt toward unionization, simply victims of our conservative natures? Or is there reason to worry that something really bad is happening?

In thinking about this question, I am profoundly troubled by the thought that residents are now eligible to join private-sector labor unions. But I am also profoundly troubled that many residents continue to face realities in their training programs that are distressing enough to warrant their even considering union representation. In fact, if residents had no alternative method for addressing their concerns, I might well approve of the NLRB's new ruling despite the devastating effects that I foresee on our profession. But residents do have alternatives for addressing their legitimate concerns. And the potential effects on our profession of unionization by residents are devastating indeed. So I do not hesitate to conclude that unions for residents are a very bad idea.

Residents as Students

I start with this premise: residents are primarily students. They provide patient-care services in the context of their educational activities, not as a consequence of employment by the institutional sponsor of the residency program. The NLRB got it right the first time around—in 1976—when it recognized in the now

From Jordan J. Cohen, "White Coats Should Not Have Union Labels," *The New England Journal of Medicine*, vol. 342, no. 6 (February 10, 2000). Copyright © 2000 by The Massachusetts Medical Society. All rights reserved. Reprinted by permission.

famous Cedars-Sinai case that residents possessed many more characteristics of students than of employees.[2] Residents are engaged in a formal educational program, subject to accreditation by an independent national body, the Accreditation Council for Graduate Medical Education (ACGME). This formal part of their education is essential for them to gain licensure to practice independently and to achieve eventual certification as specialists or subspecialists in their chosen fields.

The services they provide are assigned by the director of the training program in compliance with accreditation standards. The money they receive as residents is a stipend for living expenses during their period of training, not a salary. The level of their stipend is not set in accordance with the market value of the services they provide, but in recognition of what a suitable living standard is for students of such advanced standing. Their term of engagement within the institution is set nationally by the number of years required to complete accredited training; it is not a matter of local discretion, as is the case for typical employees. None of these characteristics of residents as students have changed one whit since 1976, notwithstanding the NLRB's recent three-to-two ruling to the contrary.

Changes in the Learning Environment

What has changed, however, is the learning environment in many teaching hospitals and the willingness of residents to acquiesce to some of the traditional but antiquated demands of residency education that are still evident in more than a few programs. As for the learning environment, anyone who has been in a teaching hospital in recent years will certainly recognize the enormous impact of market forces[3,4] and heightened concern about accountability[5] on the typical resident's educational experiences. The length of patients' hospital stay has fallen; the average severity of illness has increased; attending physicians have less time for teaching; fewer ancillary personnel are available to assist with patient care; opportunities for contemplation and study have dwindled; and the institutional commitment to education is often obscured by a preoccupation with economic survival. It is little wonder that many residents find it hard to believe us when we assert that education is the primary reason for their being there.

Compounding the negative effects of external forces on the learning environment is the seeming unwillingness of many residents to accept without challenge the often oppressive demands placed on them by their residency programs. This issue is perhaps the most contentious, and it is certainly the cause of the greatest intergenerational misunderstanding. Medical educators argue correctly that the residency experience must prepare future physicians for their uncommonly demanding responsibilities.[6] Many educators believe that limiting work hours truncates the learning experience, disrupts continuity of care, and invites a "clock-punching" mentality that is incompatible with a doctor's ethical responsibilities. Many also believe that current practices have proved effective in preparing doctors for making tough decisions under stress. By contrast, many observers believe that the residency experience is too grueling, that it is designed to haze new initiates more than to teach them valuable lessons.[7] Many also argue that exhausted residents cannot possibly learn well and, more important, that they pose a danger to their patients and to themselves.[8,9]

The Importance of Professionalism

Clearly, neither defenders nor critics of the present system would contest the importance of residents' being conscientious, being willing to work hard, placing their patients' interests uppermost, and understanding their obligation to discharge their responsibilities dutifully. But it is equally clear that residents find these essential attributes of professionalism hard to learn when they are required to put in excessively long and uninterrupted hours of duty, are assigned overly burdensome, noneducational chores, and are fearful of retaliation if they complain about their working conditions.

The present generation of residents has still more reasons to bristle at the noneducational demands of residency training. Conditioned by the major transformations that have occurred in American society over the past few decades, today's residents are, in a word, different from those in the past. Many more residents are married than was the case just a few years ago. Many have child-care responsibilities. Many more have other compelling interests that they wish to pursue outside their profession. All these healthy "lifestyle" changes should be welcomed by a profession that was long criticized as having an overly constricted outlook on the world because of its nearly monomaniacal devotion to things medical. But despite such generational changes for the better, many residency programs have not yet adjusted their expectations of trainees to conform to the needs of today's residents.

We simply have to strike a new balance between the profession's responsibility, on the one hand, to inculcate the knowledge, skills, attitudes, and behavior its acolytes must acquire and its responsibility, on the other hand, to treat those acolytes with respect as adult colleagues with their own lives to live. I think the place to begin the needed rebalancing is with a substantial readjustment of the service and education components of residency training. Hospital inpatient services, in particular, must be restructured. Reliance on residents to perform patient care services of little or no educational value demeans their status as students. We must reaffirm, with actions, the essentially educational nature of graduate medical training if we are to fulfill our obligations to our residents, not to mention our obligations to the public.[10]

House-Staff Unions Are Not the Answer

The route to rebalancing service and education and to addressing other needed changes in residency training, however, is not through house-staff unions. For openers, residents do not need labor unions to voice their concerns. Residents are not powerless. They may be unaware of their power or of how to exercise it, but residents do have the power, both individually and collectively, to improve the conditions under which they learn. Most programs with which I am familiar encourage and welcome input from house-staff members. More structured avenues for communication are widespread; they include resident-run house-staff associations, working groups comprising all the institution's chief residents, and regularly scheduled meetings between representatives of the residents and the institution's committee on graduate medical education. No doubt more needs to be done to include residents in decisions that affect their welfare. The threat of unionization could well serve as a useful impetus to make that happen.

Residents need to know that the ACGME requires all institutional sponsors of graduate medical education programs to establish formal procedures whereby house-staff members can register their complaints, grievances, and recommendations. The ACGME strengthened its call for effective representation of residents' viewpoints as recently as September 1998, when it adopted its latest revision of the *Institutional Requirements*.[11] Failure to comply with these requirements threatens an institution's accreditation status, but—to be sure —residents are understandably reluctant to aid and abet a process that could jeopardize their own program's viability. Although residents are also free to communicate with the ACGME directly (and anonymously, if they wish) about program violations,[12] the council would do well to establish some additional inducements, short of threatened extinction, to ensure that recalcitrant programs comply with established standards and that residents can communicate their ideas for improvement without fear of retaliation or abandonment.

The clincher for me, however, is the predictable intrusion of union activities into the domain of academic concerns and, with it, the inevitable degradation of the learning environment. To put it simply, the tools available to unions organized under the National Labor Relations Act are not designed to foster education. Rather, they are designed explicitly to obtain benefits for union members by pressing unwelcome demands on employers. The adversarial dynamics that frequently characterize labor-management relations in the American workplace are fundamentally antithetical to the atmosphere necessary for education. Educational objectives cannot be achieved without a firm foundation of trust between teacher and learner. The foundation for collective bargaining is, by contrast, naturally adversarial. Unions' ultimate weapon is the withholding of services through "job actions" or strikes. What could be more out of keeping with the educational setting, to say nothing of the clinical setting, than a strike—or even the threat of a strike?

Many proponents of unions for residents assert that such concern is overblown. They offer as evidence the benign behavior of house-staff unions that have operated for years in a number of state, county, and municipal hospitals.[13] The fallacy in assuming that this history predicts the future under the NLRB's new ruling is that all prior house-staff unions have operated under the framework not of the National Labor Relations Act, but of various state laws. State laws apply to government employees; such laws commonly forbid strikes and limit the issues over which collective bargaining is permissible.

By contrast, the National Labor Relations Act not only permits strikes by unionized employees; it considers the right to strike a fundamental element of the collective-bargaining process.[14] If a union, by contract, waives the right to strike, the payoff for making such a waiver enforceable is invariably the employer's agreement to final, binding arbitration of unresolved grievances.[15] And what might be the subject of such grievances? Troubling examples that leap to mind are a program director's decision not to promote a resident, to impose disciplinary action because of unprofessional behavior, to require remediation for a sub-par performance, or to dismiss a resident from the program because of repeated unsatisfactory evaluations. The prospect of such academic decisions' being subject to second-guessing by an outside arbitrator is chilling.

Broader Implications

As if these considerations were not enough, the idea of residents joining the ranks of organized labor also has problematic implications for medicine as a whole. If unions succeed in organizing physicians in their formative years of residency, they are sure to see the medical profession in its entirety as fertile ground for expanding their influence and enlarging their dues-paying rolls. At a time when the perceived triumph of cost cutting over quality has raised public suspicion of the health care system to an all-time high, the last thing our profession needs is a stampede of doctors into unions. To be sure, many practitioners (such as those who are self-employed) are currently barred by antitrust laws from joining unions, but many are not so barred. Moreover, who is to know how Congress will view this matter in the future? Indeed, the American Medical Association, in keeping with its lamentable decision to help eligible physicians form "negotiating units,"[16,17] is actively lobbying Congress to permit self-employed doctors to organize.[18]

The issue of residents' unions is thus linked firmly to the far larger issue of unions for doctors in general. If young physicians, during residency, become used to seeking redress of their grievances through the tactics of organized labor, they are less likely to see the risk entailed by doing so as fully trained practitioners. That risk, in my judgment, is no less than the loss of medicine's most precious possession: public trust. Unions flourish in an atmosphere characterized by the mistrust of employers by employees. Medicine requires trust of doctors by patients. At all times, patients must have confidence that their doctors will act in the patients' interest and in their interest alone. Nothing can protect patients as well as trustworthy physicians —no laws, no regulations, no fine print in the insurance policy, no watchdog federal agency, no patients' bill of rights, and certainly no union contract. Trust cannot be acquired through negotiation across a bargaining table. It must be earned. And the only way to earn it is to be trustworthy. Doctors seeking marketplace leverage through unions are trading their precious ethic of professionalism for commercialism's promise of a quick fix. Residents need to be fully acquainted with the perils inherent in that Faustian tradeoff.

Conclusions

Teaching hospitals are right to be troubled by the specter of residents' unions. By promising to put union muscle behind demands for shorter work shifts, more days off, fewer nights on call, and a variety of other "benefits," labor organizers are sure to find some receptive prospects among discontented residents. Residents who are training in institutions that still require excessively long duty hours and that do not fully comply with the spirit and intent of the ACGME's standards governing the treatment of trainees will, for obvious reasons, be particularly vulnerable to the organizers' appeal. Time is short, but even such institutions have the opportunity to confront the problems, both old and new, that unions will promise to address on behalf of residents. After taking a careful look at their training programs from the residents' perspective, all program directors, department chairs, deans, and teaching-hospital executives who wish to avoid having to deal with unions of residents need to offer credible assurances to their house staff that their education is of prime importance and that effective mechanisms are available for the institution to hear, and to act on, their legitimate concerns.

Finally, I want to appeal directly to residents who may be attracted to the union's siren call. Your decisions today are not without consequences for tomorrow. Before joining a union, I urge you to be absolutely certain that you have exhausted all other avenues for registering your complaints and your recommendations for improvements. You will soon inherit the responsibility for sustaining our Hippocratic tradition. As fragile as it is ancient, this priceless tradition cannot withstand the loss of public trust. As future stewards of medicine's core value of service to others, ask yourselves if affixing the union label to your white coats signals trust in your noble calling or allegiance to some lesser ideal. Unions are magnificent instruments for extracting marketplace benefits for their members. But the odds are long indeed that they will be able to shun self-interest and sustain a value system rooted in altruism.

References

1. Boston Medical Center, 330 NLRB No. 30 (1999).
2. Cedars-Sinai Medical Center, 223 NLRB 251, 91 LRRM 1398 (1976).
3. Iglehart JK. Support for academic medical centers—revisiting the 1997 Balanced Budget Act. N Engl J Med 1999;341:299–304.
4. Marwick C. AAMC analyzes 1997 Balanced Budget Act. JAMA 1999;281:1781–2.
5. Cohen JJ, Dickler RM. Auditing the Medicare-billing practices of teaching physicians—welcome accountability, unfair approach. N Engl J Med 1997;336:1317–20.
6. Marchione M. Long days and nights await medical residents. Milwaukee Journal Sentinel. July 12, 1998:1.
7. Hospitals work new doctors too hard. USA Today. May 28, 1998:12A.
8. Richardson GS, Wyatt JK, Sullivan JP, et al. Objective assessment of sleep and alertness in medical house staff and the impact of protected time for sleep. Sleep 1996;19:718–26.
9. Daugherty SR, Baldwin DC Jr. Sleep deprivation in senior medical students and first-year residents. Acad Med 1996;71:Suppl:S93–S95.
10. Cohen JJ. Honoring the "E" in GME. Acad Med 1999;74:108–13.
11. Institutional requirements. Chicago: Accreditation Council for Graduate Medical Education, 1998.
12. Procedures for dealing with complaints against residency programs. Chicago: Accreditation Council for Graduate Medical Education, 1999.
13. Boston Medical Center Committee of Interns and Residents. In Re: Boston Medical Center, petitioners' brief on review of regional director's decision, 1999:44–54.

14. In Re: State of Minnesota, 1975: 219 NLRB 1093.
15. Supra, p. 10, note 24.
16. Klein S. AMA to establish national collective bargaining unit. American Medical News. July 5, 1999:1, 34.
17. AAMC Executive Council. AAMC statement on negotiating units for physicians. AAMC Reporter 1999;9(2):7.
18. Klein S. Physician Antitrust Bill pronounced dead for now. American Medical News. November 8, 1999:5-6.

POSTSCRIPT

Should Doctors-in-Training Be Unionized?

The question of physician unionization goes beyond housestaff issues. As a result of managed care's real and perceived limitations on their autonomy and expertise, physicians in private practice are increasingly turning to unions as a way to bargain collectively. However, unlike with interns and residents, wages and working conditions are not the primary issues. Physicians want to regain what they believe is their hard-earned right to control their own patient care and practice decisions. The American Medical Association has endorsed physician unions, but many physicians are wary of the idea. They are concerned that unions are not in keeping with the traditions of medical professionalism and that unionization will negatively affect the physician-patient relationship. For more on this issue, see "Physician Unionization: The Impact on the Medical Profession," by Chris Phan in *The Journal of Legal Medicine* (vol. 20, 1999). Also see Ellen L. Luepke, "White Coat, Blue Collar: Physician Unionization and Managed Care," *Annals of Health Law,* (vol. 8, 1999).

The Libby Zion case and its aftermath is discussed in a series of articles in *The New England Journal of Medicine* (March 24, 1998). Also see Jeffrey M. Brensilver, Lawrence Smith, and Christopher S. Lyttle, "Impact of the Libby Zion Case on Graduate Medical Education in Internal Medicine," *The Mount Sinai Journal of Medicine* (September 1998). Despite the changes in New York State law and regulation, residents continue to work long shifts; however, the number of trainees has expanded.

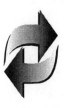

Contributors to This Volume

EDITOR

CAROL LEVINE joined the United Hospital Fund in New York City in October 1996 where she directs the Families and Health Care Project. This project focuses on developing partnerships between health care professionals and family caregivers, who provide most of the long-term and chronic care to elderly, seriously ill, or disabled relatives. She also continues to direct The Orphan Project: Families and Children in the HIV Epidemic, which she founded in 1991. She was director of the Citizens Commission on AIDS in New York City from 1987–1991. As a senior staff associate of The Hastings Center, she edited the *Hastings Center Report*. In 1993 she was awarded a MacArthur Foundation Fellowship for her work in AIDS policy and ethics. She has written several books and articles, including a "Sounding Board" essay in *The New England Journal of Medicine* entitled "The Loneliness of the Long-Term Care Giver" (May 20, 1999). She most recently edited *Always On Call: When Illness Turns Families Into Caregivers*, which was published in September 2000 by the United Hospital Fund.

STAFF

Theodore Knight   List Manager
David Brackley   Senior Developmental Editor
Juliana Gribbins   Developmental Editor
Rose Gleich   Administrative Assistant
Brenda S. Filley   Director of Production/Design
Juliana Arbo   Typesetting Supervisor
Diane Barker   Proofreader
Richard Tietjen   Publishing Systems Manager
Larry Killian   Copier Coordinator

AUTHORS

FELICIA ACKERMAN is a professor of philosophy at Brown University in Providence, Rhode Island. Her articles have appeared in various philosophy journals and anthologies, including *Philosophical Perspectives* and the *Midwest Studies in Philosophy* book series. She is also a writer of short stories, some of which deal with issues in medical ethics. She received her Ph.D. from the University of Michigan.

AMERICAN ACADEMY OF PEDIATRICS (AAP) and its member pediatricians dedicate their efforts and resources to the health, safety, and well-being of infants, children, adolescents, and young adults. Founded in June 1930, the AAP currently has approximately 55,000 members in the United States, Canada, and Latin America. Members include pediatricians, pediatric medical subspecialists, and pediatric surgical specialists. More than 36,000 of them are board-certified and called Fellows of the American Academy of Pediatrics (FAAP).

MARCIA ANGELL is the former editor-in-chief of *The New England Journal of Medicine.*

GEORGE J. ANNAS is the Edward R. Utley Professor of Law and Medicine at Boston University's Schools of Medicine and Public Health in Boston, Massachusetts. He is also director of Boston University's Law, Medicine, and Ethics Program and chair of the Department of Health Law. His publications include *Standard of Care: The Law of American Bioethics* (Oxford University Press, 1993) and *Some Choice: Law, Medicine, and the Market* (Oxford University Press, 1998).

ROBERT M. ARNOLD is an M.D. at the University of Pittsburgh's Medical Center. He is coauthor, with Charles W. Lidz and Lynn Fisher, of *The Erosion of Autonomy in Long-Term Care* (Oxford University Press, 1992) and coeditor of *Procuring Organs for Transplant: The Debate Over Non-Heart-Beating Cadaver Protocols* (Johns Hopkins University Press, 1995).

JEFFREY BLUSTEIN is an associate professor of bioethics in the Albert Einstein College of Medicine at Yeshiva University and an adjunct associate professor of philosophy at Barnard College in New York City.

SISSELA BOK is an Annenberg Visiting Fellow and Distinguished Fellow of the Harvard Center for Population and Development Studies. She is a member of the Pulitzer Prize Board and of the editorial boards of a number of journals. Her publications include *Secrets: On the Ethics of Concealment and Revelation* (Vintage Books, 1983) and *A Strategy for Peace: Human Values and the Threat of War* (Pantheon Books, 1989).

DANIEL CALLAHAN is director of International Programs for The Hastings Center in Garrison, New York. He was a cofounder of The Hastings Center in 1969, and, from 1969–1996, served as its director and president. He is an elected member of the Institute of Medicine, National Academy of Sciences. He is also a member of the Director's Advisory Committee, Centers for Disease Control and Prevention, and chair of its Ethics Committee. He won the 1996 Freedom and Scientific Responsibility Award of the American Association for the Advancement of Science.

ALEXANDER MORGAN CAPRON is the University Professor of Law and Medicine at the University of Southern California, where he also heads the Pacific Center for Health Policy and Ethics and holds the Henry W. Bruce Professorship of Law. He has also taught at Yale University, Georgetown University, and the University of Pennsylvania. He is coeditor, with Jay Katz, of *Catastrophic Diseases: Who Decides What?* (Transaction Books, 1982).

MILDRED K. CHO is assistant professor of bioethics in the Center for Bioethics and the Department of Molecular and Cellular Engineering at the University of Pennsylvania School of Medicine.

JORDAN J. COHEN is president of the Association of American Medical Colleges.

WILLIAM S. CUSTER is an associate professor in the Department of Risk Management and Insurance in the College of Business Administration at Georgia State University.

NANCY NEVELOFF DUBLER is in the Department of Epidemiology and Social Medicine at Montefiore Medical Center/Albert Einstein College of Medicine in New York City.

EZEKIEL J. EMANUEL is a professor in the Division of Medical Ethics at Harvard Medical School. He also does research in the Division of Cancer Epidemiology and Control at the Dana-Farber Cancer Institute in Boston, Massachusetts.

AMITAI ETZIONI, senior adviser to the White House from 1979 to 1980, is a professor in the Department of Sociology at George Washington University in Washington, D.C., where he has been teaching since 1980. He is also the founder of the Society for the Advancement of Socio-Economics and the founder and director of the Center for Policy Research, a nonprofit organization dedicated to public policy. His publications include *A Responsive Society: Collected Essays on Guiding Deliberate Social Change* (Jossey-Bass, 1991).

KATHLEEN M. FOLEY is attending neurologist at Memorial Sloan-Kettering Cancer Center and professor of neurology, neuroscience, and clinical pharmacology at Cornell University Medical College. She is also director of the Project on Death in America at the Open Society Institute.

THOMAS B. FREEMAN is a professor in the Department of Neurological Science at the University of South Florida.

DAVID A. GRIMES is vice president of Biomedical Affairs at Family Health International in North Carolina and a clinical professor in the Department of Obstetrics and Gynecology at the University of North Carolina School of Medicine. An advisory board member of the American Medical Association, he is board-certified both in obstetrics and gynecology and in preventive medicine. He served as an epidemiologist at the Centers for Disease Control for nine years, and he has published over 200 peer-reviewed articles, 40 textbook chapters, and several books.

JOHN HARDWIG teaches in the philosophy department and in the College of Medicine at East Tennessee State University.

DIANE E. HOFFMANN is a professor in the University of Maryland School of Law.

CHARLES N. KAHN III is president of the Health Insurance Association of America in Washington, D.C.

CHARLES W. LIDZ is a professor of psychiatry and sociology at the Western Psychiatric Institute and Clinic at the University of Pittsburgh in Pittsburgh, Pennsylvania.

JEROD M. LOEB is director of the Department of Research and Evaluation for the Joint Commission on the Accreditation of Health Care Organizations. He is also a cardiovascular physiologist, and he has published widely in areas related to the heart, the use of animals in biomedical research, science education, and science policy.

STEVEN LUTTRELL is senior registrar in the Department of Health Care for Older People at Whittington Hospital, London, England.

RUTH MACKLIN is a bioethicist at the Albert Einstein College of Medicine. She is also the chair of the Ethical Review Committee for the United Nations Programme on AIDS (UNAIDS). Most recently, she wrote *Against Relativism: Cultural Diversity and the Search for Ethical Universals in Medicine* (Oxford University Press, 1999).

GLENN McGEE is associate director for education and assistant professor of bioethics, philosophy, and history and sociology of science in the Center for Bioethics at the University of Pennsylvania. He is the author of *The Perfect Baby: Parenthood in the New World of Cloning and Genetics,* 2d ed. (Rowman and Littlefield, 2000). He is editor of *The Human Cloning Debate,* 2d ed. (Berkeley Hills Books, 2000) and *Pragmatic Bioethics* (Vanderbilt University Press, 1999).

JON F. MERZ is assistant professor in the Center for Bioethics at the University of Pennsylvania. His emphasis includes legal policies and ethical bases of clinical and research informed consent.

BERNARD C. MEYER is a psychiatrist in New York City. He has also worked as a clinical professor of psychiatry at Mount Sinai Hospital School of Medicine.

STEVEN H. MILES is an associate professor of medicine in the division of geriatric medicine at the Hennepin County Medical Center and in the Center for Biomedical Ethics at the University of Minnesota in Minneapolis, Minnesota.

BRENDAN MINOGUE is professor of philosophy in the Department of Philosophy and Religious Studies at Youngstown State University. He is also a bioethics consultant for Forum Health Care of Youngstown, Ohio, and for Sharon Regional Hospital of Sharon, Pennsylvania.

THOMAS H. MURRAY is president of The Hastings Center in Garrison, New York. He was formerly a professor of biomedical ethics and director of the Center for Biomedical Ethics in the School of Medicine at Case Western Reserve University in Cleveland, Ohio. He is a founding editor of the journal *Medical Humanities Review* and the author or editor of over 100 publications, including *Feeling Good, Doing Better* (Humana Press, 1984) and *Which Babies Shall Live?* (Humana Press, 1985), coauthored with Arthur L. Caplan.

MARK G. NEERHOF is an assistant professor of clinical obstetrics and gynecology at Evanston Northwestern Healthcare in Evanston, Illinois. He completed medical school and a residency in obstetrics and gynecology at the Chicago College of Osteopathic Medicine. His fellowship in maternal-fetal medicine was at Pennsylvania Hospital in Philadelphia, Pennsylvania.

MARY Z. PELIAS is a professor in the department of biometry and genetics at the Louisiana State University Medical Center in New Orleans. She is also a member of the Social, Ethical, and Legal Issues Committee for the Federation of American Societies for Experimental Biology.

CHARLES PETERS is an associate professor of clinical pediatrics in the Division of Hematology-Oncology and Blood and Marrow Transplantation at the University of Minnesota Medical School in Minneapolis, Minnesota.

J. RADCLIFFE-RICHARDS, a feminist writer, is a member of the British Society for Ethical Theory. She has published a number of articles on such issues as clinical genetics and euthanasia, and she is the author of *The Sceptical Feminist: A Philosophical Enquiry,* 2d ed. (Penguin, 1994).

TOM REGAN is a professor of philosophy and a department chair at North Carolina State University in Raleigh, North Carolina, where he has been teaching since 1967. He has published many books and articles on animal rights and environmental ethics, including *The Struggle for Animal Rights* (ISAR, 1987). In addition to his scholarly activities, his work as a video author and director has earned him major international awards.

UWE E. REINHARDT is James Madison Professor of Political Economy at Princeton University. He recently edited *Regulating Managed Care: Theory, Practice, and Future Options* (Jossey-Bass, 1999).

JOHN A. ROBERTSON is a professor in and the Vinson and Elkins Chair of the University of Texas School of Law in Austin, Texas. He earned his B.A. from Dartmouth College in 1964 and his J.D. from Harvard University in 1968.

LAINIE FRIEDMAN ROSS is an assistant professor of pediatrics in the McLean Center for Clinical Medical Ethics, Department of Medicine, at the University of Chicago in Chicago, Illinois. She is also director of the Ethics Case Consultation Service and codirector of the Multidisciplinary Ethics Lecture Series at the university. Her many articles have appeared in such journals as *The New England Journal of Medicine, Bioethics,* and *The Hastings Center Report,* and she is the author of *Children, Families, and Health Care Decision Making* (Clarendon Press, 1998).

DAVID J. ROTHMAN is a professor of history at Columbia University in New York City. He is the author, coauthor, or editor of numerous books, including *Low Wages and Great Sins: Two Antebellum American Views on Prostitution and the Working Girl* (Garland, 1987), coauthored with Sheila M. Rothman.

CHRISTOPHER JAMES RYAN is a consultant-liaison psychiatrist in the Department of Psychiatry at Westmead Hospital in Westmead, New South Wales, Australia.

MARK SHELDON is a professor of philosophy and an adjunct professor of medicine at Indiana University Northwest and the Indiana University School of Medicine, as well as a member of the faculty of Rush-Presbyterian-St. Luke's Medical Center in Chicago, Illinois. He has also held appointments as an adjunct senior scholar at the MacLean Center for Clinical Medical Ethics at the University of Chicago and as a senior policy analyst at the American Medical Association.

ANN SOMMERVILLE is head of the Medical Ethics Department of the British Medical Association in London, England.

M. LeROY SPRANG is a doctor at Northwestern University Medical School and Evanston Northwestern Healthcare in Evanston, Illinois. Board-certified in obstetrics/gynecology, he graduated from the Loyola University Stritch School of Medicine in 1969.

ANDREW SULLIVAN is a columnist for *The New York Times Magazine*. He is the author of *Virtually Normal: An Argument About Homosexuality* (Alfred A. Knopf, 1995) and *Love Undetectable: Notes on Friendship, Sex, and Survival* (Alfred A. Knopf, 1999).

JEAN TOAL is a justice of the South Carolina Supreme Court.

ROBERT M. VEATCH is director of and a professor of medical ethics in the Kennedy Institute of Ethics at Georgetown University in Washington, D.C.

ROBERT F. WEIR is director of the Program in Biomedical Ethics and Medical Humanities in the College of Medicine at the University of Iowa. A professor of pediatrics, he is also on the faculty of the university's School of Religion. His major research interests include ethical issues at the beginning of life, at the end of life, and in genetics. He is the editor of *Physician-Assisted Suicide* (Indiana University Press, 1997) and *Stored Tissue Samples: Ethical, Legal, and Public Policy Implications* (University of Iowa Press, 1998).

THOMAS F. WILDSMITH IV is a policy research actuary at the Health Insurance Association of America in Washington, D.C.

ERIC A. WULFSBERG is a clinical associate professor of pediatrics in the University of Maryland School of Medicine and a member of the Maryland chapter of the American Academy of Pediatrics. His area of expertise is genetics and birth defects.

ANDREW C. YACHT is a resident in internal medicine at Boston Medical Center.

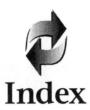

Index